"Dr. Kharrazian's material is way beyond the stuff they teach in medical school."
Ron Manzanero, MD, Austin Integrative Medicine, Austin, TX

"Dr. Kharrazian goes beyond a superficial treatment of neurotransmitters. Every new naturopath should look at his body of work."
Don Baker, DC, NMD, Mesa, AZ

"This information is critical to all practicing health care professionals and their suffering patients, which often includes the doctors themselves. It is eye-opening, relevant to any disease or pathology, and immediately applicable for all your patients. I highly recommend it for any brain owner."
Kari Vernon, DC, Scottsdale, AZ

"I think Dr. Kharrazian's presentation is extraordinary. I had a head injury and have struggled all my life with low brain function. I am looking forward to applying this knowledge to myself and my practice. I love the way Dr. Kharrazian gets excited about teaching."
Tom Groover, DC, PLLC, Boulder, CO

"Dr. Kharrazian masterfully pulls together functional neurology, endocrinology, nutrition, and physiology in a practical and immediately useable format."
Heith Root, DC, San Antonio, TX

"Fantastic! Nothing else like it—I learned so much and feel like I can look at patients from an entirely new level. Information regarding neurodegeneration is invaluable and gives us tools that no one else has."
Dana Carey, LAc, Longmont, CO

"Great! Dr. Kharrazian is as always exceptional in his concise, in-depth explanations of all the problems my patients experience. Best of all, he makes it easy to understand the most complicated of conditions. Thank you, thank you, thank you!"
Marie Starling, DC, Centennial, CO

WHY ISN'T MY BRAIN WORKING?

*A revolutionary understanding of brain decline and
effective strategies to recover your brain's health*

By Datis Kharrazian, DHSc, DC, MS

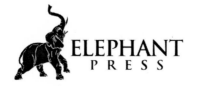

ELEPHANT
PRESS

Why Isn't My Brain Working?

ISBN 978-0-9856904-3-4

Library of Congress Control Number: 2012948479

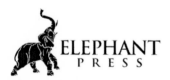

ELEPHANT
P R E S S

Elephant Press LP
7040 Avenida Encinas, Suite 104
Carlsbad, CA 92011 USA
www.ElephantPressBooks.com

Book cover, design and typesetting by Laurie Griffin / LaurieGriffin.com
Interior illustrations by Jason Norman / ThePaperProphet.com

DEDICATION

First, I would like to dedicate this book to my wife, Andrea, and to my daughter, Maizy, for their continued support and the sacrifices they have endured. Developing, writing, and teaching this information has meant many days and nights locked up in my home office writing and researching, countless hours in airports and hotels during trips all over the world, and many late nights at the office working with patients.

Second, I would like to dedicate this book to the millions of patients who have been ignored and overlooked when suffering from a head injury, brain dysfunction, or brain degeneration. Nobody understands the difficulty you face as you appear normal to those around you.

Third, I would like to dedicate this book to all the health care practitioners who are reading this book because they want to better serve their patients. The world needs more caring and passionate doctors like you.

CONTENTS

Financial Disclosure

Dr. Datis Kharrazian is a member of Apex Energetics, Inc.'s Scientific Advisory Board, is a paid consultant to Apex Energetics, and, as a researcher, developer and/or formulator, receives royalties on the sale of various Apex Energetics nutritional products. He is not an employee of and has no ownership interest in Apex Energetics.

He is also a member of the editorial board of the Journal of Functional Neurology, Rehabilitation, and Ergonomics. He receives no financial compensation for his service on the board.

Dr. Kharrazian serves on the Curriculum Advisory Committee of the Institute for Functional Medicine. He receives no financial compensation for his participation on this committee.

Dr. Kharrazian has been engaged as an industry expert by Cyrex Laboratories, LLC to assist in the development of clinical assays and to educate health care practitioners in the technology and application of its arrays. As such, he receives commissions from Cyrex as permitted by and in compliance with federal and state laws, codes and regulations, including Stark and other anti-kickback provisions. He is not an employee of Cyrex and has no ownership in it.

Intended Use Statement

The content of this book is intended for information purposes only. The medical information in this book is intended as general information only and should not be used in any way to diagnose, treat, cure, or prevent disease. The goal of the book is to present and highlight nutritionally significant information and offer suggestions and protocols for nutritional support and health maintenance.

It is the sole responsibility of the user of this information to comply with all local and federal laws regarding the use of such information, as it relates to the scope and type of the user's practice.

DISCLAIMER AND NOTICES

The information and recommendations outlined in this book are not intended as a substitute for personalized medical advice; the reader of this book should see a qualified health care provider. This book proposes certain theoretical methods of nutrition not necessarily mainstream. It is left to the discretion and it is the sole responsibility of the user of the information indicated in this book to determine if procedures and recommendations described are appropriate. The author of this information cannot be held responsible for the information or any inadvertent errors or omissions of the information.

The information in this book should not be construed as a claim or representation that any procedure or product mentioned constitutes a specific cure, palliative, or ameliorative. Procedures and nutritional compounds described should be considered as adjunctive to other accepted conventional procedures deemed necessary by the attending licensed doctor.

It is the concern of the Department of Health and Human Services that no homeopathic or nutritional supplements be used to replace established medical approaches, especially in cases of emergencies or serious or life-threatening diseases or conditions. The author shares in this concern, as replacing conventional treatment with such remedies, especially in serious cases, may deprive the patient and pose a major legal liability for the health professional involved. The nutritional compounds mentioned in the book should not be used as replacements for conventional medical treatment.

The Food and Drug Administration has not evaluated the information detailed in this book. The nutritional supplements mentioned in this manual are not intended to diagnose, treat, cure, or prevent disease.

ABOUT THE AUTHOR

Datis Kharrazian, DHSc, DC, MS, MNeuroSci, FAACP, DACBN, DABCN, DIBAK, CNS

Dr. Datis Kharrazian has spent more than a decade teaching several thousand hours of postgraduate education in non-pharmaceutical applications for chronic illnesses, autoimmune disorders, and complex neurological disorders all over the world to health care providers. He has trained thousands of health care professionals in an evidence- and physiological-based model of clinical practice. His reputation not only as an educator but also as a clinician has become renowned worldwide. Patients from all over the world fly to his practice in San Diego, California to understand his perspective regarding their condition and to apply natural medicine alternatives to help them improve their quality of life. Dr. Kharrazian has become the referral source for many doctors nationally and internationally for complex cases.

Dr. Kharrazian is one of the most sought-after educators and clinicians in natural medicine, laboratory analysis, and nutrition. His seminar schedule is booked years in advance. He lectures both nationally and internationally at major medical and scientific conferences worldwide. He conducts several professional and scientific presentations a year in addition to giving radio and television interviews and appearances in movie documentaries. Dr. Kharrazian has personally trained a group of more than a dozen exceptional doctors to lecture nationally to meet the demands by health care providers on how he clinically manages complex cases.

Dr. Kharrazian's first book, *Why Do I Still Have Thyroid Symptoms When My Lab Tests Are Normal?* quickly became the best-selling thyroid book. It has been listed as the number-one selling thyroid book on Amazon since its release in October of 2009. His book created an international explosion of interest in his detailed review of the scientific literature regarding thyroid disease and his clinical model of patient management. Hundreds of positive testimonials have been received globally from patients and doctors worldwide.

Dr. Kharrazian has published numerous professional papers, post-graduate course manuals, and professional journal articles about functional medicine, nutrition, laboratory analysis, and case studies. Dr. Kharrazian is also on the editorial board of the Journal of Functional Neurology, Rehabilitation and Ergonomics.

Dr. Kharrazian is an adjunct faculty member for Bastyr University California, where he teaches neuroscience, neuroanatomy, and human brain dissection. Several institutes and universities have asked Dr. Kharrazian to develop advanced academic programs for graduate and post-graduate programs outlining the latest information in natural approaches to various chronic disorders. He serves on the education advisory committee for the Institute for Functional Medicine that is recognized by the Accreditation Council for Continuing Medical Education (ACCME). He is currently teaching postgraduate education courses that are approved for continuing educations by the University of Bridgeport.

Dr. Kharrazian earned his Bachelor of Science degree from the University of the State of New York with honors and his Doctor of Chiropractic degree graduating with honors from Southern California University of Health Sciences, where he was distinguished with the Mindlin Honors at Entrance Award, the Dean's List, and the Delta Sigma Award for Academic Excellence. He has earned a Master of Science degree in Human Nutrition from the University of Bridgeport, a Master of Neurological Sciences from the Carrick Institute of Graduate Studies, and a Doctor of Health Science from Nova Southeastern University.

Dr. Kharrazian has completed many postgraduate specialty programs and has been board certified in numerous specialties that include Diplomate of the Board of Nutrition Specialists, Diplomate of the American Board of Clinical Nutrition, Diplomate of the Chiropractic Board of Clinical Nutrition, Diplomate of the American Board of Chiropractic Neurology, and Diplomate of the International Board of Applied Kinesiology. His contributions and devotions to clinical practice and educations have earned him several fellowships including Fellow of the American Board of Vestibular Rehabilitation, Fellow of the American Academy of Chiropractic Physicians, Fellow of the International Academy of Functional Neurology and Rehabilitation, and Fellow of the American College of Functional Neurology.

Dr. Kharrazian has been a consultant to the nutritional industry and has formulated more than 90 nutritional products, including topical creams, protein powders, liquid supplements, sublingual hormones, and sublingual nutrients. His formulations are used by thousands of health care professionals nationally for various health disorders.

Dr. Kharrazian was recognized by his peers and awarded the Clinician Trailblazer award at the 2010 Annual Conference of Functional Neurology. This award was given to him by his peers in recognition for his contributions to the practice of functional neurology. He was also given a special recognition award by the International Association of Functional Neurology and Rehabilitation for his contributions to the field of neurology in 2011.

Special Thanks and Recognition

My sincere gratitude to the readers who support and share my work.

My sincere gratitude to the talented doctors and dear friends that teach my model of functional medicine and nutritional neurochemistry all over the country: Dr. Mark Flannery, Dr. Steve Noseworthy, Dr. Tom Culleton, Dr. Shane Steadman, Dr. Sam Yanuck, Dr. Brandon Brock, Dr. Glen Zielinski, Dr. David Arthur, Dr. Nancy Doreo, Dr. Richard Herbold, Dr. Jeannette Birnbach, Dr. Kari Vernon, Linda Clark, MA NC, Dr. Chris Turnpaugh, Dr. Mike Pierce, Dr. Robert Mathis, Dr. Ben Anderson, and Dr. John Saman.

My sincere ongoing gratitude to my clinical assistant Sandra Arender who has helped make my life and the life of my patients so much easier.

My sincere gratitude to Elaine Fawcett for her help in editing my information and helping me organize this book.

My sincere gratitude to Aristo Vojdani, PhD, the undisputed "Father of Clinical and Functional Immunology," for his mentorship, friendship, and his dedication to teaching me complex immunology.

My sincere gratitude to Jeffrey Bland, PhD, the undisputed "Father of Functional Medicine," for his inspiration and devotion to changing the practice of health care and for efforts that have made functional medicine mainstream medicine all over the world.

My sincere gratitude to Frederick Carrick, DC, PhD, the undisputed "Father of Functional Neurology," for starting the concept of functional neurology that has now evolved into so many new levels of application.

My sincere gratitude to Gerry Leisman, MD, PhD and Robert Melillo, DC, PhD for their ongoing work in organizing functional neurology publications, conferences, and educational materials.

My sincere gratitude to Trish Merlin and the faculty of Carrick Institute.

BOOK ASPIRATIONS

I aspire for this book to empower and give insights to readers so they can develop strategies to improve the function of their brain and to become all they can and should be.

I aspire for this book to change the practice of functional neurology to include strategies of patient care that go beyond brain exercises and rehabilitation to truly question all of the mechanisms of brain impairment. I also aspire for functional neurology health care providers to become versed in more than just brain rehabilitation and to understand clinical relationships of the brain and autoimmunity, immunology, endocrinology, nutrition, neurochemistry, and metabolism. Without understanding these relationships they can never become clinical experts in neurology.

I aspire for this book to change the practice of functional medicine to include understanding of the gut-brain axis and the role the brain plays in various metabolic, endocrinological, and immunological conditions typically not associated with brain function.

PREFACE

After I published my first book *Why Do I Still Have Thyroid Symptoms?* I was shocked to see it become a best-selling book. I really did not think anyone would read it. After the book was released I received so many emails, faxes, phone calls, and stories from thyroid patients all over the world about how the book made such a positive impact on their lives that it completely changed me forever. Although I commonly received praise from my own patients and from doctors I taught, and I enjoyed hearing their success stories, it did not compare to the magnitude of positive impact publishing a book had on so many lives. I knew at that point I had to publish more books and bring this information directly to the public instead of just to postgraduate seminars for health care professionals. I am now on a mission to share my personal research and the insights I have gained through practicing with the general public.

I initially became interested in health care after I sustained a severe back injury in high school. The only treatment given to me was pain medication, which adversely affected my ability to focus and offered me very little help. I continued to suffer for weeks until a friend of the family took me to his chiropractor. I experienced immediate relief and knew then I wanted to be a chiropractor.

I went to chiropractic school simply expecting to learn how to adjust the spine. Instead, I was immersed in human physiology, biochemistry, pathology, histology, radiology, physical examination, laboratory analysis, and many other classes that helped me mature and become a primary care provider.

After I graduated and went into practice, I was horrified by what I discovered about the health care field. I could not believe how many patients were medically mismanaged and how poorly they were treated in the system. I was also shocked at the amount of medication patients were prescribed in the simple model of "one symptom = one drug."

As I cared for my patients, I realized many of them were not receiving direction in improving their overall health. Instead, symptoms or signs were masked with medication. Patients constantly asked me to help them as they did not know where else to go. They had all seen numerous specialists and the simple "take a pill" model was not serving them. Also, many of them felt awful but did not have a disease, so they were dismissed in the health care system.

I have never been anti-medicine, but it became clear to me patients need more than what is being offered. I remember looking at the mechanisms of the top 50 most prescribed medications and realizing almost all of them block, inhibit, or shut down a system of the body, such as beta-blockers, serotonin reuptake inhibitors, calcium channel blockers, protein-pump inhibitors, and so on. But none offered the body support.

Most patients who were suffering had impaired function but did not have disease. The health care model did very little to improve their actual health or it blatantly dismissed their complaints. These realizations inspired my passion to learn more about nutrition and pursue clinical strategies for patients who do not have a clear black-or-white model of disease or health, but instead are somewhere in a gray area.

To this day I am not anti-medicine. I have a high-degree of respect and admiration for the practice of medicine and medical physicians. However, there is no doubt a void exists in the current practice of medicine. Many areas of specialization and training are not provided to medical physicians despite being accepted models in the scientific community, such as diet, nutrition, and lifestyle changes.

I was forced into a unique position very early in my career. As I began to create efficient ways to manage my chronic patients, I wrote some papers and was given opportunities to lecture to other health care providers. This was immediately successful and I began practicing and lecturing. I alternated weeks, seeing patients one week and researching, writing, and lecturing the other week, something I continue today.

Lecturing to skilled clinicians forces me to stay current with the research and the clinical applications for the various topics I teach. Working with patients guides me to know which questions to ask when researching and developing education seminars. As I began to lecture nationally, doctors referred their failed cases and complex patients to me, which further drove me to develop the highest clinical competence I could achieve. The combination of needing to perform at a high level both as a postgraduate educator and as a clinician seeing patients with complex conditions created a demanding cycle that has led to the information I share with you now.

At this point in my career I have seen patients from literally all over the world with various complex conditions. I am not always able to help them but I can usually find strategies to improve their quality of life in some way. Sometimes it is profound and sometimes it is not. There is no question many chronic patients who cannot be helped are suffering from brain dysfunction or early brain degeneration. My aspiration to write this book is to share some fundamental concepts and strategies for those types of cases.

I really hope you enjoy reading this book and that it empowers you. I have made every attempt for this book to serve you and help you gain insights and strategies into supporting your brain health and to get your brain working again.

Datis Kharrazian, DHSc, DC, MS, MNeuroSci
Fellow of the American College of Functional Neurology
Fellow of the American Board of Vestibular Rehabilitation
Fellow of the American Academy of Chiropractic Physicians
Fellow of the International Academy of Functional Neurology
 and Rehabilitation
Diplomate of the American Board of Clinical Nutrition
Diplomate of the Board of Nutrition Specialists
Diplomate of the Chiropractic Board of Clinical Nutrition
Diplomate of the International Board of Applied Kinesiology
Diplomate of the American Board of Chiropractic Neurology

Disclosure About
Case Studies in This Book

I have included case studies in this book. Some are from my own practice and some are from health care practitioners I have trained in my brain health model. Specific case studies are intentionally chosen to help illustrate how the concepts in the book relate to actual patients and their lives.

Although many nutritional theories exist today, the concepts in this book have been used by thousands of clinicians with real patients. The model I present always begins with a review of the scientific literature; a deep appreciation for human physiology; and applications of diet, nutrition, and lifestyle. This model is not a miracle, a promised cure, or anti-medicine. Many patients may require medication or conventional medical treatment outside the concepts presented in this book in order to improve their lives.

I debated putting cases in this book because some reviewers of my thyroid book accused me of using them as a marketing tactic. However, after careful consideration of the criticisms, I am convinced the case stories are necessary to connect complex information with real-life people. I shared this book with several of my patients before its release, and they said the case studies gave them hope while facing terrifying scenarios of poor brain function.

Hope and optimism are very important to improving health. However, it is also very important to note that many patients with poor brain health do not respond to the models presented in this book. Many talented health care practitioners and I have countless failed cases.

I hope the case studies help you see how some of the concepts presented in this book have helped others, even though they are not guaranteed to help everyone. I also hope this book is never accused of promoting false promises, gimmicks, or sales. The book represents years of exhaustive research, clinical trial and error, and countless hours of work to develop strategies that help patients and their families support brain function naturally.

The case studies are there to help motivate you and connect you with the lives of real people. Although not all cases have positive outcomes, sometimes for reasons we don't understand, the vast majority do. I feel it's worth sharing them to help generate optimism and positivity to assist you on your journey.

INTRODUCTION

WHY ISN'T MY BRAIN WORKING?

• •

Jackie, 42, a mother of two children ages 4 and 6, worked as an attorney. She had a caring husband and a successful career she had worked very hard to create for herself. She had paid her own way through college and throughout life, as she had come from a modest background. Jackie had always had an incredible memory and could always count on her brain. However, over the past few years she noticed she couldn't remember phone numbers long enough to put them in her iPhone and was unable to keep up with her work and family responsibilities.

She knew she was no longer dependable at work, which really bothered her, but that was nothing compared to the guilt and frustration she felt because she wasn't able to be the mother she wanted to be. She suffered from bouts of depression and although she was never a fan of medications, her depression had gotten so bad she began taking antidepressants. The medications worked initially, but she stopped taking them when she did not notice any effect from them after a couple of months. Jackie also started to gain weight and have headaches as well as various aches and pains throughout her body.

Jackie had always been the kind of person who could read an entire book in one sitting and remember everything she read. Now she could no longer focus and she found herself fatiguing after reading just a few pages. She was also unable to remember what she had read after finishing just one paragraph.

Jackie started to worry and went to see her doctor, who performed a complete physical examination, ran routine blood work, and diagnosed her with high blood pressure and high cholesterol. He told her she was overweight and needed to eat better and exercise, but he did not give her any specifics. When Jackie explained her symptoms of declining memory and poor brain function symptoms, he laughed and told her she was just getting older and not to worry about it. Jackie left her doctor's appointment feeling embarrassed and ashamed.

After months of feeling depressed she finally decided to take control and figure out what was going on. She read an article on chronic fatigue syndrome and was convinced she was suffering from it. She then spent the next few years trying various treatments, such as bioidentical hormones, heavy metal chelation, adrenal fatigue support, and countless nutritional supplements with no effect. Her symptoms continued to progress.

Finally, a doctor who had seen me speak at a conference referred Jackie to my office. When I saw Jackie she was barely functioning. She came in with countless natural supplements and a long list of practitioners she had seen. The instant I saw her I knew her brain was not working very well. She had facial paresis (drooping of her face), she had ptosis (drooping of her eye lids), and she walked very slowly with very little arm swing. Her handwriting was terrible, and when I asked her about it she said it had been declining the past few years. These were all signs of a brain that was not working well.

Her examination demonstrated she couldn't perform cognitive tasks, such as counting backwards by sevens, or basic memory tasks, such as remembering a few numbers. She was so shocked to realize how far things had deteriorated that she started crying during the exam. She was unable to balance herself when standing with her eyes closed, she had lost her sense of smell and taste, she couldn't touch her nose accurately with her finger if her eyes were closed, and her inability to do various other tasks demonstrated that her brain was not working well.

Despite seeing so many practitioners, none took her brain health into question. One tried to give her some amino acids to support her depression, and another gave her a product for general brain support, but they were all superficial strategies and nobody ever asked why her brain was failing.

After I evaluated Jackie, I could see severe blood sugar fluctuations were impacting her brain chemistry. She was eating a poor diet and she had chronic gastrointestinal inflammation and brain inflammation. She was also suffering from significant impairment of her serotonin and acetylcholine systems. I implemented many of the concepts presented in this book and, unsurprisingly, Jackie began to emerge from the dark place she once inhabited. I checked up on her every month and within three months she said, "I am finally back."

Jackie's story is like so many others. All her symptoms were blamed on aging while both the conventional and alternative medicine models completely overlooked her brain. Most people who have brain impairment and even early brain degeneration suffer from fatigue, depression, and lack of motivation, and they eventually lose some sense of self. Jackie was expressing early signs of brain degeneration and early Alzheimer's disease symptoms. She was very lucky she was able to catch it early enough and change the expression of her brain's future through appropriate diet, nutrition, and lifestyle intervention.

Unfortunately, many people will not be as lucky as Jackie. Most people will have their brain deteriorate more every year thinking that is part of normal aging, until they become impaired enough to be diagnosed with Alzheimer's disease or dementia—with virtually no treatment options to make any difference at that point.

Datis Kharrazian, DHSc, DC, MS

● ●

The incidences of brain disorders are on the rise. Not only do one in eight senior citizens develop Alzheimer's these days, but one in eight children are also diagnosed with brain development disorders, including autism, ADD, and ADHD.[1][2][3] The global prevalence of dementia has been estimated to be as high as 24 million, and is predicted to double every 20 years until at least 2040.[4] Anxiety disorders, such as obsessive compulsive disorder, learning disabilities, and depression are much more prevalent today, while more "garden-variety" symptoms of poor brain health—sleep disorders, brain fog, mild depression, moodiness—have become commonplace.

The most often prescribed drugs in the United States are antidepressants.[5] Depression is rarely due to a direct emotional cause. Instead it is known to develop when the frontal lobes of the brain do not fire like they should. That is why most people who are depressed also can't concentrate, focus, or remember things. Depression not associated with a severe emotional trigger is a sign the brain is failing and steps to improve brain health are crucial not only for recovery from depression, but also for protecting against brain degeneration.

The vicious mood swings associated with premenstrual syndrome, perimenopause ("pre-menopause"), and menopause, the results of hormone-driven brain chemistry imbalances and brain inflammation, are so ubiquitous these days people think they're normal—they aren't. Ditto the gradual descent into andropause, or "male menopause," when a man's increasingly skewed hormonal function creates the "grumpy old man" syndrome, or triggers the stereotypical mid-life crisis. Both menopause and male hormone disorders create an environment for early brain degeneration that is initially preceded by a poorly functioning brain.

Thyroid disorders, which profoundly impact brain health and function, affect an estimated 27 million Americans, causing brain fog, depression, anxiety, and other brain-based abnormalities. But most importantly they accelerate brain degeneration and even coexist with brain autoimmunity.

Add to these factors the ingestion of newly modified dietary proteins, such as gluten, fried foods, and other foods high in free-radicals, a diet low in antioxidants and essential fatty acids, and the ups and downs of a blood sugar roller coaster thanks to too many sweets and starchy foods, and it is no wonder we have created an environment that promotes brain decay.

A high stress, sedentary lifestyle rounds out the perfect recipe for brain degeneration. Besides the dietary and lifestyle triggers that create poor brain function, previous head injuries, subtle brain autoimmunity, poor circulation, and various other factors unrelated to diet can also cause the brain to fail and degenerate quickly.

When the brain loses its ability to do its job, people have trouble learning. They lose their passion and motivation, their ability to enjoy music and hobbies, and their taste perception so they no longer enjoy food like they once did. Their balance becomes compromised, they start to get lost and become bad with directions, they lose their ability to digest food, and they basically become inefficient at running their lives. Many will lose their jobs or perform poorly at home and work. They will notice their inabilities lead to social, family, and professional strains and that over time the life they used to know is gone. In summary, a highly functioning brain leads to a highly productive and appreciative life. A poorly functioning brain leads to a life of unreachable goals, inefficiency, depression, and a continued dependence on others.

So why aren't doctors taking better care of their patients' brains? Because brain care is not part of the common health care paradigm in conventional or alternative medicine. In both branches, health care seems to be a "neck-down" practice, even though the brain can be the most fragile and susceptible organ to the health imbalances caused by poor diet and chronic stress. Practitioners aren't focused on or versed in how to recognize or manage the early stages of brain degeneration until it's progressed to a pathology past the point of return (Alzheimer's, Parkinson's, etc.).

In the current health care model you have to wait until you cannot recognize your family members or find your way home before a doctor will diagnose you with Alzheimer's disease, despite the fact you notice your sense of direction and your memory are progressively deteriorating years before the diagnosis. You have to wait to develop tremors before a doctor diagnoses you with Parkinson's disease, despite the fact the earliest stages of Parkinson's start with chronic constipation, loss of smell, and slowness of movements and mental speed years before you develop a tremor. At that point, the golden window of opportunity to make dramatic changes is forever gone. We have a health care model that does not diagnose, treat, or attend to brain health until an end-stage neurological disease develops. This is why if your brain is not working you must learn how to save it yourself.

Rare is the brain disorder that mysteriously pops up out of nowhere, or is due solely to a genetic predisposition. In most cases, one can trace the demise of a person's brain to the modern lifestyle—high-carbohydrate diets, processed foods laden with neurotoxins, brain-sapping "bad" fats, common digestive problems, wheat and gluten foods, lack of sleep, and chronic stress.

Why Isn't My Brain Working? is a guide that brings together both scientific and natural medicine approaches to help you learn how to spot weaknesses and abnormalities in your own brain function, whether they are subtle or loudly obvious. One person may notice his memory isn't quite what it used to be, or that a long day at work is more tiring than he remembers it used to be. Someone else may have a more overt neurological imbalance, such as depression, anxiety, or brain fog. Either way, you will learn how to unravel the underlying causes of your dysfunction—because the same symptom can have myriad causes—and how to go about remedying them.

For instance, you will learn how to spot your own brain function weaknesses through a list of questions at the beginning of each chapter along with examples of real-life scenarios. When specific areas that need addressing are identified, you will then be taken through an approach to restore your brain health and integrity. A sample plan, for instance, could include restoring balance to blood sugar, addressing gut inflammation, boosting dopamine levels, and restoring the integrity of the blood-brain barrier—all through natural, non-pharmaceutical means.

I explain neurotransmitters and how to support neurotransmitter pathways. Neurotransmitters are chemicals that allow brain cells to communicate with one another, although they are more popularly known for their effects on our mood, behavior, and personality. I discuss the four main neurotransmitters:

- Acetylcholine, our "learning and memory" neurotransmitter
- Serotonin, our "happy and joyful" neurotransmitter
- Dopamine, our "pleasure and reward" neurotransmitter
- GABA, our "calm and relaxed" neurotransmitter

But I go beyond common knowledge of neurotransmitters to explain the relationship between male and female hormones and these neurotransmitters, as well as the impact of inflammation, autoimmune disease, and other immune issues on neurotransmitter activity.

For example, a woman with hormonal imbalances may find her estrogen drops too low before her periods, causing a serotonin dysregulation and, consequently, irritability and depression. Addressing that would include not only restoring hormonal balance using dietary modifications and nutritional compounds, but also supporting serotonin pathways.

Or a man with chronic joint pain and stress may find ongoing inflammation and stress responses are decreasing his dopamine levels, causing a short temper, poor motivation, and feelings of worthlessness. His remedy would include not only restoring harmony to the immune system, but also supporting dopamine pathways to protect his brain health and hormonal balance.

For the majority of people, **brain nutrition**, **stress**, and **blood sugar imbalances** must be addressed first. While working with supplements to boost and balance brain chemistry is exciting since the effects can be so profound, one must tackle these three basics first for effective, lasting results.

For instance, a person with depression, inner rage, and paranoia due to a serotonin imbalance is going to have poor luck boosting serotonin pathways if she continues to indulge in pastries for breakfast, pasta for lunch, starchy, high-carb bean and rice burritos for dinner, and sugary snacks and coffee drinks throughout the day. A diet like this severely disrupts blood sugar balancing, and, hence, serotonin pathways.

Once the fundamentals of brain health are established, it's time to take on the four major neurotransmitters: acetylcholine, serotonin, dopamine, and GABA. After addressing brain nutrition, stress, or blood sugar imbalances, many people find they no longer need specialized brain support. Or, whereas they showed symptoms in all four main neurotransmitters before, they have now whittled it down to one. At that point, targeted support through specific nutrients and herbs can profoundly restore brain chemistry and, as a result, quality of life.

I then go into whether the brain is receiving enough **oxygen**. You would be surprised how many people's brains are not getting enough oxygen from conditions such as anemia or from poor circulation. I discuss the symptoms and how to restore the brain's ability to "breathe" through lifestyle and supplementation.

Then I delve into the extremely important and little known area of **brain inflammation**—the brain has its own immune system that operates quite differently from the immune system in the rest of the body (although inflammation in the brain can be triggered by inflammation in the body). The brain's immune system can be triggered by harmful substances that have snuck into the brain through its lining, which has become overly porous from degeneration. At that point, the brain's immune system launches an all-out assault to destroy the invader, unfortunately chewing up plenty of brain tissue in the process. This not only produces troubling symptoms, such as brain fog, but it also puts one at a higher risk for a brain-based autoimmune disease with consequences that run the gamut from poor balance to autism.

I have found in my practice that autism is often the result of an autoimmune attack in the brain. Addressing the underlying immune imbalances can, in some cases, significantly improve autism symptoms. Spotting the very early warning signs of dementia and addressing them can reduce the risk of Alzheimer's disease or delay its onset. I will also discuss the long-term implications of brain injury and some immediate steps one can take after a brain injury, based on exciting discoveries in neurological research, to help prevent future problems.

I also explore the direct relationship between the immune health of the brain and the immune health of the gut, and why you need to address both when one or the other is ailing. For instance, when my patient John presented with multiple food intolerances, symptoms of irritable bowel syndrome, and constant heartburn, remedying these gut issues helped significantly with neurotransmitter imbalances that were causing feelings of rage and worthlessness.

Also, hormones come into play when addressing the brain's immune system, as both male and female hormones, and thyroid and adrenal hormones, are vital to protecting and regulating the immune health of the brain. For example, hypothyroidism can activate brain inflammation and dysregulate all the major brain neurotransmitters. The same can also happen to a woman going through menopause if her estrogen levels drop too low, depriving her brain of this protective hormone.

We all experience a certain degree of ongoing brain degeneration as a natural matter of course, but the trick is to not let that degeneration go any faster than it ought to, and to learn how to compensate for it by building a healthy, active brain. Aging is a nicer term for accelerated brain degeneration, and significantly losing your memory, your alertness, your response time, and your mental stamina while getting older is neither normal nor healthy.

We all have known the octogenarian who is sharp as a tack, although they are getting rarer. Their performance signifies the maintaining of a healthy and alert brain despite advancing years, because that is actually how nature designed us to be. The human species is living longer than ever before, but it is not functioning well in later years due to progressed brain degeneration. It doesn't matter how long you live, but how highly functioning your brain is as you get older.

You are your brain; the health of the brain dictates everything about you. How you perceive events in life, your personality, how much you enjoy life, how you react to everyday occurrences, your emotional health, and so on—these are all determined by your brain's health and function.

Why Isn't My Brain Working? will teach you to take care of your brain as you would any other part of your body, and it will show you through real-life stories of others who have improved the health of their brains and the quality of their lives. *Why Isn't My Brain Working?* builds upon my work in functional medicine—medicine based on addressing health concerns before disease develops. By integrating brain health with the health of the body and identifying and addressing downward trends in brain health before they turn into irreversible conditions and diseases, *Why Isn't My Brain Working?* may not only help readers avoid debilitating brain diseases, but it may also enhance the quality of their lives through optimal brain health.

CHAPTER ONE
BRAIN BASICS 101

• •

Jack, 26, was a college graduate with a degree in anthropology. Although he managed to graduate from college it was not without great difficulty. Jack had been diagnosed with attention deficit disorder (ADD) as a child but could not take any medications because they made him hyperactive and physically aggressive. Poor mental endurance and motivation made what seemed so easy and routine for everybody else a huge struggle for Jack. Just getting out of bed and completing an ordinary day left him both emotionally and physically depleted. It took him hours and hours to read each chapter for his classes because of his poor brain endurance. When studying he was easily distracted and needed to constantly take breaks because he couldn't focus. He frequently missed homework deadlines and was always pleading with his professors to pass him.

Jack managed to finish college after six years but was so nervous about how he would compensate for his poor brain function in the real world that he moved back with his parents. He basically slept in every day and did nothing productive for more than a year. Jack's parents initially understood and gave him support and encouragement, but eventually they succumbed to disappointment and anger. Jack spent many days alone crying because he did not understand why he could not get his life started. Then one day a friend in the family mentioned my work and they flew Jack across the country for an evaluation.

When I first meet Jack I could see the deep sadness and shame in his eyes over having disappointed himself and his family. He was willing to try anything but was deeply doubtful anything would work. His parents were obviously emotionally broken and worn out by Jack's condition. An examination made it very clear Jack's frontal cortex was not working well. He was unable to perform basic math calculations. When evaluated for fast eye movements, called "saccades," they were very slow. His handwriting was already very poor and worsened the longer he wrote. He also had increased muscle tone on one side of his body. Together with his history of ADD these symptoms it was clear he had gone his entire life with poor frontal cortex function.

I now needed to find out what factors were involved. He had all the symptoms and patterns associated with poor dopamine activity (dopamine is a brain chemical important for motivation) and his lab work indicated iron-deficiency anemia. Iron is critical for dopamine production, which helps explain why anemia can cause depression and lack of motivation. Lab tests indicated his iron deficiency was related to an infection in his stomach of H. pylori, a bacterium that impairs iron absorption. Jack was also suffering from poor diet and lifestyle habits that led to blood sugar imbalances and a lack of essential fatty acids.

Jack was treated for his H. plyori infection, and I placed him on supplements to increase his iron and brain dopamine levels. I also had him follow a diet that stabilized his blood glucose and improved his essential fatty acid levels (all discussed later in this book). Jack experienced a dramatic outcome in the first 30 days, as if somebody pushed his "on button," according to his family. As his brain function and endurance improved, I introduced exercises such as Sudoku, math exercises, and coordination exercises to help develop his frontal cortex.

I share Jack's case with you because it is a great example of how lack of activity in one area of the brain can completely derail a person's life and disrupt family dynamics and relationships. It was a tragedy that nobody in the health care system could develop strategies to improve brain function early in his life. He was prescribed stimulants for his ADD but because they didn't work the health care system simply dismissed him. Unfortunately, his brain never grew out of the ADD pattern and he suffered from impair-

ment all the way through college. It is painful to imagine how different Jack's life would have been had he been given strategies to improve his brain function as a child.

There are two great windows of time to change brain function. The first window is before age nine as the brain's grey matter completely develops by then. The next window is before age 19, when the white matter completely develops. Unfortunately for Jack, he missed both developmental opportunities.

Development of brain growth, timing, and coordination in childhood are critical to proper function throughout life. If there is developmental delay in brain function in childhood, such as ADHD, autism, Tourette's Syndrome, obsessive compulsive disorder (OCD), anxiety, tics, dyslexia, learning or processing disorders, or even more subtle symptoms, it is best to aggressively rehabilitate function before adulthood. Unfortunately, the current model of health care tells parents to wait for the child to grow out of it. However, many children do not grow out of it and miss key windows of time for ideal brain development.

Unrelated to developmental delays, early symptoms of brain degeneration such as poor mental endurance, poor memory, and inability to learn new things are also serious issues when timing matters. The longer a person waits to manage their brain degeneration or developmental delay the less potential they have to make a difference.

Datis Kharrazian, DHSc, DC, MS

HOW THE BRAIN WORKS

By learning how a healthy brain is supposed to work, you gain a better understanding of why and how things break down and what to look for in your own behavior and symptoms. Rare is the patient who walks into a doctor's office and says, "Doc, I'm experiencing accelerated neurodegeneration. Can you help me?" An experienced practitioner, however, will be assessing your brain health before you even arrive. Were you late? Could you find the office? Did you have to call and ask for directions more than once because you had a hard time following them? Were you able to fill out the intake forms in a timely manner or answer questions without getting distracted or forgetting what was asked? Has your handwriting deteriorated so much that your intake form is hard to read? Are you rude and aggressive with the reception staff, or do you nod off in the waiting room? These are all clues that can alert the astute practitioner to what is going on with your brain, and these will be detailed in this book.

Before we can launch into what causes brain degeneration and poor brain function, as well as how to optimize brain health, we will cover some basics of brain anatomy and neuroscience.

The brain is the most complex tissue in all of the human body. Weighing in at about three pounds, it is one of our heaviest organs and the most oxygen-demanding, and it uses up to 30 percent of the body's glucose supply to function. This gray and white mass with the texture of tofu allows us to sense our environment, move with purpose, feel emotions and interpret them, operate all our bodily functions 24 hours a day with no conscious effort, think, and, ultimately, become who we are with our various personality traits, habits, and quirks.

The brain has become the darling of new exploration by highly specialized doctors and researchers as well as armchair enthusiasts. The 1990s were declared "The Decade of the Brain" by the U.S. Congress, and we are still more than 20 years into that "decade." The brain is divided into different lobes or sections, and if you can become familiar with the basic functions of each lobe, you will have a much better understanding of your own brain function or brain imbalance. I will give you a quick review of each major lobe and what symptoms and signs you may develop if it is not working well.

FUNCTIONAL AREAS OF THE BRAIN
Frontal lobe

The frontal lobe, or cortex, is the largest lobe in the brain. It is located directly behind your forehead and stretches between the temples. The human's large frontal lobe is what distinguishes us from other animals, and much of our personality and who we are stems from this part of the brain. This is why a severe frontal lobe injury can completely change one's personality—he or she may never be the same person again. (This is why bike helmets and other helmets should always fit snugly over the forehead.)

A healthy frontal lobe allows us to function appropriately within society, as it is involved in the ability to reason and suppress impulses. These impulses include acting on sexual desire, violent tendencies, and other types of socially unacceptable behavior. A functioning frontal lobe is what prevents you from walking up and kissing a good-looking stranger, or from shouting at or hitting someone in an angry moment.

It is now understood that children with attention deficit hyperactivity disorder (ADHD) have delays in frontal cortex development and cannot suppress their immediate desires and impulses. Parents and teachers may punish these children for bad behavior. However, the part of the brain responsible for reasoning is not developed and behavior modification is difficult to impossible.

Instead of focusing on strategies to help the frontal cortex develop, physicians prescribe these children stimulant medications similar to cocaine. These medications overstimulate the brain in an attempt to make it work better but do not help support brain development. Many ADHD children become addicted to the medications. Over time, the effectiveness of the stimulants wears off while the underlying disorder is never addressed.

Adults with impaired frontal cortex function also may struggle with impulse control. They are more likely to say things they shouldn't, cheat in relationships because they cannot dampen their sexual impulses, or use bad judgment in business and personal matters.

The frontal lobe also governs emotional drive, motivation, and planning, and frontal lobe impairment can lead to an inability to set goals or follow through on projects or plans. You no can longer commit to anything, or even want to, and as a result you may become lazy, unmotivated, and even depressed.

In the field of neuroscience, depression is considered a frontal cortex impairment. The standard model of treatment is to give a patient an antidepressant that increases activation of certain neurotransmitters, brain chemicals that relay messages between neurons. Unfortunately, the mechanisms of these medications are short-lived and fail to address the underlying issue of poor health or neurodegeneration of the frontal cortex.

Lastly, your frontal cortex is responsible for activating muscles. Impairment of the frontal cortex results in reduced amplitude (the

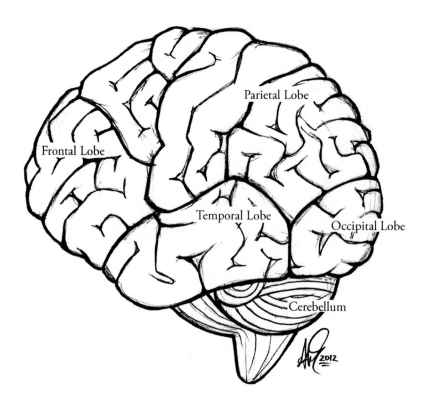

intensity and force exerted by the muscle) and speed of the muscles. It may be as subtle as just moving slower or not swinging your arms when you walk, or as severe as moving in slow motion.

The frontal cortex is also responsible for fine-motor coordination, which is needed for such activities as handwriting or embroidery. This is why it's common to see poor handwriting develop when the frontal cortex degenerates. Whenever I evaluate new patient intake forms, I always study the handwriting to look for signs of neurodegeneration. Many times I see signs of a tremor in the handwriting, or "micrographia," a condition associated with certain disease of the brain in which the handwriting becomes smaller. Or I see an angle or sway preference in the writing, which can indicate a dominance of certain eye muscles or balance-related areas of the brain. When the frontal cortex degenerates, however, it is common just to see overall sloppier handwriting.

The first question I ask when I see poor handwriting is, "Has your handwriting always been bad or has it become bad over the years?"

If they say they used to have great handwriting but it has gotten worse, I become concerned about the health of their brain. I then ask when they noticed their handwriting becoming worse. If they say it happened rather quickly in the past year that tells me they are suffering from rapid brain degeneration. If they tell me it occurred during the past five years, it indicates a much slower loss.

When evaluating frontal lobe health, you should look for all of these symptoms: Has your handwriting gotten much worse? Are you suffering from lack of motivation and general laziness? Are you having episodes of inappropriate social behavior? The frontal lobe also plays a role in cognitive function. If you also find you're not as good as you used to be with math, word searching, or other cognitive tasks, it may suggest your frontal cortex is showing early signs of degeneration.

Symptoms and signs of frontal cortex impairment

- Decreased amplitude or slower movements of muscle
- Depression
- Mental sluggishness and laziness
- Poor impulse control
- Poor social behavior and judgment
- Poor handwriting
- Poor cognitive function, such as poor math or planning skills
- Poor cognitive learning, such as math, new languages, or philosophy
- Poor muscle-coordinated learning such as dancing and playing sports

Temporal lobe

The temporal lobes are located on either side of the brain above the ears and are responsible for hearing, speech, memory, emotional responses, and distinguishing smells. Different areas of the temporal lobe perform different tasks.

The temporal lobes are critical for interpreting sound. Many times when the temporal lobes start to spontaneously fire from early neuro-degeneration, tinnitus (ringing in the ear) can occur, although not all tinnitus is due to temporal lobe degeneration. A compromised temporal lobe can make it difficult for you to distinguish different tones and cause you to have difficulty hearing someone talking if there is background noise.

Within the temporal lobes you have a very important area called the hippocampus (Latin for sea horse because of its anatomical shape). This area of the brain is involved with learning and memory, and degeneration of the hippocampus leads to poor memory and eventually Alzheimer's disease. The hippocampus must be healthy in order for you to convert short-term memory into long-term memory. Older memories are already stored in the medial temporal lobe, which is why in early stages of hippocampus degeneration a person can give you specific details about their wedding 30 years ago, but cannot recall what they ate for lunch yesterday. This area of the brain is also involved with spatial orientation and sense of direction. In the early stages of hippocampus degeneration, a person not only begins losing short-term memory but also becomes bad with directions and needs a navigation system while driving. As the degeneration progresses, one begins to lose long-term memory and will get lost driving home on well-traveled routes. These changes are associated with Alzheimer's disease.

The hippocampus is also involved with your circadian rhythm, or sleep-wake cycle, that is responsible for healthy energy in the morning and a relaxed state at night. Dysfunction in this area can lead to insomnia, an inability to get of bed in the morning, and afternoon crashes in energy.

If you notice you're losing your memory, you forget why you walk into rooms, you can't remember where you put things like your car keys, or you constantly forget where you parked your car, you may be suffering from early temporal lobe degeneration. This should be a concern for you because these are also the earliest symptoms of Alzheimer's disease.

Symptoms and signs of temporal lobe impairment
- Poor memory
- Difficulty hearing with background noise
- Episodes of tinnitus

- Abnormal shifts of fatigue throughout the day
- Ongoing episodes of insomnia

Parietal lobe
The parietal lobes are located directly behind your ears. Their primary function is to perceive sensations, such as touch or pressure, and to interpret sensation, such as texture, weight, size, or shape. Another important parietal lobe function is to integrate input from the skin, muscles, joints, and vision to become aware of the body in its environment. When the parietal lobe starts to degenerate, you have difficulty maintaining your balance in the dark and may even have difficulty perceiving where your arm or leg is.

It is really common to get reoccurring injuries such as ankle sprains when your parietal lobe is impaired and your brain cannot recognize where your limbs are in space. You may have difficulty discerning coins or other objects through touch and need to see them in order to know what they are. You may misjudge the back of the chair or try to lean on a wall and misjudge where your body is in relation to the wall. If you are a woman, you may start to feel unstable in high heels and prefer shoes that keep your feet closer to the ground.

Symptoms and signs of parietal lobe impairment
- Feeling unstable in darkness or with thick or high-heel shoes
- Misjudging where your body is in relation to your environment
- Unable to recognize objects through touch
- Difficulty perceiving where your limbs are and becoming prone to falls and sprains

Cerebellum
Your cerebellum, or "little brain," is comprised of two distinct lobes and sits at the back of your head directly above your neck. The cerebellum calibrates muscle coordination of movement when you perform basic actions, such as putting a spoon to your mouth. One symptom of early cerebellar degeneration is termination tremors—a couple of beats of shakiness at the end of a movement, such as pointing or reaching for a pen. There is no tremor at rest as with Parkinson's disease, but just a couple of subtle shakes at the end of a movement.

The cerebellum also helps calibrate and interpret information responsible for balance coming from the inner ear. As the cerebellum begins to degenerate, a person may walk and stand with their feet wider apart for more stability. They also have difficulty walking down stairs without holding on to the handrail, walking in a straight line with their eyes closed, or standing on one foot. They would basically fail a DUI test.

In fact, DUI tests are cerebellum tests because alcohol suppresses the cerebellum. It is not uncommon for patients with cerebellum degeneration to feel wobbly at times as if they are drunk. These people cannot handle alcohol very well because they cannot afford any further suppression of the cerebellum. Being a "cheap date" can be a sign of poor cerebellar health.

While the cerebellum receives information from the muscles and inner ear, it also must filter that information before sending it to the brain. If the cerebellum degenerates, it loses the ability to do this adequately, with sometimes unpleasant consequences. People who have poorly developed or impaired cerebellums will typically get carsick and seasick very easily. They may become nauseous from staring at wallpaper, shirts, or rugs with stripes or complex patterns. Cerebellum problems are so common in my practice that I never wear pinstriped shirts or ties with complex patterns because they make many of my patients sick.

Symptoms and signs of cerebellum impairment
- Episodes of dizziness or vertigo
- Nausea from visual inputs (car sickness)
- Poor balance
- Subtle shakes at the end stage of movement

Occipital lobe
The occipital lobe is located in the back of the brain. It processes visual information, such as recognizing shapes, colors, and motion, and distinguishing between colors. People with depressed occipital lobe function have difficulty distinguishing borders of lines with similar colors, or fail to appreciate vivid colors in art. They may also see occasional flashes of light, have visual hallucinations, or persistence of a visual image after it has been removed.

Symptoms of occipital lobe impairment
- Difficulty processing visual information and recognizing shapes, colors, and motion
- Visual hallucinations
- Visual floaters
- Visual persistence or reoccurrence of the visual image after it has been removed

As you finish reading this chapter you should ask yourself if you or any of your family members have any of the symptoms I covered. In adults these symptoms usually mean degeneration in those specific areas of the brain. In children these symptoms indicate brain developmental delay in those areas. You may have many of these symptoms if your overall brain is not functioning. Or you may have only a few symptoms but you are having issues with overall brain endurance.

HOW A HEALTHY BRAIN RUNS YOUR BODY

To conclude this chapter on neuroscience basics, it's important to look at the relationship between the brain and autonomic control. This section of the book can get a little complicated, so if you don't get it, that's OK. You can even skip it if you'd prefer.

The autonomic nervous system runs our organs, blood vessels, glands, and other bodily functions of which we have no conscious awareness. This is an important consideration because if we lose brain function due to accelerated degeneration, we risk digestive problems, high blood pressure, dry eyes, incontinence, erectile dysfunction, and more.

The autonomic system can be roughly divided into two categories: the sympathetic system, more simply known as our "fight or flight" system, and the parasympathetic system, known as the "rest and digest" system. The sympathetic system originates from the upper third of the brain stem, in what is called the mesencephalic reticular formation (MRF), while the parasympathetic system rests primarily in the lower two-thirds of the brain stem, in the pontomedullary reticular formation (PMRF).

If the MRF fires, you get a sympathetic response, such as startling in reaction to a loud bang. If the PMRF fires, you get a parasympathetic response, such as digesting a nice meal while leaning back in your chair

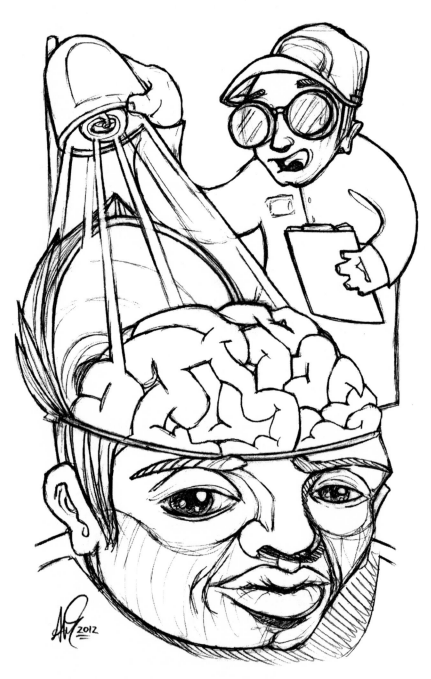

*A healthy brain ensures strong digestion, normal blood pressure,
sufficient saliva and tears, good bladder function, and more.*

to relax and talk with friends. These two systems cannot simultaneously dominate, so when one fires, it inhibits the other. For most stressed-out Americans, unfortunately, this means digestion and other important parasympathetic actions all too frequently take a back seat to the action-oriented, get-up-and-go sympathetic system.

In a healthy brain, 90 percent of information from the brain exits through the PMRF, which in turn stimulates parasympathetic activity. It also inhibits sympathetic activity, which exits through the intermediolateral cell column (IML) in the spinal column.

When the brain is operating optimally, normal brain output generates a parasympathetic response while at the same time dampening the sympathetic system. This ensures, among other things, that digestion is strong, blood pressure is normal, and that there are enough tears, mucus, and saliva in your body. When one or more of the brain regions explained above starts degenerating, there is less input into the PMRF, leading to a decline in parasympathetic activity and a simultaneous increase in sympathetic activity.

WHAT OLD PEOPLE AND NEWBORNS HAVE IN COMMON

The brains of newborn babies and old people are similar in how their parasympathetic and sympathetic systems function. When a baby is born, its parasympathetic system hasn't yet developed. Babies can't digest well, they have high heart rates, and their pupils are huge—all aspects of sympathetic dominance. As their brain develops and they learn to move and walk, the brain increasingly fires into the PMRF, generating more parasympathetic activity. Their heart rate goes down, pupil size shrinks, and their digestive system can take on foods more complex than breast milk.

On the other hand, as people get older, their brain degenerates and they start reverting to the sympathetic dominance of a newborn. They develop constipation, an inability to digest foods, an inability to produce digestive enzymes, and an elevated heart rate due to poor brain function. The sympathetic response also restricts blood flow to the extremities and they have cold hands and feet, and chronic fungal growths on their nails. They also fatigue quickly and struggle with other breakdowns in autonomic function. They may lose their sense of smell and taste because there is not enough mucus in their nasal passages, which in turn causes the brain's olfactory pathways to decline. In fact, a common cause of death of seniors is eating rotten food because they have lost their ability to smell or taste.

PROTECTING YOUR MOST PRECIOUS ORGAN

The scenario I painted above doesn't belong just to infants and the aged. I also see it in my chronically ill patients and even in children with developmental delays in brain function as indicated by writing, speaking, and social development. Even if you are not chronically ill, brain degeneration can suppress your parasympathetic system and lead to insomnia, high blood pressure, or chronic digestive issues, despite the fact that you otherwise function normally.

Regardless, it's always important to address the fundamentals of brain health. Are the neurons receiving enough oxygen, glucose, and stimulation? Are blood sugar issues, poor liver function, inflammation, hormonal imbalances, or lack of neurotransmitter activity promoting brain degeneration? Is plasticity (the ability of your brain to learn and adapt to change) being promoted in a positive or negative direction? These are the principles we'll discuss in this book.

Incorporating these fundamentals prevents health care from being a strictly neck-down approach or, as is often the case in neurology, a strictly neck-up approach. It is impossible to separate the health of your body or mind from the health of your brain, and health care that ignores the brain will always be incomplete care.

In this chapter I introduced you to important fundamentals of neurology that pertain to brain health and brain degeneration. With that under our belts, we will now begin to explore the particulars of these dynamics and how to address them.

● ●

James, 43, was a perfect example of someone slowly succumbing to a rapidly aging brain brought on by his diet and lifestyle. True, he was a marathon runner who ran 30 to 40 miles a week and looked like the picture of health. But when he came to see Dr. Kari Vernon, DC, a Scottsdale, Arizona practitioner who was trained by Dr. Kharrazian, he suffered from anxiety, panic attacks, sleeplessness, chronic pounding headaches, and hands that constantly shook. The more anxious he became, the worse his hands shook. He was taking medications for high blood pressure and an experimental drug to help with his shaking hands.

James always skipped breakfast and drank a few triple-caffeine drinks or took caffeine pills every morning to get going. When the tremors started he stopped the caffeine, but to no avail. In fact, they were steadily getting worse.

I put him on herbal and nutritional compounds to stem the damage and begin restoring health to his brain. I also addressed a bacterial gut infection by giving him a detoxifying protein powder and recommended a powerful antioxidant in the form of a glutathione cream. This helped reduce the inflammation from the infection that was taxing his brain health.

He followed a strict diet for three weeks that eliminated all the major allergens and inflammatory foods, such as wheat, dairy, and eggs, while I ran adrenal tests, a comprehensive blood panel, and a gluten intolerance test.

Before the results were in, James already noticed significant improvement. His headaches vanished and his anxiety and tremors abated. His testing revealed adrenal fatigue, no doubt brought on by a combination of poor diet, excess caffeine, food intolerances, and marathon training. The adrenal test also revealed an abnormal circadian rhythm, a brain-based sleep-wake cycle that ideally has us feeling alert in the morning and tired at night. James' circadian rhythm was backwards; he had a hard time waking up in the morning and was up late at night with insomnia.

Other lab testing revealed he had celiac disease, while an at-home GABA challenge (explained later in the book) showed the lining of his brain had become overly porous. This can allow pathogens into the brain, triggering inflammation and accelerating brain degeneration.

I tailored nutritional compounds to counteract James' conditions (the specifics will be discussed in this book), and based on the feedback from his allergen-elimination diet, put him on a diet free of gluten, corn, and dairy. After a year of faithfully following this protocol, James is off his medications and completely symptom-free.

Dr. Kari Vernon, DC
Scottsdale, Arizona
www.karismaforlife.com

• •

CHAPTER SUMMARY

• The brain is one of the heaviest organs in the body, is the most oxygen-demanding, and uses up to 30 percent of the body's glucose supply.

• The frontal lobe, or cortex, stretches between the temples. Much of our personality stems from this part of the brain. The frontal lobe governs impulse control, emotional drive, motivation, planning, and fine motor coordination. It is involved in ADHD, depression, and loss of fine-motor control, such as deterioration of handwriting.

• The temporal lobes are located on either side of the brain above the ears and are responsible for hearing, speech, memory, emotional responses, and distinguishing smells. It contains the hippocampus, which is involved in learning and memory and the sleep-wake cycle. Symptoms of temporal lobe issues include poor memory, difficulty hearing with background noise, tinnitus, disturbed sleep or daytime energy levels, and insomnia.

• The parietal lobes are located directly behind your ears. Their primary function is to perceive sensations, such as touch or pressure, and to interpret sensation, such as texture, weight, size, or shape. Another important parietal lobe function is to integrate input from the skin, muscles, joints, and vision to become aware of the body in its environment. Symptoms of parietal lobe impairment include feeling unstable in darkness or with thick or high heel shoes, misjudging where your body is in relation to your environment, being unable to recognize objects through touch, and having difficulty perceiving where your limbs are and being prone to falls and sprains.

• Your cerebellum, or "little brain," is comprised of two distinct lobes and sits at the back of your head directly above your neck. The cerebellum calibrates muscle coordination of movement when you perform basic actions, such as putting a spoon to your mouth. Symptoms of cerebellar impairment include episodes of dizziness or vertigo, nausea from visual inputs (car sickness), poor balance, and subtle shakes at the end stage of movement.

• The occipital lobe is located in the back of the brain and processes visual information, such as recognizing shapes, colors, and motion, and distinguishing between colors. People with impaired occipital lobe function have difficulty processing visual information and recognizing, shapes, colors, and motion, visual hallucinations, visual floaters, and visual persistence or reoccurrence of the visual image after it has been removed.

• A healthy brain stimulates "rest and digest" activity while dampening "fight or flight" activity.

• It's always important to address the fundamentals of brain health. Are the neurons receiving enough oxygen, glucose, and stimulation? Are blood sugar issues, poor liver function, inflammation, hormonal imbalances, or lack of neurotransmitter activity promoting brain degeneration? Is plasticity (the ability of your brain to learn and adapt to change) being promoted in a positive or negative direction? These are the principles we'll discuss in this book.

Chapter Two
BRAIN PLASTICITY AND HOPE

● ●

Ryan was a passenger in an Isuzu Rodeo on the way to a high school formal dance when the driver lost control of the vehicle and it rolled over three times. Three passengers were ejected from the car and two died. Ryan was wearing a seat belt that restrained him; however, the roof of the car came down on his head very violently and he suffered a severe head injury. At the hospital, he was intubated and kept on the respirator until he could breathe on his own, which happened two and a half days later. He has no memory of the accident. His last memory was about 15 minutes before the accident.

After one week he went home from the hospital with a neck brace and was given a cane for balance. He suffered chronic pain from ongoing muscle spasms. Three years after the accident, Ryan was sitting on the couch at his aunt and uncle's house when he had a severe seizure. He remembers feeling a tug on his right foot and then his entire right side lifted and he dropped a drinking glass he was holding. He made a noise and, according to the family, his face turned gray and he went unconscious.

Paramedics were called and he was taken to the hospital. He was released the following evening with a prescription for seizure medication. Once out of the hospital, Ryan noticed intermittent tingling and loss of feeling in his arms, legs, hands, and feet—sensations that had never occurred before. It was more prominent in his right foot and leg, happened at different times, and was unprovoked. Ryan suffered from several other seizures and was given various anti-seizure medications with varying results. His last two seizures occurred during rehabilitation treatments.

Ryan came into my office with his parents three and a half years after the accident suffering from continued progression of his initial head trauma. He was no longer able to drive and needed to be watched at all times in case he had another seizure. He was also suffering from numbness and tingling sensations in his extremities and severe muscle tightness and spasm in his shoulders.

When I examined him I found his left frontal and parietal lobe were significantly damaged. He had difficulty sensing a metal pinwheel rolled across his skin or vibration on the right side of his body. He also suffered from spasticity in his right lower leg. He had abnormal pupil responses to light, and light made his entire brain fatigue.

What was most concerning about Ryan was that too much stimulation just from the examination would cause muscle spasms in his right lower leg, one of the earliest signs of an impending seizure. I had to be very careful examining him as I did not want to induce a seizure. I placed him on a heart rate monitor and constantly watched his right leg muscle tone to make sure he was not going to go into a seizure.

During the examination I found that having him perform eye movements called "optikinetics" in a specific direction stimulated the injured areas of his brain to relax his muscle tightness and regain his ability to better perceive sensation on the right side of his body. However, if I continued the therapy for too many repetitions he would get worse, which was a sign his brain chemistry was not ready to handle aggressive brain therapy. I needed to use brain rehabilitation therapy to rebuild, or develop positive plasticity, in the injured areas of his brain. But the brain inflammation from his trauma was so severe it was compromising the ability of his neurons to respond.

What was most concerning about Ryan's case was that he had become worse since his injury three years earlier. Typically after a severe head injury, there is swelling in the brain, and as the swelling goes down many functions return. However, the consequences of a head injury for many people do not appear until years after the trauma. This is because a brain injury activates the brain's microglia cells, which create inflammation. This inflammation *can persist long after the injury. This continued microglia inflammatory cascade leads to ongoing neuron loss and the possible progression to neuron death.*

My first and immediate goal with Ryan was to dampen his microglia brain inflammation. I placed him on a protocol of high-dose flavonoids that have been shown in peer-reviewed studies to dampen microglia brain inflammation. I also placed him on several natural compounds to improve blood flow to his brain. These strategies will be discussed in the next few chapters. I taught him how to stabilize his blood sugar levels to keep energy levels in his brain consistent while we taught him how to rehabilitate his brain.

Within a couple of months, Ryan's leg spasm and tingling sensations were completely resolved and his ability to function in daily life began to return quickly. Within a short period of time he was able to attend college and get involved with theater productions. After a couple of years of being seizure-free, he was able to travel to Europe on his own. It has been more than three years now that he has been seizure-free, and he is attending college full time.

I share Ryan's case with you because it is a great example of the brain's potential to regain function even years after a severe brain injury. You need to know the brain has amazing potential to change. Despite any loss of brain function, there is always potential to change your brain to some degree.

You may not have a brain injury, but perhaps you have some level of brain degeneration or impaired brain function. Despite the level of brain impairment there is always great potential and hope to improve the function of your brain, and hence the quality of your life. The brain is considered plastic, meaning it is has the capacity to be remolded. Just as plastic can be melted and changed, so can your brain.

Datis Kharrazian, DHSc, DC, MS

● ●

PLASTICITY: THE USE-IT-OR-LOSE-IT PRINCIPLE OF BRAIN HEALTH

From the minute we are born we are losing neurons and synapses. The older you are, the fewer neurons you have. You have already lost hundreds of neurons just since you have been reading over the past few minutes. So why are adults so much more capable than infants? For that matter, why are some seniors sharper and more quick-witted than the catatonic teen waiting on you at the coffee shop, when the teen has so many more neurons and synapses? Because it is not just about the number of neurons you have, but how well they communicate with each other.

In a healthy brain, as neurons become stimulated they create more branches into each other so they can communicate more efficiently. The more developed your neuronal communicating network becomes the more function you have. So even though you have fewer neurons as you get older, you also have more branches and improved communication. Compare the brain of a six-year-old child to that of a 40-year-old adult. The child has more neurons and greater synapses, but the child has less coordination, focus, and cognition because his brain has not yet developed efficient neuron communication. However, if both the child and the adult were to learn a new language at the same time, the child will have greater learning potential because he has more neurons and synapses to work with.

The healthier your neurons are, the more potential they have to develop a strong communication network with one another. As neuron communication improves, your brain becomes more efficient and functional. In Ryan's case, his severe brain injury led to an immediate loss of a large amount of neurons. Those damaged neurons are dead and forever gone. However, Ryan's function improved because we were able to change his brain chemistry and stimulate his brain so that the remaining neurons could communicate better with each other.

If you look at Ryan's brain on an MRI before and after treatment it will look exactly the same. His ability to regain function after treatment was not related to gaining new neurons, but to his ability to encourage existing neurons to communicate better with each other. He had spent several years in rehab without any improvements and with further progression of brain degeneration because the chemical environment

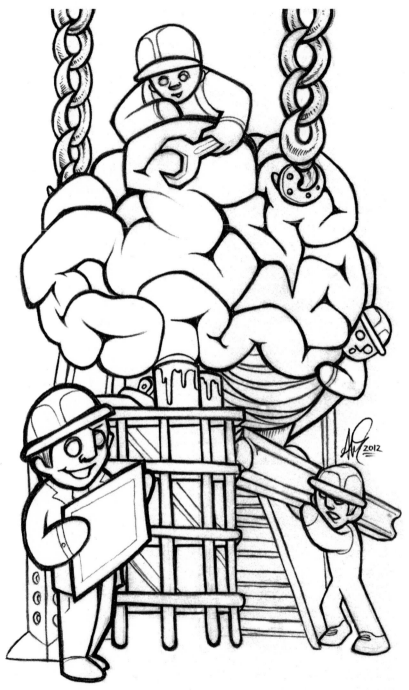

To preserve brain function and maintain a passion for life into old age, protect your neurons and continually develop plasticity.

of his brain was not conducive to the development of a good neuronal communication network.

As you stimulate neurons, their branches, called dendrites, grow outward into surrounding neurons, just as the roots of plants grow to find water. This branching leads to greater communication between neurons and better brain function. This is called plasticity, or the ability to build a pathway in the brain. Brain plasticity is dependent upon two factors. First, it needs **stimulation** to activate branching into other neurons. Second, it needs the **appropriate chemical environment** in order to be able to branch out. Both factors are important for change to occur. This is why there is so much variation when you look at brain recovery.

Let's take for example a stroke patient who has been a smoker for 30 years, has led a sedentary lifestyle, and eats fried or processed foods every day. Compare this person's potential for recovery to that of a stroke patient who has eaten a healthy diet and been an athlete his entire life. It is likely the active patient with a better diet will have a better recovery since he probably has a healthier environment for neurons to develop communication, or plasticity, with each other.

How do you know what your level of potential brain plasticity is? It's easy—just ask yourself if it is easier or harder for you to learn something new or acquire new skills than it was five years ago. If it is easier, then you have developed a brain with greater plasticity potential. If it is harder, then you have developed a brain with inefficient plasticity and you are also probably losing neurons more rapidly.

Remember, your brain function is not directly related to your age. As you get older you have the potential to develop either greater neuron plasticity or greater neuronal death and degeneration. I know for myself it takes me about one-third of the time it did five years ago to read research papers and write educational materials. Over the years my brain has become more plastic and efficient at these tasks. I have not declined in my function despite being five years older. This is an indication my brain plasticity has improved.

If you notice a decline in your brain function and if it has become harder for you to learn new things, you need to shift the chemical environment in your brain to regain function. If your brain is not working properly, it means the environment is such that it cannot gain plasticity and that there is accelerated neuron loss or neuron degeneration. Do not blame your declining brain function on aging.

I was recently fortunate enough to see an interview with 85-year-old Eric Kandel. He is considered one of the leading neuroscientists in the world and was the recipient of the 2000 Nobel Prize in physiology and medicine for his contributions to neuroscience research. I was completely blown away by the integrity of his brain. He was mentally sharp, fast, and articulate. Despite his age, his brain functioned at a very high level because of the plasticity he has developed as a devoted academician his entire life.

The same day I went to a Starbucks to order some tea. The young man behind the counter, in the prime of his life, could not calculate the proper change to give back to me because his register was malfunctioning. Although the younger man had more neurons than Professor Kandel, he had not developed plasticity so his brain was not very efficient.

In order to maintain the health of your brain, you must maintain as many neurons as you can during your lifetime. You also need to create a brain chemical environment conducive to the development of plasticity. If you can do these things, you will live into your old age with a high level of function and passion for life. In this book I will share with you the key concepts you need to evaluate your brain health and strategies to optimize your neuronal health and positive plasticity.

* *

Forty-three-year-old Chloe decided to take a tap dancing class. She found tap class challenging and was amazed to see how easily it came to the teenage girls 30 years younger. However, Chloe's teacher, who was in her mid-50s, could out tap both the adults and the young girls. A lifetime of learning, performing, teaching, and choreographing tap had developed many highly efficient patterns of synapses for tap dance in the teacher's brain. She could tap faster, jump higher, and stomp louder than the most accomplished teen student. She stored hundreds of tap sequences in her brain for ready recall and could handily put together routines for four or more classes at the same time for the spring recital, never having to write them down.

If you were able to take a PET scan of her brain while learning a new tap routine and compare it to a PET scan of Chloe's brain learning the same routine, you would probably see far less activity in the teacher's brain. Why? Because thanks to plasticity, her synaptic communicating pathways were so efficient that learning a new tap routine did not require that much energy from her brain. By firing less of her brain, Chloe's teacher would not be fazed by learning a new routine, while it might tire Chloe out as her neurons began to fatigue.

⦿ ⦿

Studies of "asymptomatic Alzheimer's disease" point to some exciting possibilities for the role of plasticity in preserving brain function. A person with asymptomatic Alzheimer's disease shows all the plaques and lesions associated with memory disorders, but none of the symptoms, even well into old age. A 2008 study showed 21 percent of study subjects with physical signs of dementia showed no symptoms.[1] The Nun Study of 2001 followed the lives of more than 600 nuns, including one who was more than 100 years old, and demonstrated how healthy plasticity could possibly prevent Alzheimer's disease, even in a brain full of plaques and lesions.[2]

Both these studies suggest better language skills and cognitive abilities are correlated with less risk of Alzheimer's disease in later life. In the Nun Study, all the nuns were required to write an autobiographical essay in their early 20s when they joined the convent. The essays ranged from being dense with insight and observation to the boring and mundane ("I went to the post office and then put gas in the car.") The nuns who had written more complex essays were more likely to escape Alzheimer's disease in their later years.[3] Could it be that a predisposition to more cognitive ability and an intellectual curiosity kept plasticity alive and well in their otherwise degenerating brains, so that they could remain sharp into old age? Although much has yet to be discovered in this realm, it is certainly food for thought.

Colin, 28, came to me about nine months after falling 20 feet from a water tower onto a rooftop in Brooklyn, New York. Although he did not fracture his skull, he suffered a significant traumatic brain injury (TBI). Brain MRIs revealed diffuse axonal injury and bruising of the left temporal lobe. While recovering in the hospital, he suffered a stroke on the right side of his brain, resulting in paralysis of the left side of his body.

When I met Colin, he had exhausted the medical and rehabilitative services that were available to him. He presented to my office with an unsteady gait (ataxia), an inability to coordinate the movements of his left arm and leg (dyspraxia), and double vision. Less obvious to him was his "leaky gut." TBI causes gastrointestinal dysfunction and increased intestinal permeability (leaky gut), which promotes multiple food sensitivities and autoimmunity.

I created a specific neuro-rehabilitative routine that targeted his deficits and activated his brain cells. However, in order to maximize Colin's recovery, I had to improve his leaky gut by mitigating the inflammatory chemical cascade that lingers after a TBI. I began supporting Colin with nutrients to support his gut and brain health and dampen inflammation.

After a few months of care, his ataxia improved dramatically! He is now able to swim and do jiu jitsu, and we even have him riding a bicycle outside. His double vision has improved, and his ability to have smooth, coordinated function of his left arm and hand have allowed him to begin playing the guitar once again. Colin, affectionately known as "Mr. Bounce," is a TBI survivor and inspirational speaker. He continues to amaze me with his progress!

Dr. Thomas Culleton, DC, DACNB, FACFN
Austin, Texas and New York, New York
www.CNWcenter.com

NEGATIVE PLASTICITY

Plasticity can be a good thing or a bad thing. Just as we can develop plasticity to learn new skills, so can we develop it to ingrain a bad habit or negative condition. Examples of negative plasticity include post-traumatic stress disorder, chronic pain disorders, phantom pain, or anything else in which neuronal communicating pathways have become more efficient at creating negative responses.

Many individuals develop chronic pain thanks to negative plasticity. These are conditions in which a person's neuronal pathways that perceive and generate pain signals become more developed and efficient.[4] For example, a person's herniated disk could cause pain for years. The pain further activates the pain signal, in essence making these pathways very efficient in generating pain. Additionally, pain-receiving fibers increase in number and branch out to further activate pain perception. Over the years these new pathways heighten the pain response, even though the tissue injury is no longer sufficient enough to actually generate pain.

Some people may eventually opt to have surgery and have the disk removed. But the disk removal does not change the negative plasticity for pain perception they developed. So even though they had the surgery, they still experience pain.

Another example of negative plasticity is phantom pain syndrome. In these cases, a person may have his arm crushed in an accident, leading to an amputation. Once the arm is amputated, the person still feels burning pain in the fingers and wrist that no longer exist. The trauma is so intense it profoundly influences the generation of pain perception pathways in the brain, which still send pain signals as though the limb were still there.[5]

Negative plasticity can involve any part of the brain, such as the limbic system, which governs emotion and survival. If a person goes to war and sees his fellow soldiers die, he may develop post-traumatic stress disorder. In post-traumatic stress disorder researchers have found increased plasticity in a part of the brain called the amygdala, which is responsible for fear, anger, and rage.[6]

Everyday stress responses unrelated to war can also induce negative plasticity. In other words, the more practice your brain has generating a stress response, the more efficient and better it gets at it. Over time, the negative plasticity from everyday stress can develop to the point where a person cannot handle minor stress without insomnia, hypertension, or anxiety.[7]

An all-too-common example of negative plasticity can occur with children who play video games constantly and never exercise. For instance, a 10-year-old boy who has been playing video games since the age of five for hours every day after school. These games are violent and require looking at things quickly and blowing them up. This type of activity develops negative plasticity of the brain's survival-oriented limbic system. The limbic system is directly involved in stimulating the flight-or-fight response when you feel something may be attacking you, which can be triggered by a quick movement in your visual field or an abrupt noise. Basically, playing video games that cause you to respond quickly to attacks increases the negative plastic development of your limbic system.

In the meantime, this child has not been running around outside, reading, playing with friends, or doing other activities that would develop his frontal lobe, the area of the brain in the forehead that governs reasoning and controls the limbic brain. The limbic brain is very reactive and primitive, while the frontal lobe makes sure you react appropriately by reasoning through and assessing situations.

For instance, if you see someone attractive you may have immediate primitive thoughts generated by your limbic system; however, the frontal lobe prevents you from walking up to that person and kissing him or her. The child who has been playing video games for more than half his life—and neglecting other brain development activities—may find his frontal lobe is not sufficiently developed to moderate his emotional responses. The result in these children is poor behavior and impulsivity. He may act aggressively or violently to get his way because he has not developed the ability in his frontal lobe to reason through things. Instead, he just reacts in a reflexive, primitive way, and constantly gets in trouble for misbehaving.

Now let's say the parents finally take the video games away from the child and work with him to start reading, exercising, and socializing with his peers. These activities will develop the frontal lobe while dampening the limbic system, in essence changing the wiring structure of his brain and consequently improving his behavior. So, in summary, the effects the long hours of playing video games had on his limbic system could be seen as negative plasticity, while the later development of his frontal lobe through reading, exercising, and playing could be considered positive plasticity. As the child's brain regains positive plasticity, the parents may even claim he is a totally new person.

The goal in maintaining a healthy brain is to avoid activities and a lifestyle that promote negative plasticity and activate centers of the brain that develop positive plasticity. This is especially important for children.

MAINTAINING POSITIVE PLASTICITY

Not only do you want to be able to develop positive plasticity, but you want to be able to maintain it over the long run. This is referred to as "long-term potentiation," which means a long-lasting ability of neurons to communicate better with each other. The process results in not only becoming more efficient at learning and memory tasks, but also maintaining that efficiency as you get older.

Our much admired Professor Kandel of 85 years of age, who has the brain function of a 20-year-old, has developed both positive plasticity and long-term potentiation of his learning and memory centers.

For instance, learning a new sport or skill can be painstakingly slow in the beginning, but with continued practice you become more efficient at, say, tennis or knitting because the neurons involved develop long-term potentiation. The exact mechanisms of how long-term potentiation occurs aren't yet fully understood, but it appears the receptors on the postsynaptic neurons become more sensitive, so that over time fewer neurotransmitters are needed for the same effect.[8]

In early long-term potentiation, the activity, such as a mouse trying to find the cheese at the end of the maze, increases sensitivity of the synapses involved in the task. As the mouse repeatedly performs the maze task, it excels at getting to the cheese quickly because the receptors on the postsynaptic neurons have increased in number and sensitivity.[9] Hence it is "long-term" because the changes in the brain's neural pathways to complete the task don't vanish as soon as the task is done, but instead remain in place long afterward.

A more interesting example of long-term potentiation comes from a breakthrough study in 2004 that compared the effects of meditation on 10 novice meditators and 10 Buddhist monks by evaluating their brain waves during and after meditation. Both groups were told to meditate on compassion and love. During the meditation, two of the novices and all of the monks experienced an increase in the number of gamma waves, a high brainwave state associated with deep meditation. However, as soon as the subjects stopped meditating, the novices' gamma wave production returned to normal, while the monks, who by then had completed thousands of hours of meditation, did not return to normal but rather stayed in the gamma wave state.[10]

By entering into meditation, the novices who were successful in reaching a gamma state delivered a signal that triggered the beginnings of long-term potentiation. However, it lasted only as long as the meditation. The monks had been triggering those synapses repeatedly over many years, slowly but surely creating the neural pathways, or plasticity, to achieve a lasting gamma state. Long-term potentiation had so refined the process that the effects of the meditation were felt after the synaptic "trigger," the meditation, had ceased. When a neuron fires over and over again through a pathway, those neurons get healthier and coordination in the sequence of firing becomes more efficient. Eventually you need fewer neurotransmitters for the same effect.

If you want to maintain a high level of function throughout your life, you need to develop plasticity. As you continue activating these pathways they become more efficient and require less energy to communicate, which is called long-term potentiation. The best thing you can do is challenge your brain constantly with both cognitive and physical activities. In order to maintain your brain you need to be a scholar and an athlete.

WHY A HEALTHY BRAIN HELPS YOU LIVE LONGER AND SMARTER

Although we can all develop long-term potentiation and plasticity, success depends on the health and chemistry of the brain. This means the neurons must receive enough oxygen, glucose, and stimulation. Neurotransmitters used in the synapses must be sufficient, the post synaptic receptors must be receptive but not overly receptive, the neurotransmitters must clear after the synapse has occurred, and the brain must not be battling ongoing inflammation or degeneration, which compromise neuron health.

As we go through each chapter, I will explain all of these crucial mechanisms and offer effective strategies you can do to optimize brain function.

Although the brain gradually loses neurons and synapses as we age, we can keep it in peak function by developing healthy and abundant synaptic function.

Ozzy Osbourne is a fascinating study in neurology. Whenever I watched his reality television show several years ago, I was amazed at how he slurred his speech, needed to wear sunglasses indoors, and shuffled around. The years of drug abuse and life on the road had clearly taken their toll. However, once he got on stage in front of 50,000 people, all his finely tuned synaptic pathways for singing kicked back into gear, and he performed as if he were still in his 20s.

We can do better than Ozzy and not only perform well at the tasks that matter to us, but also stay sharp and active well into old age. By keeping our brains healthy we can keep our bodily functions purring along instead of succumbing to disease and degeneration.

This is why it is so vital to attend to your brain health before it's too late and symptoms of dementia or Parkinson's disease set in, a stroke occurs, or function is increasingly lost to accelerated brain aging. By maintaining a healthy brain, you maintain the ability to maximize your brain's plasticity, and by maximizing your brain's plasticity, you maintain the good health and function of your brain.

In this book you will learn the necessary steps to do that, such as ensuring proper neurotransmitter and synaptic function, avoiding brain inflammation and accelerated degeneration, and learning how and why addressing your bodily health—gut, hormones, immunity, and more—can so profoundly affect brain health.

I will discuss the following areas critical to brain health and plasticity:

- The importance of neurotransmitters, the brain's messenger chemicals, and lifestyle factors that impact their function
- How stress affects neurotransmitters, immunity, and blood sugar levels, all of which in turn affect brain health
- The importance of circulation and oxygen delivery to brain tissue
- The effect of the brain's immune system on brain tissue
- The connection between gut health and brain health
- How hormonal imbalances affect brain health and vice versa

CHAPTER SUMMARY

• Although a younger person has more neurons, an older person has more branches and improved communication. The key to good brain function as you age is maintaining the health of this communication, or plasticity while also maintaining as many neurons as you can.

• Brain plasticity is dependent upon **stimulation** to activate branching and the **appropriate chemical environment**, or your brain health.

• The Nun Study of 2001 demonstrated how healthy plasticity could prevent Alzheimer's disease, even in a brain full of plaques and lesions.

• Plasticity can be positive or negative. Examples of negative plasticity include post-traumatic stress disorder, chronic pain disorders, phantom pain, or anything else in which neuronal communicating pathways have become more efficient at creating negative responses.

• Long-term potentiation is the long-lasting ability of neurons to communicate better with each other. The process results in not only becoming more efficient at learning and memory tasks, but also maintaining that efficiency as you get older. A study of Buddhist monks showed they maintained a gamma brain wave state induced by meditation long after the meditation ended thanks to long-term potentiation. For novice meditators, the gamma brain wave state lasted only as long as the meditation.

CHAPTER THREE

THE FAILING BRAIN

●　●

My eyes are closed, the air is filled with the smell of formalde-hyde, and I feel a wide bumpy groove under my fingertips that horrifies me. I am in a post-graduate human brain dissection course at Touro University School of Medicine in California and I just felt a brain with such advanced degeneration that I couldn't stop my emotions and imagination from going all over the place. Before the dissection course began I had been privileged enough to palpate about 50 different brains in the anatomy lab. When you palpate a human brain, you should be able to feel multiple small, tight convolutions that are spongy yet offer resistance to pres-sure. When you a feel a degenerated brain, you feel wide spaces between the convolutions, and the brain feels very soft.

As I felt brains that were degenerated in specific areas, I imag-ined the disabilities the person must have had, and specific tasks that must have been difficult. I remember feeling a degenerated frontal cortex (behind the forehead) and knowing this person must have had personality changes and an inability to focus and concentrate. She probably had lost motivation for life, and her "spark," as the decayed part of the brain under my fingertips was once responsible for those functions. I had no doubt she developed these symptoms slowly over time, and that the consequences of her degenerated brain were identified as personality and mood changes instead of a degenerative brain disease.

I imagined she began first losing her motivation and passion for life, and her family and friends thought she was just moody.

35

Perhaps she was diagnosed with depression and given various antidepressants, which did nothing to slow down her brain degeneration. She probably then started to have difficulty focusing and remembering directions and simple phone numbers.

With such significant degeneration, I guessed she also lost her bladder tone and suffered from incontinence. I imagined her doctors told her that she was just getting old and that she had nothing to worry about. If she was like millions of other people, she was never diagnosed in the early stages of her brain degeneration or given strategies to improve her brain health.

Datis Kharrazian, DHSc, DC, MS

● ●

CATCHING BRAIN DEGENERATION, IF YOU CAN

Just as we make conscious efforts to eat right and exercise to lower the risk of cardiovascular disease, so should we make conscious efforts to protect our brain health. We all have some degree of brain degeneration, but the symptoms can become very scary if it advances unchecked. However, the problem with brain degeneration is that it is hard for us to recognize it in ourselves when it happens slowly. What's worse, brain degeneration prevents us from being able to recognize when it's happening, or to get motivated enough to do something about it.

When I travel around the country teaching, I reconnect with friends and acquaintances in multiple cities every six months to a year. This is an interesting way to assess brain function in people, as any decline is more apparent than it would be if I saw them every day. I can see evidence of facial paresis, a mild form of paralysis caused by unchecked degeneration that causes one side of or the whole face to droop somewhat. I see their mental processing slow, that they repeat themselves, or their mood becomes more negative.

It is not because they have gotten chronologically older; it is because they have neurologically degenerated. The fact that half of their face has lost tone means the neurons that innervate the facial muscles on that side of the brainstem have lost integrity. That their mental processing speed has slowed down is also not related to a chronological age but to degenerative changes.

36

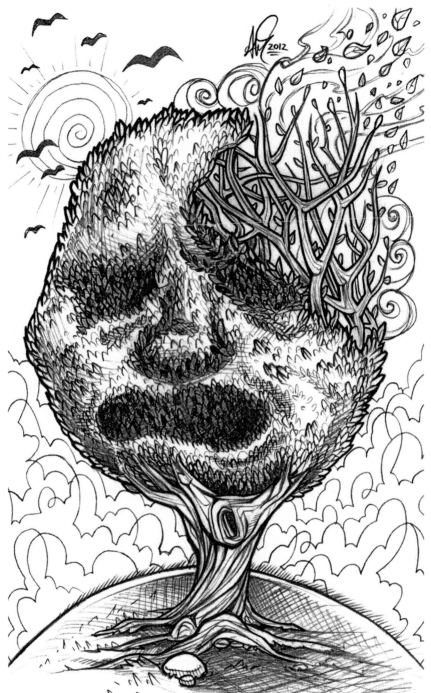

It is difficult to recognize brain degeneration in ourselves or get motivated to address it.

The scary thing is people don't see this in themselves. When your brain degenerates, you don't typically realize it. Most people think forgetting things is a normal part of getting older, as is dozing off every time they read, or no longer finding joy in the things or relationships that used to delight them. But it's not age. It's brain deterioration.

If you have a really good day at work where you perform well, it means your brain is firing well. If you have a poor day where you can't focus or remember things, those are days of poor brain function. We all have good and bad days. But some people end up having more and more bad days until those become normal and they don't remember the good days anymore. So not only is your brain deteriorating, but consequently so is your career and other aspects of your personal life.

FATIGUE, DEPRESSION, AND GASTROINTESTINAL PROBLEMS — MORE TROUBLESOME BUT OVERLOOKED BRAIN-BASED CONDITIONS

Not all brain-based problems come down to Alzheimer's disease, autism, or Parkinson's disease. In fact, three of the more common outcomes of brain degeneration problems are fatigue, depression, and gastrointestinal problems, though they are rarely treated as such.

Fatigue

Chronic fatigue syndrome is often brain-based. As the brain degenerates, brain cells develop poor endurance for ordinary tasks. In essence, they begin to fatigue, and if the brain fatigues, the entire body fatigues. In these people trivial stimulation to the brain triggers exhaustion.

For instance, reading causes fatigue, as does driving, or being in a loud, noisy restaurant. Watching an action movie with lots of quick flashes of light and constant screen changes fatigues them, as does the drama of the movie. All these various inputs to the brain overwhelm the degenerated and exhausted neurons so that they fatigue quickly. Consequently, the brain's output to the rest of the body is compromised, and the body fatigues as well.

A 49-year-old male with an apathetic presentation was referred to my office after having completed a one-month stay at a prestigious rehabilitation facility for alcohol abuse. He was hesitant to try alternative medicine, having felt no change after urinary neurotransmitter testing and a protocol of vitamins and popular adrenal glandular supplements at the rehab facility.

The patient's primary symptoms were depression, fatigue, lack of appetite, and an acid feeling in his stomach at night. The patient also reported taking antidepressants five years ago, which led to an increase in his alcohol intake.

On his barely completed assessment forms, the patient noted he drank four cups of coffee per day and usually skipped breakfast, lunch, or both. Blood chemistry, saliva, and stool testing confirmed insulin resistance, adrenal fatigue, and a disturbed sleep-wake cycle.

The testing also indicated an H. pylori infection (bacterial overgrowth in the stomach that causes indigestion, ulcers, and is linked to heart disease), yeast and parasite infections, hypothyroidism, poor liver and gallbladder function, insufficient stomach acid, vitamin D deficiency, B-12 anemia, and suppressed immune function. A GABA challenge confirmed a leaky blood-brain barrier.

I put the patient on a regimen of nutritional compounds to address his H. pylori infection, as well as additional anti-parasitic herbs and probiotics for his gut infections. I taught him how to stabilize his blood sugar through diet and decreased caffeine intake, and also addressed his liver function, inflammation, and vitamin D deficiency with additional nutritional compounds.

Just three weeks after starting this program the patient reported a significant increase in energy, return of his appetite, and no need for an over-the-counter antacid medication for the first time in years. He also noted his rectal itching, which he was too embarrassed to tell me about, was gone. He told me, "When you feel bad for so long, that becomes your normal… I feel dumb for dealing with those symptoms for so long."

The patient's care continued to include a three-week detoxification program with a hypoallergenic detoxification and anti-inflammatory compounds. The patient noted adverse symptoms after returning wheat and other gluten grains to his diet, and thus remains on a gluten-free diet. Given that this patient had a gluten intolerance, one can only imagine the inflammation to his body and brain caused by his daily habit of drinking 30 beers, which contain gluten.

Not only has the patient noted a dramatic change in his mood on this protocol, but his daughter has also noticed he is "less angry, more patient, and happier."

This case clearly depicts the impact of the gut-brain connection. For this patient, a gut infection, gluten intolerance, and leaky gut undoubtedly contributed to his alcohol abuse and depression. It is also unfortunate that a rehab facility charging $25,000 per month could have overlooked such important factors.

We continue to support his adrenal function, blood sugar balance, anemia, and neurotransmitter activity, but it is amazing the transformation this patient experienced just in supporting the gut-brain connection. He continues to remain sober. Every rehab facility should learn this work.

Alexis Daniels, DC, CSCS
Woodland Hills, California
www.dralexisdaniels.com

● ●

Depression

Depression is another common outcome of poor brain health and brain deterioration. From a neurological standpoint, depression is simply decreased firing of the frontal lobe, the area at the front of the brain that gives us motivation and a sense of well-being. Many different things can cause this decreased firing, including imbalances in brain chemicals or hormones.

For instance, we know men need sufficient testosterone and women estrogen for good frontal lobe function, and a deficiency in those hormones alone can cause depression. Messenger chemicals, called neurotransmitters, significantly influence the frontal lobe. If they are deficient or their pathways are not functioning properly, this too can cause depression. Of course many other factors can affect frontal lobe firing, but these are two possible examples, neither of which would be appropriately addressed by antidepressants.

When gastrointestinal problems are brain problems

Chronic gastrointestinal issues such as indigestion, acid reflux, constipation, burping, gas, bloating, diarrhea, pain, or irritable bowel syndrome are a third common clinical presentation of brain degeneration. Brain issues aren't always the cause of gastrointestinal problems, so don't rush off in a panic to your local neurologist if you pop antacids regularly (which you shouldn't do anyway, as you'll read later in this book). But when gastrointestinal problems seem to be irresolvable, breakdowns in brain function should be considered.

Your brain outputs communication to the body through the brainstem on an ongoing basis. Normal firing of the brain stimulates the centers of the brainstem to control your heart rate, your breathing, your digestion, and other vital functions that keep you alive.

The brainstem contains a group of nerve bundles called the vagal nuclei, which branch out into the vagus nerve. The vagus nerve then branches out like roots of a plant from your brainstem to your intestines. When the vagus is working well at its job of transmitting information from the brain, a person has good bowel movements, good enzyme output from the pancreas so their food is properly broken down, and overall good digestion. When the brain functions poorly due to degeneration and inflammation, output through the brainstem lowers. This in turn decreases the firing rate of the vagus nerve. With less input into the vagus nerve, people can suffer from poor digestion, constipation, and an inability to tolerate many foods because they can't digest them.

For instance, Lea had been battling chronic digestive issues, in particular severe indigestion and acid reflux. Despite her advanced knowledge in alternative health therapies, she never seemed to be able to resolve her gastrointestinal problems. She ate a gut-healing diet, took digestive enzymes and other digestive herbs and nutrients, had lab panels done to assess the health of her digestive tract, and yet nothing brought her relief. It wasn't until a doctor addressed her brain health that she began to experience some progress in addressing her gut issues. (I will review in detail the connections of the brain with digestive functions in Chapter Nine.)

It's this connection between the brain and body—not to mention the brain and one's general well-being—that is ignored today. When brain function improves, it's also common to see a person's bodily functions improve while they gain more energy, have more motivation, and enjoy better relationships with friends, family, and coworkers. Performance in any sport can be improved through better brain function, as can performance on the job. We all have room to enhance our brain health.

Much has been discovered recently to further our understanding of the two-way street between brain health and general health, which will be discussed in this book. But in order to understand how to best support the brain, you must start with the neuron. The next chapter will discuss the needs of the neurons.

CHAPTER SUMMARY

• When you palpate a human brain, you should be able to feel multiple small, tight convolutions that are spongy yet offer resistance to pressure. When you a feel a degenerated brain, you feel wide spaces between the convolutions, and the brain feels very soft.

• Just as we make conscious efforts to eat right and exercise to lower the risk of cardiovascular disease, so should we make conscious efforts to protect our brain health. We all have some degree of brain degeneration, but the symptoms can become very scary if it advances unchecked. However, the problem with brain degeneration is that it is hard for us to recognize it in ourselves when it happens slowly. What's worse, brain degeneration prevents us from being able to recognize when it's happening, or to get motivated enough to do something about it.

• Most people think forgetting things is a normal part of getting older, as is dozing off every time they read, or no longer finding joy in the things or relationships that used to delight them. But it's not age. It's brain deterioration.

• Three of the more common outcomes of brain degeneration problems are fatigue, depression, and gastrointestinal problems, though they are rarely treated as such.

• Normal inputs to the brain can overwhelm the degenerated and exhausted brain so it fatigues quickly. Consequently, the body fatigues as well.

• From a neurological standpoint, depression is simply decreased firing of the frontal lobe, the area at the front of the brain that gives us motivation and a sense of well-being. Many different things can cause this decreased firing, including imbalances in brain chemicals or hormones.

• When gastrointestinal problems seem to be irresolvable, breakdowns in brain function should be considered.

CHAPTER FOUR

THE NEEDS OF THE NEURON

● ●

Kevin was a 12-year old boy who had been having difficulty in school for most of his young life. He was also very uncoordinated and not good at sports and spent most of his time playing video games. His father privately told me Kevin could not kick a soccer ball if his life depended on it and he was always fidgeting and making snorting noises. He also suffered from chronic allergies, asthma, and bouts of depression and had been prescribed an asthma inhaler and antihistamines by his doctor. Kevin's father was worried his son would not do well academically or socially in high school. Although he didn't say it, I detected that despite loving his son very much, Kevin's father was also embarrassed by him.

The first time I saw Kevin in my office it was clear his brain was not healthy. He walked in with a stooped posture and his arms swinging all over the place. These are signs of poor muscle tone, or "hypotonia." He also could not keep still and needed to move all of the time while sitting in the chair. This is called akathisia and is associated with dysfunction in a part of the brain called the basal ganglia. The snorting noises and head jerks are categorized as simple motor and vocal tics, which also occur from a basal ganglia dysfunction. Unfortunately, such established signs of brain impairment go overlooked in the health care system, as most physicians today are unfamiliar with brain function and neurology.

An examination revealed Kevin had abnormal deep tendon reflexes and muscle tone. He also failed most of his balance and coordination neurological tests. However, most striking was that

*when I measured his oxygen saturation levels with a pulse oxim-
eter his levels were below normal by 10 percent, meaning his brain
and other tissues were not getting sufficient oxygen. We could also
see this by his white fingernails from lack of oxygen and blood
reaching his fingertips. Using a stethoscope I could hear severe
wheezing from his asthma, which explained why his brain was not
getting enough oxygen.*

*In these situations it is important to oxygenate the brain, which
meant we needed to address his asthma and poor breathing. I put
him on an anti-inflammatory diet, boosted his lung antioxidant
levels, and supported his adrenal and blood glucose levels. I also
had him perform breathing exercises with a heavy book on his
abdomen to strengthen his diaphragm. Within the first few weeks
he had cut down use of his asthma inhaler by 50 percent and by
the end of two months he rarely needed it.*

*Over time we did many more things to help improve Kevin's
brain, such as giving him many coordination and balance exercises to improve his brain integration. But it would have been very
difficult without boosting oxygen delivery to his brain first. As we
stabilized his blood sugar levels he was also able to loosen his
dietary restrictions.*

*I share Kevin's story with you because there is no magic supple-
ment or treatment for the brain, but the brain needs three essential
things to function at its best: oxygen, glucose, and stimulation.*

Datis Kharrazian, DHSc, DC, MS

NEURONS—HOW BRAIN CELLS TALK WITH ONE ANOTHER

As you know, the brain acts as a central command center for all functions of the body, including digestion, hormone production, immune
function, learning, memory, mood, and sleep.

The key players in the brain are neurons, cells that use electrical
charges to transmit information. Neurons are the workers of the
nervous system, and if their health becomes compromised, neurological
disorders develop.

The basic neuron is composed of a soma, dendrites, and an axon.
The soma is the central part of the neuron and contains the nucleus

(the neuron's "control center"). Dendrites are extensions that resemble a tree and are used to receive input from other neurons. The axon is a projection that transmits signals to other neurons or cells. So in essence, every neuron is a one-way street with information coming in through the dendrites and leaving through the axon, all propelled by electrical charges generated in healthy, active neurons.

Many neurons only have one axon, but the axon typically develops an extensive network of branches, so it can communicate with many other cells simultaneously. Neurons communicate by discharging a small messenger chemical called a "neurotransmitter," which is picked up by the target neuron. The neuron that sends the neurotransmitter is the "presynaptic neuron" and the neuron that receives the neurotransmitter is the "postsynaptic neuron." A presynaptic neuron releases neurotransmitters from its axon that are then picked up by the dendrites of the postsynaptic neuron. To get from the presynaptic to the postsynaptic neuron, the neurotransmitter must travel across a small empty space, called the "synaptic cleft."

This whole process is called a synapse. The word synapse comes from the Greek word "synaptin." "Syn-" means together and "haptein" means to clasp, so synapse means to "clasp together" neurons.

In order for a synapse to occur, something must stimulate the neuron. This stimulation sets off a series of chemical and electrical impulses via synapses to reach various areas of the brain and nervous tissue.

If synaptic activity decreases, this can impair brain function and, consequently, bodily function. However, synaptic activity naturally declines as we age. Young children have an estimated 10 quadrillion synapses going on at any one time, whereas an adult's activity is estimated at between one to five quadrillion synapses at one time.

As neurons degenerate there is a gradual decline in synaptic activity. This is one reason it's hard "to teach an old dog new tricks," and why stimulating the brain in a positive way, such as through intellectual challenges, social support, good diet, and physical activity will help slow brain aging.

Much can go wrong during a synapse in an unhealthy system. For instance, there can be sufficient neurotransmitters, but a problem with the presynaptic or postsynaptic receptors. Or the neurotransmitter doesn't break down or get reabsorbed as it should after the synapse

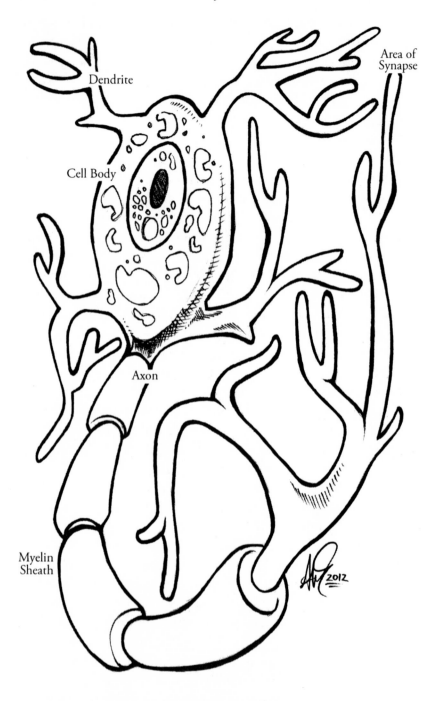

Dendrite

Area of
Synapse

Cell Body

Axon

Myelin
Sheath

Neurons are cells that use electrical charges to transmit information.
Every neuron needs oxygen, glucose, and stimulation.

is complete, disrupting future synapses. Neurons may fire too many neurotransmitters at once, or too few, and so on.

Inflammation, hormone imbalances, and poor blood sugar handling are some of the factors that can sabotage neurotransmitter function. In this book I will cover not only nutritional compounds to boost neurotransmitter activity, but also the many other factors necessary for good synaptic activity.

IMPROVING YOUR BACKHAND OR PREVENTING ALZHEIMER'S DISEASE—THE THREE THINGS EVERY NEURON NEEDS

It doesn't matter if you simply want to perform better at your favorite sport, gain a competitive edge at work, or address something more serious, such as depression, autism, healing from a head injury or stroke, or reducing your risk of Alzheimer's disease. When addressing any aspect of brain health you have to start with whether your brain's neurons are getting enough of the three things every neuron needs:

- Oxygen
- Glucose
- Stimulation

Brain degeneration happens when any one of these three is compromised. For instance, reduced blood flow to the brain, such as from poor circulation, reduces the amount of oxygen it receives, and this problem is more common than you would think. Lack of glucose is common in those who suffer from poor blood sugar stability, especially hypoglycemia—it's the reason people become spacey and lightheaded when they go too long without eating.

Stimulation such as physical activity and mental challenges "exercise" the neurons and are necessary to keep them healthy and active. Neuron stimulation is also dependent upon healthy neurotransmitter activity.

Oxygen

Just because you breathe doesn't mean your brain is getting enough oxygen. Anemia, for instance can rob the brain of oxygen, as red blood cells are not healthy enough to deliver sufficient oxygen to it. People with blood sugar disorders, such as hypoglycemia, insulin resistance, or diabetes, can also deprive their brains of oxygen.

Blood sugar disorders create a state of chronic stress in the body, which inhibits blood flow to the brain. For this reason, just being stressed out all the time will steal oxygen from your brain, sending it instead to the organs and limbs that prepare you for "fight or flight."

Certain metabolic disorders, such as low blood pressure or hypothyroidism, can also inhibit oxygen flow to the brain. Poor lifestyle choices such as smoking and being sedentary can dramatically reduce blood flow to the brain.

Whenever overall blood flow in the body is reduced, the tissues of the body that are farthest from the heart are hardest hit. These are the hands, feet, and brain. Unfortunately, our brain does not have gravity working for it as do our hands and feet.

In fact, when you see evidence of poor blood flow in the hands and feet, you can be assured the brain is affected too. Chronic nail fungal growth, the kind that doesn't respond to antifungal treatments, is one such symptom. This occurs because your blood carries immune cells to your toes. When circulation is compromised, your immune system cannot fight the fungal growth that would normally be suppressed from wearing shoes every day.

Weak nails and poor capillary refill time are other signs of poor circulation. Weak nails occur because the blood is not delivering enough hormones and vital nutrients for healthy nail development. You can test your own capillary refill by pushing on one of your fingernails. It should instantly return to its pink color once the pressure is taken off. In the case of poor blood flow that pink color returns slowly or the nail beds were never pink to begin with. Also, in a person with poor blood flow a simple touch will reveal their hands and feet are colder than their forearms and calves.

People who have poor circulation will experience cramping in their hands and sore feet because they cannot get blood to those tissues very well. Basically, if a person cannot get healthy blood flow to their feet, we know they probably suffer from poor blood flow to the brain.

If a person's brain is not working properly we need to focus on improving blood flow to their brain. Don't forget, your blood is carrying everything neurons need to work—glucose, oxygen, nutrients, hormones, and neurotransmitters. We will discuss specific strategies to improve blood flow to your brain in Chapter Seven.

●●●●●●●●●●●●●●●●●●●●●●●●●●●●●●●●●

Janet was always freezing, especially her hands and feet. She always wore thick, woolly socks, even on warm days, and never left the house without a pair of warm gloves in her purse. She chalked it up to her hypothyroid condition for which she was being treated by her doctor. But when she started using herbs that have been shown to be effective in promoting blood flow to the brain, not only did she enjoy more alertness and a sharper intellect and memory, but her hands and feet became much warmer.

●●●●●●●●●●●●●●●●●●●●●●●●●●●●●●●●●

To slow the rate at which the brain degenerates and to enhance brain performance, it's vital to make sure the neurons are receiving enough oxygen from healthy circulation. In addition to seeking out and addressing conditions such as anemia, which steal blood from the brain, exercise is an excellent way to keep the brain oxygenated. Also, desk jockeys take note—being hunched over at a computer all day, drawing the shoulders forward and caving in the chest, can also restrict the flow of oxygen to the brain.

Glucose

While Sudoku or crossword puzzles are good brain food, doing them while eating a frosted pastry and slurping down an extra-large caramel latte with whipped cream works against you. All that sugar will upset glucose levels in the brain and create conditions that ultimately deprive the brain of energy.

Up to one third of the body's glucose supply fuels the brain. If you are hypoglycemic (low blood glucose levels) and you've gone too long without eating, no doubt you have experienced the effects of low glucose in the brain, such as feeling spacey, lightheaded, dull, and slow-witted. Perhaps your hands shook because there was not enough glucose for the brain to support good muscle control. If you give a hypoglycemic person a math quiz after breakfast and then six hours after their last meal, they're going to perform much better on the after-breakfast quiz because their brain is sufficiently fueled.

On the other hand, give a person who is prediabetic or has insulin resistance (high blood glucose levels) a math quiz after breakfast, and they're more apt to perform better on the quiz given several hours after a meal, as they'll be too sleepy to think straight right after eating. In insulin resistance, glucose can't get into the body's cells, including the brain cells, and one feels sleepy and slow as a result.

Unfortunately, appropriate glucose levels aren't about doing better on math quizzes. What people don't understand is that every time they "bonk" and get into those spacey, hypoglycemic episodes, or every time they go into a mini-coma and need a nap after eating due to insulin resistance, they're killing off massive amounts of neurons and speeding along their brain degeneration.

Insulin resistance, which is a precursor to diabetes, delivers too much glucose and insulin into the brain, which is extremely damaging to the brain's tissue and circulatory system, to the point where neurologists have dubbed Alzheimer's disease "Type 3 diabetes."[1]

One of the most essential things a person can do for the health and performance of the brain is work toward keeping blood sugar balanced. For a person with hypoglycemia, this means eating frequently enough to avoid "bonking." And for both hypoglycemia and insulin resistance, it means scaling back carbohydrate consumption so that blood sugar levels stay on an even keel.

* *

I first met this young client when he was eight years old. He was very shy with a calm disposition. He had been diagnosed with a sensory processing disorder and his parents had hired a special tutor. His mother and father were already clients of mine, and his mother was very conscientious with his diet. She was most concerned about his extreme fatigue, how difficult it was to get him up in the morning, and how difficult it was for him to fall asleep. He was also falling asleep at school.

In addition, she was concerned he was having difficulty remembering his schoolwork. With sensory processing disorder, children may have difficulty concentrating, planning and organizing, and responding appropriately to external stimuli. It is considered to be a learning disorder that fits into the autism spectrum of disorders.

To target his diet and nutritional supplementation, I recommended a comprehensive blood panel, an adrenal profile, a food sensitivity panel, and an organic acids profile to determine vitamin, mineral, and energy deficiency status. His blood panel indicated low thyroid function, iron deficiency, and autoimmune thyroid. His adrenal profile indicated adrenal fatigue. His organic acids test indicated low B vitamins and zinc, low detoxification capacity, and low levels of energy nutrients, particularly magnesium. He was also low in omega-3 fatty acids and sensitive to gluten, dairy, eggs, and corn.

Armed with all of that information, he and I worked together to develop a diet based on his test results. I like to involve children in the designing of their diet. That way they get to include the foods they like, learn how to make healthy substitutions for foods they love but can no longer eat, and learn how to improve their overall food choices. He also learned he needed to include protein at all meals, have snacks throughout the day, and what constitutes a healthy snack.

I recommended he start with a gut restoration protocol along with iron support; food sensitivities often go hand in hand with leaky gut issues. This would also impact brain function.

In the second phase of his program, I added inositol and serotonin support for sleep, thyroid support, DHA, glutathione support (to help regulate autoimmunity), a vitamin and mineral complex, fish oils, B-12, licorice extract for his adrenals, and dopamine and acetylcholine support to improve his concentration, energy, and memory.

Within a month, his parents reported that he was falling asleep easily and would wake up with energy in the morning. His concentration improved, as did his ability to remember what he had learned at school. He started to play sports in the afternoon and took the initiative to let his mom know what foods not to include in his diet. He is still on his program three years later, and the improvements in his energy, sleep, and brain function continue.

Linda Clark, MA, CN
Fair Oaks, California
www.uwanutrition.com

Stimulation

Because neurons communicate using electrical charges, they can be looked at as little batteries. The basic requirements of oxygen, glucose, and stimulation are what keep these batteries "juiced." When a properly nourished neuron is stimulated, the internal machinery within the neuron produces energy for function, maintenance, and repair. In an improperly nourished neuron, this machinery falters and energy production slows. The neuron becomes fatigued and easily overwhelmed by constant input, eventually causing it to burn out.

A good example of this is the 35-year-old who is bored by his job, always follows the same routine, and watches several hours of television each day. One day he decides to go back to college and is surprised to find studying is not as easy as it used to be. When he first hits the books, he becomes fatigued and sleepy after only 20 minutes of reading. This could be because the neurons responsible for reading and learning have poor energy production thanks to years of insufficient stimulation, and if the brain fatigues the body fatigues.

Just as you wouldn't want to suddenly run 10 miles after years of couch surfing, neither would you want to overwhelm the long-neglected brain with too much activity. Otherwise you risk "burning out" neurons of poor endurance. Our older college student must take frequent breaks to avoid fatigue during the first few weeks. As times goes on, the repeated stimulation of reading improves the internal machinery of his neurons, and they produce more energy, leading to greater endurance for reading without fatigue.

If, however, he developed headaches after 20 minutes of reading due to this fatigue but decided to push on and keep reading, he may overwhelm the poorly functioning neurons, causing many of them to fail, and wind up experiencing poor concentration and focus the next day. Also, as explained earlier, he can better his chances of rehabilitating those neglected neurons with a brain-healthy diet that won't spike his blood sugar and regular exercise to improve blood flow to his brain, and by addressing any stressors that might compromise his ability to learn new information. He would also need healthy levels of neurotransmitters to sustain this increased stimulation.

In fact, healthy stimulation of the neurons is strongly dependent upon neurotransmitter activity. If our older college student is deficient

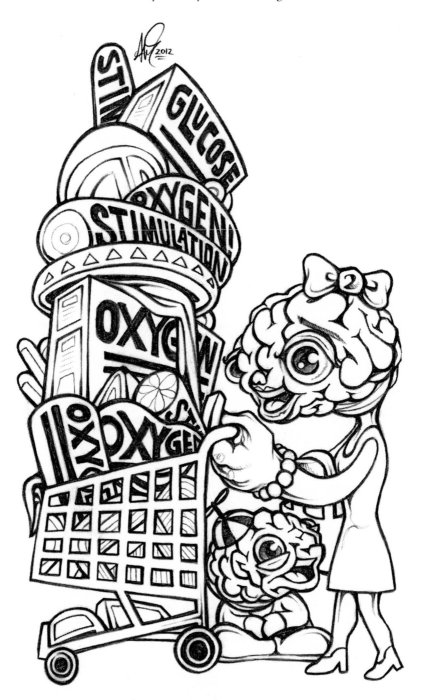

*If neurons receive sufficient oxygen, glucose, and stimulation,
your brain will function well and stay healthier longer.*

in some key neurotransmitters, such as acetylcholine for learning and memory, he may struggle for a long time in building his reading endurance. If he is dopamine deficient, he may feel a lack of motivation and poor self-worth and drop out, feeling he is not capable enough to go to college. Also, the input of all the new stimulation without sufficient neurotransmitters to handle it could lead to accelerated brain degeneration. I will discuss neurotransmitters beginning in Chapter Twelve.

• •

When I first met Charles, he was a 27-year-old man suffering from Tourette's syndrome and some mental delays. These manifested as a severe tic disorder and inappropriate social skills. His mother had taken him to every major (and minor) hospital and medical center up and down the East Coast over a period of 21 years. Charles had been to dozens of natural medicine doctors, alternative medical professionals, classic neurologists, and allopathic doctors.

After carefully examining him and his blood work, we decided to support some pathways via nutrition in an effort to improve overall brain function. Over the next three weeks, Charles' mother saw what she characterized as an amazing improvement.

During a family gathering some months later, the extended family wanted to know what the new medication was that "fixed Charles." His mother replied that it was no medication at all but a properly applied nutritional support program.

Today Charles works and is able to drive. He does continue to have the occasional tic and some residual mental delays. However, it is worth noting that prior to this intervention, his parents had made arrangements to support him and have him live at home for the remainder of his life.

His mother rates her son's improvement at 90 percent and feels he will certainly be able to live independently. Charles' parents recently went on a two-week vacation, leaving Charles at home alone. This is the first time since he was born that they have felt comfortable doing so!

Chris Turnpaugh, DC, DABCN
Mechanicsburg, Pennsylvania
www.drchristurnpaugh.com

• •

In the next several chapters, I will discuss the symptoms you may have if your neurons are not getting proper glucose, oxygen, or stimulation. I will also give you strategies to improve those systems. If you cannot supply your neurons with their basic needs, not only will your brain not function well, but it will also degenerate much faster.

In addition to the needs of the neuron, I will discuss other mechanisms that can degenerate your brain, such as brain inflammation, poor gastrointestinal function, gluten intolerances, autoimmunity, poor diet, and environmental pollutants. I will also give you strategies to deal with each of these issues so you can improve your brain function and slow brain degeneration.

CHAPTER SUMMARY

• The basic neuron is composed of a soma, dendrites, and an axon. The soma is the central part of the neuron and contains the nucleus. Dendrites are extensions that resemble a tree and receive input from other neurons. The axon is a projection that transmits signals to other neurons.

• Neurons communicate by discharging a small messenger chemical called a "neurotransmitter," which is picked up by the target neuron. The neuron that sends the neurotransmitter is the "presynaptic neuron" and the neuron that receives the neurotransmitter is the "postsynaptic neuron." The neurotransmitter must travel across a small, empty space, called the "synaptic cleft." This process is called a synapse.

• As neurons degenerate there is a gradual decline in synaptic activity. This is one reason it's hard "to teach an old dog new tricks," and why stimulating the brain in a positive way, such as through intellectual challenges, social support, good diet, and physical activity will help slow brain aging.

• Much can go wrong during a synapse in an unhealthy system. For instance, there can be sufficient neurotransmitters but a problem with the presynaptic or postsynaptic receptors. Or the neurotransmitter doesn't break down or get reabsorbed as it should after the synapse is complete, disrupting future synapses. Neurons may fire too many neurotransmitters at once, or too few, and so on.

• Inflammation, hormone imbalances, and poor blood sugar handling are some of the factors that can sabotage neurotransmitter function.

• Every neuron needs oxygen, glucose, and stimulation. Brain degeneration happens when any one of these three is compromised. Factors that affect oxygen include blood sugar disorders, chronic stress, anemia, low blood pressure, hypothyroidism, and smoking. Blood sugar disorders affect glucose supply to neurons and brain health.

• The effect of blood sugar on the brain is so profound that some researchers refer to Alzheimer's as Type 3 diabetes.

• Stimulation of the neurons requires healthy neurotransmitter activity.

Chapter Five
BLOOD SUGAR IMBALANCES

This chapter deals with blood sugar imbalances, whether your blood sugar is chronically too low, too high, or swings between the two. It is not uncommon to have symptoms of both, as many people with blood sugar imbalances have glucose levels that shoot up and down like a roller coaster.

SYMPTOMS OF BLOOD SUGAR IMBALANCES
Reactive hypoglycemia symptoms (drops in blood sugar)
- Increased energy after meals
- Craving for sweets between meals
- Irritability if meals are missed
- Dependency on coffee and sugar for energy
- Becoming light headed if meals are missed
- Eating to relieve fatigue
- Feeling shaky, jittery, or tremulous
- Feeling agitated and nervous
- Become upset easily
- Poor memory, forgetfulness
- Blurred vision

Insulin resistance symptoms (high blood sugar spikes)

- Fatigue after meals
- General fatigue
- Constant hunger
- Craving for sweets not relieved by eating them
- Must have sweets after meals
- Waist girth equal to or larger than hip girth
- Frequent urination
- Increased appetite and thirst
- Difficulty losing weight
- Migrating aches and pains

• •

Melissa was a 25 year-old graduate student suffering from mood swings, her symptoms having developed during her past year of graduate school. She suffered bouts of depression, was tired all of the time, and her personality changed so that she was irritable and angry at times, which was nothing like her former self. A psychiatrist diagnosed her with depression, then with bipolar disorder and prescribed several different medications, which only made her feel worse. The psychiatrist wanted her to continue trying different medications, but both Melissa and her mother were hesitant.

Her mother was worried about her and brought Melissa in for an evaluation. She felt the stress of graduate school was too much for Melissa and wanted her to drop out and come home, something Melissa would not consider. Melissa felt graduate school was not that stressful and although it had been very taxing for her, she had been able to maintain good grades.

Although Melissa tried different medications that impact the neurotransmitter pathways, nobody asked her about her diet, the most basic approach. What a tragedy! In talking to her about her diet it was obvious to me she was doing all the wrong things. She skipped breakfast but then consumed a dessert at Starbucks loaded with sugar, whipped cream and caramel (also known as a coffee). She typically skipped meals during the day but snacked on fruit and high-sugar foods. She crashed in the afternoon, had difficulty waking up and did not feel rested in the morning, and she had difficulty staying asleep during the night.

When you see somebody as young as Melissa develop symptoms within a year of moving it is easy to blame stress. Our physiology should be able to handle stress, but Melissa's diet and lifestyle had already put her blood sugar on a very stressful roller coaster ride. Graduate school further taxed her blood sugar and adrenal stress-handling system, which was already depleted.

I was able to help Melissa commit to a diet that stabilized her blood glucose. She took nutritional supplements to help stabilize her blood sugar system as well as "adaptogens," herbal compounds that help the body better adapt to stress. The combination of her new diet and nutritional support completely changed her energy levels and brain function. She was able to sleep through the night and no longer crashed in the afternoon. Her mood swings, irritability, and depression all came under control once she started to stabilize her blood glucose levels.

Datis Kharrazian, DHSc, DC, MS

• •

I have seen so many patients like Melissa since beginning my practice. The management of their cases is so fundamentally basic and easy. However, health care professionals do not emphasize the importance of stable blood glucose levels, especially if fasting blood glucose levels are in the normal reference range. It is not uncommon for patients like Melissa to be put on psychotropic drugs, sleep medications, or labeled as a having bipolar disorder. It is also not uncommon for these individuals to seek alternative health care and have countless supplements thrown at them, while completely ignoring the importance of blood glucose fluctuations associated with diet and lifestyle. If you do not stabilize your blood glucose levels, you compromise fuel to the brain.

Glucose is the brain's fuel source, making stable blood sugar vital to healthy, balanced brain chemistry and the prevention of neurodegeneration. When blood sugar is unstable, not enough glucose gets to the brain and the brain will degenerate and not function well. This is why you see people with low blood sugar "bonk," or become spacey, lightheaded, shaky, and irritable if they go too long without eating—their brains aren't getting enough fuel to operate.

Also, stable blood sugar is necessary for the synthesis of neurotransmitters in the brain. The large fluctuations in blood sugar that accompany a blood-sugar imbalance can lead to altered neurotransmitter metabolism and disrupt neurotransmitter production and function in the brain. I will discuss these concepts for each neurotransmitter in detail in the upcoming chapters.

Low blood sugar promotes surges of the adrenal fight-or-flight hormones epinephrine and norepinephrine, which is stimulating. On the other hand, high blood sugar promotes surges of serotonin and GABA, which can make you sleepy after you eat. A classic example of this is the overproduction of serotonin and GABA after eating a potato, a bowl of white rice, or some other starchy meal, which create changes in your mood and brain function, often causing drowsiness. This also partly explains why starchy foods are, neurologically speaking, comfort foods (although if eaten all the time they create neurotransmitter serotonin dysfunction).

● ●

When Gary first came to see me he had been suffering from migraines for many years. In addition, he had low energy, anxiety, and frequent bouts of brain fog. After a thorough work-up that included health questionnaires, a consultation, a physical exam, and blood and saliva tests, I concluded a blood sugar imbalance was causing Gary's migraines, fatigue, anxiety, and brain fog, as well as an imbalance in his cortisol levels (an indicator of an adrenal imbalance) and neurotransmitter activity. He also had some detoxification issues.

We addressed his blood-sugar imbalance through a customized diet and nutritional compounds. We also smoothed out the cortisol surges with some botanical herbs to improve his resiliency to the stressors in his life, as well as discussed ways he could manage his stress. Finally, we addressed his detoxification issues with a cleanse.

After only a few months on this protocol, Gary was virtually migraine-free. His energy levels and concentration skyrocketed. He is now less anxious and his brain fog has lifted. And to top

it off, he lost 15 pounds! Once his blood sugar imbalance was under control, we used new nutritional compounds for deeper neurotransmitter support. Working with Gary was a testament to the extraordinary healing powers of the mind and body.
Titus Chiu, DC, MS, DACNB
Chicago, Illinois
www.drtituschiu.com

● ●

HYPOGLYCEMIA

Do you become irritable, shaky, lightheaded, nervous, or upset between meals or if you go too long without eating? That is because your blood sugar is dropping too low and depriving your brain of fuel.

Do you feel energized after meals? This is actually not a good sign, as it means you were feeling run-down before eating.

The only effect eating should have is to remove hunger. With ideal blood sugar function, your energy levels and mood are sufficiently maintained between meals. Do you have difficulty eating large meals in the morning, or eating at all? Do you feel nauseous in the morning? Does your energy level drop in the afternoon, sending you for sweets and coffee? Do you wake up in the middle of the night, say, around 3 or 4 a.m., full of energy or anxiety? Does your concentration falter between meals or do you have to drink coffee to keep yourself going? These are all symptoms of low blood sugar, or hypoglycemia.

Hypoglycemia is also often linked with adrenal fatigue, a condition in which the adrenal glands do not produce enough cortisol. Cortisol, a hormone that helps us cope with stress, is responsible for raising blood sugar levels when they drop too low, as they do in hypoglycemia. However, when cortisol levels are low the body is not able to boost blood sugar up to a healthy level. The result is the familiar symptoms of feeling shaky, lightheaded, spaced out, and irritable. At this point it is necessary to eat to raise blood sugar back to a level that isn't causing brain degeneration.

Certain nutrients and dietary changes have shown to be very supportive for people with hypoglycemia. Additionally, nutrients that slow the breakdown of cortisol, an important stress-regulating hormone, can also be beneficial, as many people with hypoglycemia tend to have low cortisol, which is why their bodies can't raise low blood sugar levels.

When blood sugar levels drop too low in a healthy person, such as during the night, the adrenal glands release cortisol. This triggers the breakdown of glycogen stored in the liver and muscles to release glucose into the bloodstream. However, if a person's cortisol is low the release of glycogen cannot be sufficiently triggered to raise blood sugar. Instead, the adrenals release epinephrine and norepinephrine as a backup.

These are the fight-or-flight hormones that cause one to wake up at 3 a.m. filled with anxiety or to be nauseous in the morning. Glycyrrhiza, a component of licorice, has been shown to slow the breakdown of cortisol so that it circulates longer in the system and can thus help keep blood sugar levels steady. It may be helpful for individuals whose low cortisol causes their hypoglycemia.

* *

Ruby, 19, came to see me for help with anxiety, depression, fatigue, and inability to sleep through the night. Her previous doctor had prescribed an anti-anxiety medication for her anxiety and told her he wanted to put her on a trial of antidepressants. Her mother did not want her to go on antidepressants, which prompted her to consult with me.

Her blood work revealed she was hypoglycemic (she was not eating enough protein or eating often enough throughout the day). We also ran a salivary adrenal panel, which showed elevated cortisol levels and an abnormal circadian rhythm. She was also experiencing symptoms of poor serotonin activity.

I placed her on nutritional support and began managing her hypoglycemia properly. Within 45 days her symptoms had completely turned around. She was sleeping through the night and had good energy throughout the day. Her MD took her off the medication and told her he felt she no longer needed to be on antidepressants.

John A. Warren, DC
Fountain Valley, California
www.warrenchirocenter.com

* *

INSULIN RESISTANCE

The other end of the blood sugar spectrum is insulin resistance, a condition in which the blood sugar is chronically too high. This most often occurs due to a diet high in carbohydrates—sugars, sweets, sodas, pastries, bread, pasta, rice, potatoes, corn, grains, beans, and other starchy foods. The body rapidly breaks down these foods into simple sugars that can send blood sugar levels soaring. In response, the pancreas secretes the hormone insulin to carry the sugar out of the bloodstream and into the body's cells, and to convert it into fat for storage. When this happens repeatedly, as it does for many Americans, the cells develop a resistance to the constant onslaught of insulin and refuse it entry. As a result, too much sugar and insulin circulate throughout the bloodstream causing inflammation, skewing hormones, and throwing off neurotransmitter balances, all of which lead to rapid degeneration of the brain.

Do you feel fatigued after meals, do you crave sugar and sweets after meals, or do you need a stimulant, such as coffee, after meals? Do you have difficulty losing weight, and is your waist girth equal to or larger than your hip girth? Do you urinate frequently, or has your thirst or appetite increased?

These are all symptoms of insulin resistance, red flags the brain is under attack and aging rapidly.

• •

I was diagnosed with severe depression many years ago and was prescribed various antidepressants. I was told I would have to be on medication for the rest of my life.

Recently my husband and I decided that we wanted to have children. After much research, we discovered that continuing my medication would be unsafe to our unborn child. I was apprehensive about decreasing or even stopping my medication, since I had such severe symptoms of anger, isolation, sadness, worry, and an inability to handle stress. It was at this time that I was referred to Dr. Flannery.

Dr. Flannery explained how my blood sugar imbalance affected my health—I was suffering from insulin resistance. He also said the medication I was taking only masked my symptoms and didn't fix my problems. I began to reduce my antidepressants with medical guidance, during which time I also needed dopamine support.

With Dr. Flannery's knowledge and expertise, I am now completely off all my medication and am feeling as good if not better than I did while I was on my medication. I am currently free of all symptoms of depression and my husband and I are now expecting our first child in a few months.

a patient of Dr. Flannery
Mark Flannery, DC, MS, BS, FAAIM, DCBCN, DCCN, CNS
Woodland Hills, California
www.DrFlannery.com

● ●

The person with insulin resistance typically feels drowsy after meals and may even need a nap. She also may have an insane, relentless craving for sugar after meals, making dessert a necessity (and perpetuating the problem). This is also the person who carries a lot of fat on her belly and complains of insomnia. Insulin resistance also promotes testosterone production in women, fostering the growth of facial hair while the hair on the scalp starts to thin. In men, insulin resistance promotes excess estrogen so that they grow breasts and hips, and suddenly find themselves crying at movies. It is estimated more than one-third of the U.S. population has insulin resistance, which is a stepping stone to diabetes.

Various herbs and nutrients have proven very effective at increasing the sensitivity of cells to insulin (so more sugar can get out of the bloodstream and into the cells). Additionally, phosphatidylserine can be helpful in lowering high cortisol levels that often accompany insulin resistance.

● ●

Carl, 52, was a retired firefighter. He was almost 100 pounds overweight, had diabetes, and struggled with depression and chronic pain. He was taking several medications for his diabetes, blood pressure, depression, and constipation. Carl's wife was very concerned about him and brought him to my office for a consultation. I asked Carl if he wanted to be there and he said, "I would rather be dead." I thanked Carl and his wife for coming and told them there was nothing I could do unless Carl was ready.

Almost a year went by and Carl became much worse. He scheduled an appointment with me himself.

He was a different person this time and told me he would do whatever I asked; he just needed direction. He had already been eating better and trying to exercise, but admitted his bouts of depression made it difficult.

As I evaluated Carl's case I noticed he had lost his sense of smell, his speech was monotone, and he had hypokinesia (slow movements). These are all early signs of Parkinson's disease. He did not have any tremors, but tremors do not occur until the disease progresses. He also had lost sense perception for vibration in his feet, an early finding for diabetic neuropathy, and he had many early symptoms of Alzheimer's disease. His brain was in bad shape thanks largely to his poorly managed diabetes.

Further lab testing indicated he had antibodies to his islet cells. This is a condition in which the immune system attacks the pancreas. Although he had the classical symptoms and markers of Type 2 diabetes, which is lifestyle-induced, the islet cell antibodies indicated an overlapping autoimmune condition contributing to his diabetes. This meant he needed to control not only his blood glucose but also his autoimmunity.

I immediately placed him on the leaky gut diet program, which I will discuss in Chapter Nine, for two reasons. The diet removes all grains, starches, and heavy sugars to control elevated blood glucose, and it is an anti-inflammatory program. Animal studies have shown leaky gut can lead to Type 1 diabetes. I also supported his dopamine and acetylcholine pathways and provided him with supplements to help improve his insulin receptor sensitivity.

Carl immediately dropped weight. As his weight came off his energy improved and his overall body pain reduced. He transformed into an entirely different person and rarely had episodes of depression anymore.

Carl's case is important because it shows once an individual's blood glucose becomes elevated that individual is at major risk for neurodegenerative conditions. High glucose in the bloodstream converts to glycosylated end products, a type of free radical that destroys neurons in the brain and in the nerves in the feet. Carl was already suffering from this, and I am sure if he continued down the path he would have developed diabetic neuropathy, Parkinson's disease, and/or dementia.

Datis Kharrazian, DHSc, DC, MS

● ●

THE HYPOGLYCEMIA/INSULIN RESISTANCE COMBINATION

Hypoglycemia and insulin resistance are not mutually exclusive. If you have one you most likely have some degree of the other. Either way, both are a sign your blood sugar is unstable and either dropping too low, spiking too high, or both. Both cause the insulin surges that skew so many other systems in the body.

In this case, you have to determine which nutritional compounds you need and at which time. For instance, you may need insulin resistance support with your meals to help sensitize your cells to insulin so blood sugar levels don't climb too high. However, between meals and before bed you may need support for hypoglycemia so that blood sugar doesn't drop too low.

Also, regardless of whether you have one, the other, or both, the most fundamental change you can make is to your diet, which I outline at the end of this chapter. All the herbs and special nutrients in the world cannot fully support you until you make the necessary, brain-friendly dietary and lifestyle changes.

● ●

I had a male 35-year-old patient whose energy swung up and down. Before meals he could barely communicate due to poor brain function. Within his first few bites he became coherent again. After meals, however, he was listless again and had brain fog. Both his father and grandfather succumbed to Alzheimer's disease, and he was worried he was going down the same path. He snacked between meals but reported a raging appetite by dinner.

He is physically active, biking and doing yoga, and he said keeping busy helped improve his brain fog. He also suffered from insomnia, would forget emails after reading them, and had trouble functioning at work. He had symptoms of poor brain function, stress, and blood sugar imbalances. He also had symptoms involving all of the major neurotransmitters, with major issues with acetylcholine, the learning and memory neurotransmitter.

I gave the patient nutritional compounds for insulin resistance with meals and put him on a diet of 70 grams of carbohydrates per day. I also gave him other nutritional compounds to support his general brain health and adrenal function, and treated him with acupuncture.

Two weeks later at his next visit, he reported heightened energy and improved mental clarity. His insomnia was much improved if he ate a snack at bedtime. However, he said the low-carb diet made it harder to exercise.

One month later he still had mild insomnia some nights, but his energy was improving, especially if he was diligent with his diet (it can take time for the body to adapt to a low-carb diet). He reported "tons" of mental energy, meaning his brain health was improving dramatically, and he had become very productive and was able to get a lot of things done.

After another month he was eating 130 grams of carbohydrates a day. If he slacks on nutritional compounds to support his adrenal health, he feels his energy dip. If not, however, he said his overall mental energy is fabulous, and his memory is like it was in his 20s.

Dagmar Ehling, Mac, LAc, DOM
Durham, North Carolina
www.orientalhealthsolutions.com

● ●

SO WHAT DOES THIS HAVE TO DO WITH YOUR BRAIN?

If you've read my thyroid book *Why Do I Still Have Thyroid Symptoms?* all of this information will sound familiar, as balancing blood sugar is imperative to thyroid health. As it turns out, it's critical for brain health, too.

Some of the reasons to avoid sugary, high-carb diets and the resultant blood sugar swings are better known. The most obvious is the effect of low blood sugar in the person with hypoglycemia. As the brain is deprived of fuel when blood sugar drops too low, it stops functioning well, producing shakiness, headache, blurred vision, difficulty concentrating, and other neurological symptoms.

More poignant, however, is that excess sugar and starchy foods are a major promoter of inflammation in the brain, and when inflammation affects the brain, neurons die rapidly and in great numbers, speeding up brain aging and increasing the risk for neurological diseases such as Alzheimer's. Like sugar, inappropriate levels of insulin are also pro-inflammatory in the brain.

• •

Jonathon, 33, struggled with lethargy, memory problems, and cloudy thinking when he went to see Dr. Flannery. It bothered him that he couldn't remember things, and he was having difficulty with motivation and focus at his job as a software developer. He tried exercise, more sleep, and more coffee, but it seemed nothing helped. Actually, the only time he felt his best was after getting a sweet coffee drink and a pastry at Starbucks, but then he would crash four to five hours later. He had been on antidepressants for about a year, although they didn't seem to work.

I started him on a diet of gluten-free and dairy-free foods, no sugar, low-glycemic foods (foods that are not too starchy or sugary), and a strict schedule of three meals a day with protein snacks between meals. Because a blood panel showed him low in vitamin D, I also started Jonathon on emulsified vitamin D, along with nutritional compounds to support hypoglycemia and adrenal adaptogens to support adrenal function.

Within 30 days, Jonathon was feeling great. He stopped taking his antidepressants after two weeks on the new diet and nutritional support, and now, six months later, he still does not take them nor suffer from any of his old symptoms. He says his memory is much better, his focus and energy are back, and his mind does not feel cloudy anymore. He also finds he no longer needs to snack anymore, although he sticks to a lower carb diet.

Mark Flannery, DC, MS, BS, FAAIM, DCBCN, DCCN, CNS
Woodland Hills, California
www.DrFlannery.com

• •

Whenever you consume something sugary or starchy, your body must release plenty of insulin to remove the extra sugar from the bloodstream and escort it into the cells. If you are insulin resistant and sugar is not able to get into the cells, your brain hears the hungry cells crying for energy and releases more insulin in an effort to deliver glucose into the cells. Now you have too much sugar and too much insulin circulating in the bloodstream. These insulin surges promote inflammation both in the brain and in the body.

Lastly, one of the more obvious consequences of a diet too high in sugars and starches is that thick roll of belly fat the majority of Americans and many children now wear. That fat itself produces pro-inflammatory compounds and inflammation, which causes inflammation in the brain.

Scientists have known all of this for years. In fact, the deleterious effects of sugar and insulin surges on the brain are so well known that many have dubbed Alzheimer's disease "Type 3 diabetes." In addition to the inflammation-promoting properties of sugar, excess insulin, and excess abdominal fat, insulin surges also reduce the brain's ability to clear out amyloid plaques, the plaques that are the hallmark of Alzheimer's disease.[1]

People with diabetes are twice as likely to succumb to Alzheimer's disease as non-diabetics. Those diabetics who are insulin dependent have a fourfold risk of developing Alzheimer's dementia—a massive 400 percent increase—thanks to all the excess insulin. This higher risk is also linked to the tendency of the insulin-dependent Type 1 diabetic to use insulin as a license to eat a high-carbohydrate diet.

Although these facts alone are alarming, they don't take into account the effect of sugar, starchy foods, and insulin surges on hormonal balance, gut health, thyroid function, and adrenal health. By skewing function in those areas, brain degeneration is promoted even further. A brain free of inflammation and degeneration requires balanced hormones, a healthy gut, good thyroid function, and good adrenal function. Those are topics I will cover later in the book.

HOW BLOOD SUGAR IMBALANCES AFFECT NEUROTRANSMITTER ACTIVITY

As if all that wasn't enough (it's just the tip of the iceberg really), what further interests me about blood sugar imbalances is how they impact the brain's ability to make neurotransmitters. As it turns out, neurotransmitter synthesis depends upon an appropriate insulin response, not too little and not too much. A person with hypoglycemia, insulin resistance, or a combination of the two rarely has that appropriate insulin response necessary for healthy neurotransmitter activity. This in a large part explains why brain chemistry imbalances are such a huge issue in our society—blood sugar issues are too.

Let's look at how the neurotransmitter serotonin is made in the brain as an example, since serotonin deficiencies are estimated to affect a large percentage of the U.S. population. Deficiencies in our "happy and joyful" neurotransmitter serotonin are linked with a variety of ills, including depression, winter blues, PMS, lack of enjoyment or appreciation for things, inner rage, paranoia, and poor sleep. You'll see why so many Americans struggle with poor serotonin activity—because serotonin production is so closely linked to the all-important blood sugar balancing act.

Serotonin synthesis starts with protein consumption. Although that may be a problem in impoverished parts of the world, the average American eats plenty of protein necessary for neurotransmitter synthesis. Proteins are broken down into various amino acids, including tryptophan, a precursor to serotonin.

For tryptophan to be made into serotonin, it must cross the blood-brain barrier. Other amino acids called "branch-chain amino acids" (BCAA) also play a part in this transport, based on a proper BCAA-to-insulin-ratio. They are leucine, isoleucine, and valine, and they are involved in signaling an insulin release necessary for the transport of tryptophan. However, they also compete with tryptophan to get into the brain. If there is a proper insulin response—not too much or not too little—the insulin will send the BCAA into body tissue so that more tryptophan can get into the brain to be made into serotonin.

If this all happens the way it should, tryptophan hitches a ride across the blood-brain barrier on a transporter protein called a "large neutral amino acid transporter" (LNAA). If you take supplements made from 5-HTP, a popular serotonin precursor, this same action is used to transport it through the blood-brain barrier and into the brain where it is synthesized into tryptophan.

To simplify this concept, pretend the LNAA is the bus that ferries amino acids into the brain, where the best paying jobs are. When foods containing tryptophan are eaten, tryptophan would really like to get

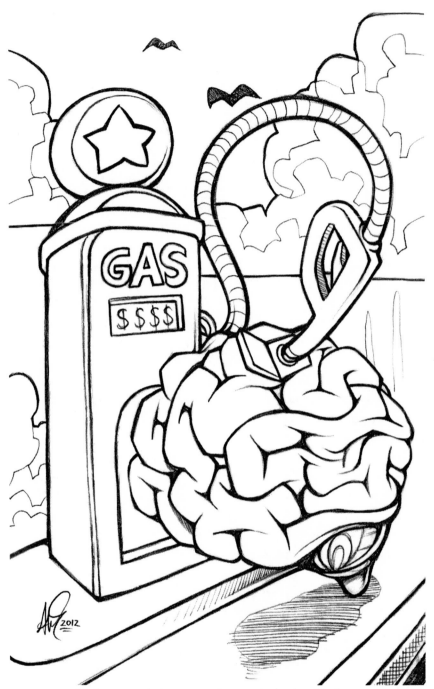

Blood sugar imbalances can deprive the brain of fuel, cause inflammation, and disrupt neurotransmitter activity.

into the brain for those good jobs. The BCAAs leucine, isoleucine, and valine want a seat on the bus, too. When the right amount of insulin is released, however, some of the BCAA aren't allowed on the bus. Instead, they're told to go to work in other tissues in the body. This makes space on the bus for more tryptophan to cross the blood-brain barrier and go to work making serotonin, so you can enjoy the things in life that give you pleasure, have an overall sense of well-being, and not succumb to depression during dark winter days.

Unfortunately, this scenario doesn't go as intended for many Americans. The problem is too much insulin is overseeing this bus transport into the brain. Sweets, sugary coffee drinks, pastries, pasta dinners, meals consisting only of toast and jam or a bag of chips—these all require surges of insulin to prevent blood sugar levels from skyrocketing too high. These insulin surges are common with insulin resistance, diabetes, and the use of insulin medications. When insulin gets too high, the following happens:

As tryptophan and the BCAAs line up for a spot on the LNAA bus, the surge of excess insulin makes it overzealous at its job. It refuses entry to almost all the BCAAs, sending them into other tissues. As a result, the bus is overcrowded with tryptophan. Once all this tryptophan gets into the brain, it is made into more serotonin than the person needs. Since serotonin is calming for most people, this surge of serotonin often causes drowsiness and sleepiness.

This partly explains why so many people with insulin resistance or diabetes feel sleepy after they eat—the excess insulin promotes the production of excess serotonin in the brain. This is also why indulging in sugary or starchy foods can give you that calming high that makes you want to lie down and snooze. But after the serotonin levels drop, people may feel depressed, spurring once again those cravings for sweets and starchy foods for that "high" they get from the serotonin surge.

It's worth mentioning here a couple of other factors that contribute to the post-meal drowsiness associated with insulin resistance. First, one of the ways the body removes excess glucose from the blood is to convert it into fat for storage. This is a very energy-demanding process that robs you of your ability to stay alert and focused after eating. Second, because the body's cells are resistant to the insulin that escorts glucose into the cells, it means the cells are not getting enough glucose, which they need for energy production. That too causes feelings of tiredness and poor mental function. So, between excess serotonin production in the brain, lack of energy in the cells, and the very demanding process of converting glucose to fat to lower blood sugar levels, the person gets a triple-whammy cocktail of post-meal sedation.

Fatigue after meals is a textbook symptom of insulin resistance for these reasons. This is the person who has a fasting blood sugar over 100 mg/dL, whose waist circumference is greater than the hip circumference, and who may struggle with insomnia. It's important to note that overeating, high stress, and lack of exercise can contribute to this cascade of events. Also, this pattern can explain why supplementing with tryptophan or 5-HTP to boost serotonin activity may not be as effective until blood sugar issues are addressed.

If excess insulin produces excess serotonin, why would a serotonin deficiency or poor serotonin activity be the end result? In Chapter Twelve I will talk about homotropic modulation and how neurons protect themselves from an oversupply of neurotransmitters by reducing their sensitivity to them. It's a concept that explains why a person needs to increase the amount of cocaine, nicotine, or even antidepressants to achieve the same effect. As high amounts of the same neurotransmitter, in this case serotonin, consistently bombard the neurons, the neurons lose their sensitivity to it so that it has less of an effect over time.

Also, the constant over-activity in the serotonin pathways eventually leads to depletion and deficiencies. This is because various other cofactors are required for serotonin synthesis, such as B vitamins and methyl donors, and over stimulation of these pathways eventually depletes these cofactors. The end result over time is a loss in effective serotonin activity and symptoms of low serotonin, such as depression, loss of interest in life, seasonal affective disorder, and more.

● ●

I have been working with migraine patients for many years using a functional neurology and functional medicine approach. Each patient is unique with his or her own type of prescription, triggers, auras, and sensitivities. However, a common thing among many of them has been the impact of blood sugar and adrenal function on the brain.

Jackie came into the office complaining of three to four migraines a week. She found herself putting together a cocktail of drugs to rid the pain. She also would inject herself at least once a week with an abortive drug for relief. She did not know her triggers since the migraines came on so frequently and sporadically.

After a comprehensive exam and history it was clear blood sugar was a main factor. She would eat dinner around 6 p.m. and her next meal would be around 1 p.m. the next day. Jackie was always on the go with a busy work schedule and low energy.

A laboratory analysis showed she had hypoglycemia, low cortisol, high CRP (an inflammatory marker), and high red blood cell values. Jackie's treatment plan consisted of eating every two hours and taking nutritional support for hypoglycemia and to increase adrenal function. She was also given methylcobalamin for B-12 support and to help with any brain inflammatory responses.

Within a week, she had not used any injectable medications and had only one migraine. Over the course of the month she had reduced her oral medications, was able to function at work, and had more energy. Follow-up testing showed an increase in cortisol and blood sugar to a normal range.

Shane Steadman, DC, DACNB, DCBCN
Englewood, Colorado
www.integratedhealthdenver.com

• •

HYPOGLYCEMIA AND NEUROTRANSMITTER ACTIVITY

With insulin resistance, the LNAA bus crossing into the brain is overloaded with tryptophan. In the case of hypoglycemia, when too little insulin is present to facilitate this process, just the opposite occurs. People with hypoglycemia are the ones who skip breakfast or are prone to missing meals, only eat sugary or starchy snacks with no protein, or perhaps, ever weight-conscious, they don't eat enough. They produce too little insulin to bring tryptophan into the brain and as a result too little serotonin is made.

Again, even supplementation with tryptophan or 5-HTP may fail to achieve the desired results due to this blood sugar problem. The issue isn't getting enough serotonin precursors into the body, but rather insufficient insulin isn't allowing these substances to make it into the brain to raise serotonin levels. Another factor is that hypoglycemia lowers overall glucose levels in the brain. Adequate glucose is necessary to fuel energy in the brain, including the energy to produce serotonin from its precursors. It should also be noted that many people with hypoglycemia suffer from many of the abnormal mechanisms discussed with excess insulin—when blood glucose is low the pancreas secretes insulin in an attempt to deliver available glucose into cells for energy production.

BLOOD SUGAR IMBALANCES AND DOPAMINE

In the examples above I used serotonin to illustrate how precursors get into the brain to be made into neurotransmitters. This same principle applies to dopamine, our "pleasure and reward" neurotransmitter. As with a serotonin deficiency, a dopamine deficiency can produce symptoms of depression. Other symptoms include feelings of hopelessness and worthlessness, lack of motivation, and a tendency to snap or fly into a rage over little things. In fact, because the transport system works the same for both, it's common to see a deficiency of both in people.

Further aggravating a dopamine deficiency is the fact that serotonin production can edge out dopamine production when blood sugar imbalances are an issue. If a person eats a meal that is higher in carbs than protein, there is a greater tendency for LNAA to carry more serotonin precursors than dopamine precursors into the brain. Higher amounts of carbs tend to activate LNAA to favor tryptophan over the dopamine precursor tyrosine. Meals richer in protein than carbs will favor the transport of tyrosine over tryptophan into the brain. Practitioners who understand this will see patients who tend toward serotonin deficiency crave more carbs, while those who tend toward dopamine deficiency crave meats and fish. Either way, a healthy blood sugar system will ensure the transport of the right levels of precursors for both serotonin and dopamine into the brain.

• •

When the thyroid book came out Michela wanted to find a prac-
titioner to help her with seemingly irresolvable thyroid problems
that were also causing poor brain function. She was perpetually

exhausted, going to bed tired and waking up tired. In fact, waking up was so difficult she asked to come to work a half hour later. She also suffered from brain fog, an inability to focus or concentrate well, an increasing loss of short-term memory, and irritability. Understandably, she had no joy in life and did not like the person she had become.

Because Michela lived in another country, I worked with Michela on diet alone. I had Michela eliminate all potentially allergenic foods, such as gluten, dairy, and corn, and eat a lower carb diet of mostly meats, nuts, seeds, produce, healthy fats, and a modest amount of rice and potatoes. I also had Michela eat a protein-rich snack every several hours, eat a good, protein-rich breakfast, and quit drinking coffee.

Quitting coffee was hard and gave Michela a headache at first, but she felt much better after a few days without it. I also had her quit watching television before bed and set a strict schedule of when she went to bed. She also added vitamin D and DHA to her regimen.

Michela began feeling increasingly better with each passing day, and after about a month she was back to her old self, having successfully regulated her blood sugar and removed foods that were causing an inflammatory response, which further disrupts blood sugar balances. "Now I can say I feel normal, like couple of years ago," Michela says.

Yolanda Loafer, DC
Phoenix, Arizona
www.dryolandaloafer.com

● ●

EATING TO BALANCE YOUR BLOOD SUGAR AND BOOST YOUR BRAIN HEALTH

Whether you have hypoglycemia or insulin resistance, you must make changes to your diet if you want to improve your brain health; there are no exceptions to this. Although flooding the brain with neurotransmitter supplements popular today may buy you a little time or a little relief, as long as blood sugar imbalances dominate brain function you will never enjoy lasting success. With insulin resistance, you can no longer simply eat what you please when you please. With hypoglycemia, you cannot continue missing meals or snacking on something sugary or starchy. The worst thing a person with insulin resistance can do is overeat or eat more carbohydrates than he or she can tolerate. (If you feel sleepy or crave sugar after a meal, you just ate too many carbohydrates.) A hypoglycemic person should never skip breakfast or eat starchy/sugary snacks, especially before going to bed. (A person with insulin resistance should avoid these habits, too).

Sticking to a diet that stabilizes blood sugar is challenging, due to intense cravings and the addictive nature of certain foods, and how ubiquitous these foods are in our culture. Also, unidentified food intolerances stimulate the adrenals so that people actually get an "adrenaline rush" from the foods to which they are sensitive, which also creates intense cravings. However, support with the right nutritional compounds that stabilize the blood sugar and the determination to weather the hardest period—that is, the first three days after changing the diet—will make it easier and more rewarding for you to follow a healthier way of eating.

• •

Lawrence, 34, presented with a major complaint of exertion headaches. He was a strapping and intelligent young man, a self-employed landscaper who did heavy labor outdoors and was well respected for the quality of his work. But his headaches significantly impacted his ability to work. His secondary complaint was an anal fistula that began six years prior and regularly became inflamed and painful, although he didn't have much faith that it could be helped.

The headaches were severe and primarily came on when the weather was hot or humid, which was often considering he lives in North Carolina. The pain would start in the early morning or by mid-day when the temperature rose and it would leave him exhausted and needing to lie down for several days to let the pain subside. Occasionally he woke with headaches. Significant neck pain accompanied the headaches.

Since Lawrence woke with his headaches fairly often, I suspected reactive hypoglycemia. I asked him to eat a carbohydrate-free snack every two hours and before bed to maintain his blood glucose levels.

Thankfully this one simple recommendation completely eliminated his headaches. Now he never wakes with a headache and can work long hours in high heat and humidity without a problem. The reduction in overall inflammation from stabilizing his blood sugar also significantly improved his fistula discomfort. We recently had temperatures over 100 degrees with high humidity. Lawrence worked from 9 a.m. to 6 p.m. in the sun moving boulders and felt great.

From a functional medicine point of view, our adrenals must produce enough cortisol to free glycogen from the liver and muscles to stabilize our blood glucose levels between meals and especially overnight. This is a critical process since blood glucose is imperative for all tissues to function—our brains are the biggest consumers of glucose.

From the perspective of Oriental medicine, the adrenals are associated with the water element, which represents the deepest aspect of our physical being. As such, Lawrence can expect a gradual improvement in his hypoglycemia over weeks or months as his physiology "fills the well" and his adrenal function returns to optimal levels with proper diet and supplementation. Once this occurs, he won't need to snack between meals to be symptom free.

Lawrence only made three visits to our clinic. No testing was needed. Simple. Elegant. Beautiful.

Kenneth Morehead, MSOM, LAc, DAONB
Durham, North Carolina
www.orientalhealthsolutions.com

• •

Whether you are hypoglycemic or insulin resistant, a few basic rules apply to boost your brain health and balance your brain chemistry:

1. Eat a breakfast of high-quality protein and fat. When you wake up in the morning, you have gone a long time without eating. Chances are your adrenal fight-or-flight hormones have been called into action (particularly if you woke up at 3 or 4 a.m. feeling anxious). You need to calm down your system by eating a low-carbohydrate breakfast of high quality proteins and fats. I realize eating breakfast is difficult when you have dysglycemia (abnormal blood sugar levels). You may wake up with

no appetite or even feeling nauseous. That is a side effect of your adrenal hormones, and that cup of coffee is only making the problem worse.

You simply must force yourself to eat some protein, even if it's a little bit. It will dissipate your nausea, and in just two to three days of stabilizing your blood sugar you will no longer wake up feeling nauseous. Supporting blood sugar issues is futile unless you eat breakfast. If you like to work out first thing in the morning, just make sure you eat within one hour of waking up.

2. If you have hypoglycemia, eat a small amount of protein every two to three hours. This does not mean eat a full meal every two to three hours—a few bites will do. The name of the game is to keep your blood sugar stable and leave the adrenal glands out of the picture. Going for long stretches without eating when you have dysglycemia exacerbates your blood sugar issues, which can accelerate degeneration of the brain and contribute to brain chemistry imbalances. Nuts, seeds, a boiled egg, or meat, or a low-carbohydrate protein shake are some examples of protein snacks. As your dysglycemia improves, you will find you can go longer between snacks.

3. Find your carbohydrate tolerance and stick to it. A high-carbohydrate diet is at the root of blood sugar imbalances and accelerated brain degeneration. How many grams of carbohydrates should you eat each day? I follow this simple rule: If you feel sleepy or crave sugar after you eat, you have eaten too many carbohydrates.

Sometimes insulin resistance causes you to feel sleepy even if you haven't eaten anything starchy or sweet. In this case, you need to work with a qualified health care practitioner to reverse the problem using specific nutritional compounds. What are carbohydrate-rich foods? Grains (remember, corn is a grain), legumes, starchy vegetables like potatoes and peas, and, of course, sweets, including natural sweeteners like agave. The more processed the grain, the more likely it is to trigger a surge of insulin into your bloodstream.

Many symptoms of blood sugar imbalances, such as sleep issues, irritability, and energy crashes start to diminish on a lower-carbohydrate diet. Also, unidentified food intolerances can create sugar cravings or fatigue after meals, so it's important to find out if that's an issue for you.

4. Never eat high-carb foods without some fiber, fat, or protein. These will slow down the rate at which the glucose is absorbed into the bloodstream and help prevent "insulin shock."

5. Do not eat sweets or starchy foods before bed. This is one of the worst things the hypoglycemic person can do. Your blood sugar will crash during the night, long before your next meal is due. Chances are your adrenals will kick into action, creating restless sleep or that 3 a.m. wake up with anxiety.

6. Avoid all fruit juices and carrot juice. These can be more sugary than soda, and will quickly have you crashing.

7. Avoid or limit caffeine. The energy boosting drinks on the market should also be avoided. Blood sugar imbalances are hard enough on the adrenal glands, the glands that handle our stress response, and adding in adrenal stimulants fatigues them further.

8. Eat a well-balanced diet consisting mostly of vegetables, and quality meats and fats. A diet of junk food, fast foods, and other processed foods works against you. To restore your brain health you must find ways to restore your diet closer to what our ancestors ate. A diet dominated by leafy, green vegetables and adequate in quality protein and fats is enormously restorative.

9. Eliminate food allergens and intolerances. Whenever a food creates an immune response, such as an allergy or intolerance, it also creates blood sugar instability and insulin surges. Common food intolerances are to gluten, dairy, eggs, corn, soy, and yeast. Eating these foods can create sugar cravings and fatigue after meals. To stabilize blood sugar and promote brain health, problem foods should be eliminated and the gut repaired. This will be explored further in Chapter Nine.

In addition to the dietary protocol outlined above, I also recommend the following to help balance blood sugar:

Nutrients to support a healthy response to insulin resistance
Certain nutrients help the cells to regain their sensitivity to insulin so that it can bring glucose into the cells for energy. Key ingredients

include chromium, vanadium, alpha lipoic acid, mixed tocopherols, magnesium, biotin, zinc, inositol, and gymnema sylvestre.

Nutrients to support a healthy response to hypoglycemia

Key ingredients include chromium, bovine adrenal gland, choline bitartrate, bovine liver gland, bovine pancreas gland, inositol, L-carnitine, co-enzyme Q10, rubidium chelate, and vanadium aspartate.

Sometimes a person will swing back and forth between insulin resistance and hypoglycemia. In these cases, I recommend taking nutritional compounds for insulin resistance with meals, and nutritional compounds for hypoglycemia between meals.

It's important to work with a qualified health care practitioner so you take the right nutrients and botanicals in the right amounts. Taking the wrong nutrients for your blood sugar condition has the potential to make your condition worse.

Special considerations for insulin resistance

Insulin resistant folks are those who become drowsy after meals or even need to lie down and take a nap, especially after a meal heavy in rice, pasta, bread, or other carbohydrates. Women with insulin resistance tend to have excess facial hair and a large belly. Men may also have a large belly, as well as "breasts" or a tendency toward being more emotional. The rule of thumb for insulin resistance is that if you feel sleepy after you eat, you just ate too many carbohydrates. What if your meal was virtually carbohydrate-free, say a chicken breast and green beans drizzled in olive oil, and you still feel sleepy after eating? It means your insulin resistance has advanced to such a degree that you may need specialized nutrients to correct insulin resistance.

RESEARCH ON COMPOUNDS TO SUPPORT INSULIN RESISTANCE

Gymnema sylvestre

Gymnema sylvestre has demonstrated positive impacts in supporting healthy insulin receptor sensitivity. It has demonstrated the ability to support efficient insulin use, healthy blood sugar balance, and pancreatic cell health.[2][3][4][5] It does not encourage the endogenous production of insulin and if given to healthy volunteers, does not produce any blood sugar-lowering or hypoglycemic effects.[6][7]

Banaba leaf extract

Banaba leaf extract contains triterpenoid, lagerstroemin, flosin B, reginin A, and corosolic acid. Studies indicate that these compounds support healthy glucose levels by supporting peripheral glucose utilization.[8][9]

Maitake mushroom

Grifola frondosa, better known as maitake mushroom, supports healthy glucose levels by supporting peripheral insulin receptor site sensitivity. This response has been shown to support a healthy amount of circulating insulin and glucose.[10][11] It also appears that maitake contains soluble fiber in the form of beta-glucan, which may support healthy glucose absorption in the gastrointestinal tract.[12] There are no recognized serious adverse side effects.[13]

Bitter melon

Mormordica charantia, better known as bitter melon, is the most popular plant used worldwide to support blood sugar balance and pancreatic health.[14][15][16] Several clinical studies have been published demonstrating the glucose-supporting effect of bitter melon.[17][18][19] It has also demonstrated blood sugar balance support in animal studies.[20] Bitter melon is well tolerated and does not appear to demonstrate adverse side effects, but it may not be appropriate for pregnant women.[21]

Opuntia streptacantha Lemaire

The compounds in *Opuntia streptacantha Lemaire* support healthy glucose utilization. It is theorized that this compound from cactus stems supports healthy levels of glucose. No adverse side effects are evident with this plant compound.[22][23]

Guar gum

Guar gum is a dietary fiber from the ground endosperm of the seeds of *Cyamopsis psoralioides*. It has been shown in numerous studies to support healthy blood glucose levels. It seems to support healthy insulin levels and healthy pancreatic function.[24][25][26][27][28] Guar gum has also been shown to support healthy lipid metabolism and healthy cholesterol levels.[29][30][31]

Pectin

Pectin is a natural component of plants. It is especially abundant in fruit, such as apples and citrus. Pectins have shown to support healthy glucose and cholesterol levels. Pectin reduces the rate of gastric emptying, which in turn slows the release of glucose into the bloodstream. It also appears to thicken the gut wall's mucosal layer, reducing intestinal absorption of glucose. [32] [33] [34]

Chromium

Chromium is an essential nutrient to support healthy insulin receptor sensitivity, especially when one considers the evidence that chromium deficiencies are common in the United States and that chromium levels are depleted by a diet of refined carbohydrates and sugars. There is evidence that chromium deficiency results in insulin resistance. [35] [36] [37] Chromium, also known as "glucose tolerance factor," appears to support the impact of insulin on receptor sites and supports healthy glucose uptake. [38] [39] Studies have demonstrated that chromium supports healthy postprandial glucose and insulin levels, glycated hemoglobin, and healthy cholesterol levels. [40] [41] [42] [43] [44]

Vanadium

Vanadium is an important mineral when it comes to supporting healthy insulin receptor sensitivity. It appears to support the transport of glucose to the cell membrane to allow cells to intake serum glucose. [45] [46] [47] This physiologic impact is of great importance. Numerous studies have demonstrated the positive role vanadium plays in supporting healthy insulin receptor sensitivity. [48] [49] [50]

Alpha lipoic acid

Alpha lipoic acid is a sulfur-containing substance that seems to support healthy insulin receptor sensitivity by supporting the proper activation of glucose transporters, which support glucose disposal through healthy insulin sensitivity. [51] [52] [53] [54] Alpha lipoic acid has also shown to support glucose metabolism, healthy levels of serum lactate and pyruvate, and to support healthy mitochondrial oxidative phosphorylation. [55] Alpha lipoic acid is also a powerful antioxidant.[56][57] Numerous studies have shown the positive impact of alpha lipoic acid for supporting healthy insulin receptor sensitivity.[58][59][60]

Vitamin E (tocopherols)

Vitamin E (tocopherols) has been shown to support healthy insulin receptor sensitivity, healthy serum triglycerides and LDL, blood sugar balance, and pancreatic function.[61][62][63][64][65][66]

Magnesium

Magnesium has been shown to support healthy insulin receptor sensitivity. It appears to support healthy insulin secretion, glucose transport for insulin-mediated glucose uptake, and insulin intercellular transcriptional response.[67][68][69] Furthermore, insulin resistance has been reported in individuals with low magnesium status.[70][71][72]

Biotin

Biotin supplementation has been shown to support a healthy insulin response to glucose load, healthy post-prandial glucose levels, and healthy levels of glucokinase, which is responsible for the first step in glucose utilization by the liver.[73][74][75][76]

Zinc

Zinc is an important mineral to support healthy insulin receptor sensitivity. Zinc supports beta-cell health, healthy insulin sensitivity, and healthy insulin metabolism.[77] There have been strong correlations with low zinc status and increased risk for insulin resistance, as well as evidence that diabetics excrete large amounts of zinc and therefore require supplementation.[78][79][80]

Inositol

Inositol has shown the ability to support normal myoinositol levels.[81]

Niacin

Niacin is a component of glucose tolerance factor, which helps support healthy insulin receptor site function.[82] Several studies have also shown that niacinimide has the potential to support blood sugar balance and pancreatic health.[83][84][85] Niacinimide has also been shown to support beta-cell health.[86]

L-carnitine

L-carnitine has the potential to support healthy insulin receptor sensitivity by supporting healthy whole-body glucose uptake and supporting healthy glucose storage.[87 88 89] L-carnitine has been shown to support the health of both peripheral nerves and vascular function.[90] In addition, it has been shown to support healthy total serum lipid and HDL cholesterol levels.[91]

● ●

I saw Bill about one year ago, just after taking the Brain and Neurotransmitter course taught by Dr. Kharrazian. He was unmotivated, depressed, and had lost joy in just about all activities. He had a good family life, good job, exercised regularly, and was active in his church.

Based on his responses on some questionnaires, it appeared he suffered from multiple neurotransmitter issues; however, it was clear his main problem was a blood sugar imbalance. I supported his hypoglycemia with nutritional compounds, tweaked his diet and eating patterns, and supported his serotonin.

He started feeling better within two weeks, and once his blood sugar imbalance was corrected and he was eating properly, he no longer needed to support his serotonin pathways. Thanks to Dr. Kharrazian's protocols, Bill was able to get his life back and was not forced to rely on antidepressants for the rest of his life.

Joe Alaimo, DC
Wilmington, North Carolina
www.drjoealaimo.com

● ●

CHAPTER SUMMARY

• It is not uncommon for people with blood sugar disorders to be put on psychotropic drugs, sleep medications, or labeled as a having bipolar disorder. If you do not stabilize your blood glucose levels, you compromise fuel to the brain.

• Glucose is the brain's primary fuel source, making stable blood sugar vital to healthy, balanced brain chemistry and the prevention of brain degeneration.

• Appropriate levels of glucose and insulin are needed for the synthesis of neurotransmitters. Glucose and insulin imbalances can lead to altered moods.

• Hypoglycemia is often associated with low cortisol while insulin resistance is often associated with high cortisol.

• Some people suffer from signs and symptoms of both hypoglycemia and insulin resistance.

• A high-carb diet promotes brain inflammation and degeneration.

• A high-carb diet also skews neurotransmitter production and can promote excess tryptophan, which may cause drowsiness or sleepiness after meals. Converting excess glucose to fat also may cause drowsiness.

• Eating a lower-carb diet with sufficient fat and protein and avoiding food intolerances will prevent blood sugar swings, energy crashes, inflammation, and degeneration. It is essential for brain health.

Chapter Six

STRESS AND THE BRAIN

UNHEALTHY STRESS SYMPTOMS

- Always have projects and things that need to be done
- Never have time for yourself
- Not getting enough sleep or rest
- Not enough time or motivation to get regular exercise
- Not accomplishing your life's purpose

• •

Clark came into my office almost 10 years ago and was one of the most stressed out individuals I have ever met. He ran a large public relations company and his job was to constantly put out fires for his clients. He once said his favorite thing to do in life was to be on a long airplane flight because nobody could call him.

Clark came to see me because he was suffering from memory lapses, insomnia, and mild depression. These all result from imbalances in brain chemistry, and in Clark's case it was caused primarily by the stress he placed on himself. Despite his high stress lifestyle he did exercise daily and ate a healthy diet. When we first discussed his case I brought up the issue of his stress load and I made him commit to taking one day a week off. His off day was still more stressful than most people's regular days of work. Despite this he did lower his workload and he did not take on new projects. I also placed him on various supplements to help his stress response, as discussed in this chapter. He started to notice improvements in memory and was starting to sleep better at night. This only lasted for about three weeks, and then he dropped out of my office and went back to his hectic lifestyle again. Years later I ran into him at the airport. I almost did not recognize him because of how much older he looked. He had aged very rapidly. He told me that was now on several hypertensive medications and sleep medications, and was starting to have regular migraines. I tried to ask about his lifestyle, but he did not want to talk about it.

I have not seen Clark since then, but a stress-based lifestyle will not only age you faster but will also promote ulcers, shrink the brain, and increase the risk of Alzheimer's and other brain chemical disorders. Unfortunately, many people with increased stress responses do not make the right decisions and suffer the consequences.

I share Clark's case with you because he is like many people who do not understand the toll chronic, unrelenting stress can have on the body and, more specifically, the brain. In this chapter I will present these concepts to you.

Datis Kharrazian, DHSc, DC, MS

● ●

Nothing is more damaging to the brain than stress. Stress atrophies the entire brain, meaning it literally shrinks the brain.[1] It promotes brain inflammation and upsets brain function. Stress also degrades the blood-brain barrier, the precious lining that protects the brain from infectious agents, whether they come from the outside world or within our own bodies.[2]

Today the word stress conjures images of running late while sitting in rush-hour traffic, rushing the kids from one activity to the next, and then scrambling to get dinner made, working two jobs, juggling a full college course load with a full-time job (and maybe raising children at the same time), or enduring a stressful work environment with an awful boss. Or sometimes stress comes in the way of bad surprises, such as a job loss, a car accident, the death of a loved one, or the unexpected news that your spouse is leaving you.

While these are all significant stressors, the most common form of stress for most Americans is the kind people aren't even aware of, despite the slow but devastating toll it takes on their brains. This is the stress from chronically poor diets and marginal health. Just because you can walk upright, talk, and maintain a job does not mean you are healthy. In fact, when I'm at an airport, a place where I spend much of my life, I people-watch and see how many Americans suffer from degenerative health conditions that slowly eat away at brain health. This can include obesity, poorly managed thyroid conditions, or chronic joint inflammation, just to name a few. Frankly, given the condition of the average American, I can state confidently that the American brain is in crisis.

The most common way people damage their brains in this country is through blood sugar imbalances due to high-carbohydrate diets. A common American breakfast is oatmeal, cereal, or pancakes, all high-carbohydrate starts to the day that will send blood sugar and insulin levels skyrocketing. Typical lunches include plenty of bread, pasta, or rice, triggering another major spike in blood sugar. Dinner is not only equally as starchy, but also usually followed by dessert. Daytime snacks include sweetened coffee drinks and sweets.

For a species that has spent the majority of its evolutionary cycle eating what it could hunt or forage, the modern high-carbohydrate diet produces a series of shocks to the body day in and day out. The human body was designed to lower blood sugar on only an occasional basis, not on an hourly basis. Eventually the stress of these chronic shocks manifest as hypoglycemia, insulin resistance, or diabetes—all of which take their toll on the brain.

Although I talked about blood sugar in more detail in Chapter Five, it's important to know these blood sugar imbalances impede brain function by taxing the body's stress-handling hormones, which in turn taxes brain function. They also lead to obesity. Excess fat is pro-inflammatory and a chronic stressor for the body and brain.[3]

Other common forms of physiological stress that contribute to brain degeneration include smoking, food intolerances and food allergies, anemia, bacterial gut infections, gut parasites, autoimmune diseases, joint pain and inflammation, poor digestion, and many more. Any time your body must struggle to compensate for imbalances and poor function, it creates a physiological stress response. If these metabolic issues go on unattended long enough, the brain becomes the ultimate victim.

Granted, none of us is in perfect health. Such perfection is likely not possible as the body is constantly adjusting to shifting variables from the environment. However, our culture's paradigm is based on ignoring health until disease develops, and then treating merely the symptoms of a disease after it does develop. Enslaved by the addictive and immediate gratification of modern foods hawked by subversive and powerful marketing, Americans are eating themselves into ever-worsening brain function and an ever-increasing risk for Alzheimer's disease, dementia, and other neurological disorders.

STRESS HORMONES AND BRAIN FUNCTION

In order to generate the energy to adapt to stress, the body's two adrenal glands, which sit atop the kidneys, produce stress hormones. The primary stress hormone is cortisol. Studies show that high cortisol in response to high stress is very detrimental to the brain, especially the hippocampus—the seat of learning and memory that is the first to be affected by Alzheimer's disease and dementia.[4][5]

The hippocampus is rich with receptor sites for cortisol, as it depends on cortisol to regulate many systems in the body. For instance, the hippocampus is what regulates our sleep-wake cycle, or circadian rhythm. A healthy circadian rhythm produces highest cortisol in the morning that gradually tapers off during the day until it is lowest at night. This has us feeling alert and refreshed in the morning and sleepy and ready to turn in at night.

However, chronic stress continually pumps out high levels of cortisol, which over-activates the hippocampus and can cause it to falter at its functions. An out-of-whack circadian rhythm is the common fallout of poor hippocampus function. Gradually the stressed-out person suffers from insomnia, energy crashes during the day, being a "night owl," not being able to stay asleep, and other sleep disturbances.

Although sleep disorders can have myriad causes, the effect of chronic stress and high cortisol on the hippocampus is perhaps the most common. In fact, recent studies point to a disrupted circadian rhythm as an early indicator of increased risk for Alzheimer's disease.[6] How many people do you know who struggle with insomnia or have a hard time getting going in the morning? Studies show 30 percent of people experience insomnia and that the 50 most-prescribed drugs include several sleep-enhancing medications.[7] These are signs the integrity of the hippocampus is at risk.

The hippocampus is also the area of the brain that converts short-term memory to long-term memory so we can learn and remember. Chronic over activation from high cortisol affects the ability to learn and remember.

When it comes to statistics for the final stages of memory loss, they are sobering and getting worse. According to the Alzheimer's Research and Prevention Foundation, one out of every eight people age 65 and older has Alzheimer's disease, and for those over the age of 85, this number jumps to almost one out of every two. What's worse, numbers are expected to skyrocket higher as the Baby Boomer generation ages en masse.[8]

When patients complain to me that they have trouble sleeping or are not remembering things as well as they used to, I realize these are common complaints today. But I also realize they are symptoms of a brain that is degenerating too fast and a warning bell for Alzheimer's disease risk that must be heeded immediately.

• •

Mark Flannery, a student of Dr. Kharrazian, teaches his material to other health care practitioners and incorporates the principles into his own clinical nutrition practice in Woodland Hills, California. However, the more he learned the more quickly he realized he needed to be a patient himself. By 10 a.m. on workday mornings he was already succumbing to mental fatigue and was wiped out by the end of day, barely able to muster the energy to give his family attention when he got home. He struggled with headaches, brain fog, and learning new information—a vital skill for practitioners who follow Dr. Kharrazian's work.

Multiple concussions, an emotionally traumatic event, and a gluten intolerance all played a part in Mark's declining brain health at such a young age. "In my teens and 20s I sustained a number of concussions playing football, skiing, snowboarding, and even whacking my head on the top of my car while getting in," he says. "I always seemed to recover just fine."

But then Mark had a significant falling out with his father with whom he ran a family business before getting into health care. This made him chronically miserable and he felt nearly paralyzed by stress. He drank more and, because this was back before he discovered a healthier lifestyle, ate at McDonald's two to three times a day. "I thought ordering McDonald's fish sandwich was being healthier. I just didn't have the ability to get to a grocery store and cook something good for myself."

Eventually, Mark got out of the family business and into massage school, and then chiropractic school. Although this new direction got him healthier, he still struggled with a "tightness" he felt in his head, a struggle to learn and retain the new information, and chronic muscle twitches throughout his body. It wasn't until Dr. Kharrazian delved into Mark's neurology that his life turned around.

"Dr. Kharrazian literally grabbed me at a seminar and told me I had to address the brain inflammation," says Mark. "Right away I started taking nutritional compounds to tame brain inflammation, help with brain activity, and increase blood flow to the brain. All of the symptoms I had been struggling with for years stopped completely within a few days. I had gone gluten-free and was doing all the right things with my diet and lifestyle, but I needed this added step of addressing the inflammation for the improvement I needed."

Mark's boost in brain health has allowed him to take on more patients, and he's now able to work a full day easily and still have plenty of energy at the end of the day for his family. More importantly, he knows intimately what so many of patients struggle with, even though they've been told by their doctors that nothing is wrong with them.

"Doctors tell these people nothing is wrong with them, their tests are normal, and they should see a psychiatrist," says Mark. "I had a patient the other day who started crying when I was able to point out through lab tests what had been causing her brain issues for so many years. People are so thankful to know there is something wrong when they've been feeling so crappy for so many years, and they're not making it up. It always helps to empathize with someone in a health crisis when you've been in one yourself."

Mark Flannery, DC, MS, BS, FAAIM, DCBCN, DCCN, CNS
Woodland Hills, California
www.DrFlannery.com

• •

STRESS AND THE BRAIN'S CONTROL OF BODILY FUNCTION

Stress also impacts the brain's command over the autonomic nervous system, that part of our nervous system that regulates breathing, digestion, heartbeat, organ function, and more—basically all the bodily functions that happen without your conscious input. When autonomic function falters, conditions such as dry eyes, incontinence, and high blood pressure can arise. I have already introduced this mechanism somewhat in previous chapters. I will go into more detail here as to how stress can affect autonomic function.

In its communication with the body, the brain constantly receives and sends information. Ninety percent of the information the brain sends goes through an area in the lower two-thirds of the brainstem called the "pontomedullary reticular formation" (PMRF). Reticular is a Latin word that means network, and the PMRF is basically a net of neurons in the brainstem. When the brain's output travels through the PMRF on its way to deliver communication to the body, the PMRF stimulates the parasympathetic system.

The parasympathetic system, also known as the "rest and digest" system, oversees digestion, enzyme production, mucus secretion, and other related bodily activities. Good brain output from a healthy brain means good stimulation of the PMRF, which means adequate stimulation of the parasympathetic system. As a result, one experiences good digestion, good enzyme production, eyes and mouth that stay moist, good bladder and bowel control, and so on.

Not only does the PMRF stimulate the parasympathetic system, but it also dampens the body's sympathetic, or fight or flight, system. An area of the spinal cord called the intermediolateral cell column (IML) stimulates the sympathetic system. The sympathetic system is what allows us to react to stress by increasing the heart rate, dilating the pupils, and sending blood away from the organs and to the extremities in preparation for fight or flight. The sympathetic system is useful to help us flee from a charging bison or react quickly to avoid a car accident; however, we don't want it engaged all day because it is stressful.

In optimal brain function, the PMRF not only stimulates a parasympathetic response (i.e., good digestion) but also dampens the IML so as to inhibit sympathetic activity (i.e. lowers stress). The result is an individual who generally moves through life in a calm, relaxed manner, enjoys good digestion and other body functions, and does not suffer from a hair-trigger stress response.

As you may have guessed by now, traffic, hectic schedules, domineering bosses, bad marriages, high-carbohydrate diets, food intolerances, and so on keep the sympathetic system engaged too often. In short, American life is filled with tiny, stress-provoking bison charging at us all day long.

Many Americans live in a state of chronic sympathetic activity, always ready to fight or flee. This sets a person up for a downward spiral of brain function, which in turn generates ever higher levels of stress.

As the brain degenerates, overall firing in the brain decreases. This means output into the PMRF decreases. Hence the PMRF's stimulation of the parasympathetic system lags, along with its ability to dampen sympathetic stress from the IML. As a result, the rest-and-digest functions of the body continue to lose power while stress powers up. You see this in people who struggle with dry eyes, dry mouth, chronic digestive issues, incontinence, and other related symptoms.

Meanwhile, the untethered IML allows the sympathetic system to increasingly spin out of control, keeping the individual in a state of heightened stress. The result may be high blood pressure, anxiety, irritability, and a general state of being stressed out. It's a self-perpetuating cycle that harms brain health and one's quality of life.

THE EFFECT OF STRESS ON THE MIDBRAIN

Another area affected by stress is the midbrain reticular formation, also called the mesolimbic system, which is located at the top of the brainstem. This is an area of the brain concerned with survival, mating, and primitive emotions such as anger and love. One of the jobs of the midbrain reticular formation is to stimulate a sympathetic response through the IML.

In the previous section I explained how a degenerating brain lowers input into the PMRF, thus lowering parasympathetic activity and failing to dampen sympathetic activity. Unfortunately, that's not all. Brain degeneration further contributes to stress by *exciting* the midbrain reticular formation, which in turn activates sympathetic stress. So not only does brain degeneration fail to dampen sympathetic stress, it also

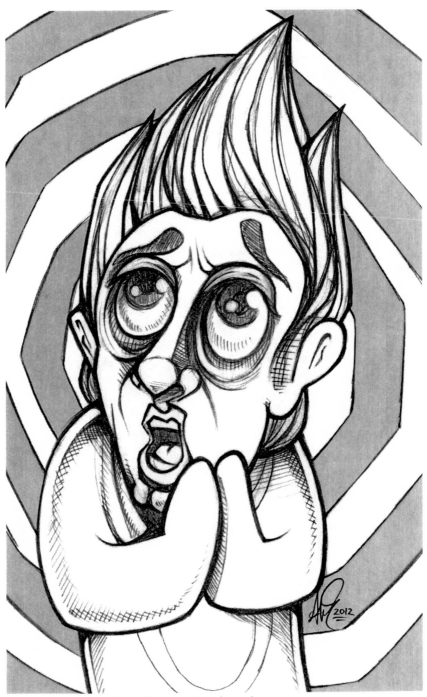

Inflammation from factors such as heated arguments, over exercising, or lack of sleep can activate the midbrain and increase stress.

creates more stress by activating the midbrain. In other words, chronic stress creates more stress. As you can see it's a vicious cycle, and this is why it's so important to avoid this loop in the first place.

One thing that has been shown to activate the stress-provoking midbrain reticular formation is inflammation. Studies show the midbrain is rich with receptors for a cytokine, or immune messenger, called interleukin-6 (IL-6).[9] IL-6 spikes in response to emotional, chemical, or physical stress, saturating IL-6 receptors in the midbrain. This in turn stimulates the IML, generating a sympathetic response. For instance, just getting into a heated argument with your spouse will raise IL-6 levels and hence the sympathetic stress response. The spike in IL-6 just from an angry argument can last up to several days.[10] Over-exercising can also spike IL-6, as can inflammation or lack of sleep.[11] [12] [13]

• •

Randy is a college student who was the victim of an assault that left him with multiple head injuries and profoundly impaired cognitive function. He had tried to continue with school but had to leave mid-semester because he couldn't function cognitively. Because his brain was so fatigued, he slept most of the time. His movements were uncoordinated as his brain's image of his body was inaccurate, and he had difficulty carrying on a conversation.

An assessment of Randy's cognitive functions revealed evidence of neurodegeneration and diminished memory related to poor acetylcholine activity. Direct trauma to the brain like the one Randy sustained can create an inflammatory response. As with any inflammatory response in the body, this inflammation should resolve itself. In Randy's case, however, it did not. Instead, the inflammation continued on, interfering with normal brain function and preventing brain cells from making energy. As a result, his movement and speech coordination were poor, and simple mental functions like reading and conversing left Randy exhausted.

I gave Randy nutritional compounds to improve blood flow to his brain, reduce brain inflammation, and improve the metabolic integrity of his brain cells. I also gave him nutritional compounds to support the brain's ability to make acetylcholine, the neurotransmitter involved in short-term memory.

I also asked Randy to change his diet to balance his blood sugar and eliminate gluten and fried foods, and I gave him a program of neurological rehabilitation tailored to the specific features of his brain function.

Within two months Randy was completely transformed. He was cognitively intact, able to carry on normal activities, and asking me for a letter to send to his college so he could return to his life as a student.

Samuel F. Yanuck, DC, FACFN, FIAMA

Chapel Hill, North Carolina

www.yanuckcenter.com

● ●

If the midbrain reticular formation gets bombarded with IL-6 too frequently, it develops negative plasticity for stress.[14] In other words, when stress repeatedly activates the midbrain reticular formation, the midbrain becomes increasingly efficient at responding to stress, so that it takes less stress over time to create the same response. Obviously, this is not a good thing as it means you'll get stressed out more easily over smaller stuff. Eventually it becomes permanently active and easily generates a stress response with very little stimulus.

We see this with post-traumatic stress disorder (PTSD). The midbrain gets flooded with IL-6 during a long period of extreme stress responses, such as war, making it increasingly sensitive to stimuli.[15] Eventually something as benign as a loud sound, a flash of bright light, or a strong emotion can trigger an inappropriately huge stress response. In the case of childhood abuse or molestation, symptoms of this mechanism may not manifest until the person is in their 40s or 50s. At this point, the brain may begin to degenerate, lowering the input into the PMRF. As a result, rest-and-digest functions falter and stress levels rise as the PMRF is no longer able to dampen the sympathetic response.

WHEN THE BRAIN BECOMES TOO GOOD AT STRESS

What do you do when the midbrain has developed plasticity for an extreme stress response that can be triggered by a relatively minor stimulus? From a nutritional perspective, the key is to go after brain inflammation. When this vicious cycle of stress overcomes the brain,

brain inflammation is the outcome. Dampening the inflammation is one way to start unwinding the self-perpetuating stress cycle.

As I explained earlier, as the brain becomes increasingly sensitive to stress, the overactive IML creates a chronic sympathetic stress response. Unfortunately, this response not only makes a person more stressed out, but it also promotes systemic inflammation. This mechanism is called neurogenic inflammation.[16] [17] Systemic inflammation then promotes brain inflammation, which in turn promotes more systemic inflammation. This essentially means the brain becomes chronically inflamed, just as a knee, a knuckle, or a shoulder can become chronically inflamed.

As the brain becomes more plastic for stress—or more efficient at responding to stress, as with PTSD for instance—this fosters chronic inflammation. This is important because chronic inflammation in the brain not only can impair neurological function, but also contributes to inflammation in the body, such as in the joints or the gut. This is most commonly seen with chronic abdominal inflammation, which actually can have its roots in brain inflammation.

• •

Theresa, 33, was on top of the world. An award-winning producer and writer for CNN in Washington, DC, her career was flourishing and her dreams were coming true. But all of that changed on the morning of September 11, 2001. She was working in a building across from the Pentagon when she heard the plane crash into it. She was sent to cover that story and then later New York City's Ground Zero. Immersing herself in these tragedies consumed her with stress and powerful emotions.

As her stress levels continued to rise her brain function began to decline. Things that used to be easy became a struggle. She began to suffer from a large number of symptoms, including brain fog, memory loss, headaches, insomnia, anxiety, uncontrollable sweating, weight gain, cold hands and feet, fatigue, dizziness, depression, and digestive complaints. She was in and out of doctor's offices searching for a common link to all her symptoms, but came away with nothing but a diagnosis of post-traumatic stress disorder (PTSD).

She struggled like this for 10 years before coming to my office. During the previous two years her health declined so rapidly that life had become almost unbearable. However, Theresa was determined to get her life back. Nothing was going to stop her from beating these devastating health issues.

We began by addressing her neurological, hormone, and immune imbalances with an anti-inflammatory diet and a program to address gastrointestinal inflammation and leaky gut. It was paramount we manage her digestive challenges to have any luck managing her PTSD, depression, anxiety, fatigue, and insomnia. I gave her powerful flavonoids to dampen brain fog, and her mental clarity quickly returned. As we improved her gut and brain health her entire outlook on life began to improve as well, and she felt a glimmer of hope for the first time in a decade.

We also used nutritional compounds to address her cortisol levels and circadian rhythm—PTSD can devastate adrenal function. Her memory returned, the anxiety and insomnia began to melt away, and her ability to handle the business of life wasn't the crushing challenge it had once been. I also used functional neurology rehabilitation to address the weaknesses within her nervous system.

By addressing the underlying causes of her symptoms, Theresa reported her former symptoms had become a distant memory and that her outlook on life turned from negative and dispirited to positive and hopeful.

Lucas Gafken, DC
Indianapolis, Indiana
chironeuroindy.com

● ●

RECOGNIZING BRAIN INFLAMMATION

How do you recognize whether you're a victim of neurogenic inflammation or brain-based inflammation? Simple. As the brain fatigues, an inflammatory response follows.

For instance, take the doting grandparents who decide to drive five hours to visit their son and grandchildren. Typically, they drive no more than 15 to 20 minutes a day doing errands around town. After driving for one hour, the grandfather notices he is feeling very tired all of a sudden, but decides to push on. Remember, his fatigue is brain fatigue, not fatigue from exercise. Once they arrive, he is exhausted from the five-hour drive, his joints are achy and inflamed for the rest of his stay, or his gut is inflamed and suddenly he can't digest anything. He also spends most of his trip resting to recover from the drive. Basically, his degenerated brain received more stimulation than it could handle and it fatigued as a result. When the brain fatigues, it can't fire sufficiently into the PMRF, parasympathetic activity and autonomic function suffer, and the sympathetic stress response goes up.

WHY THE ADRENAL GLANDS ARE THE WRONG TARGET

You don't have to be a grandfather; plenty of younger people suffer problems when they push their fatigued, inflamed brains too far, whether it's by getting too little sleep, working more hours than they can handle, or driving too long.

When this level of stress becomes a problem for people, the first instinct of both the lay public and the majority of natural medicine practitioners is to target the adrenal glands for support (truthfully, the first instinct for most Americans and doctors is a prescription drug—drugs for stress and anxiety sit at the top of the 50 most-prescribed drugs in the United States). Adrenal glandulars, minerals, B vitamins, and a variety of herbs are all attempts to restore the adrenal glands.

There are times when this is a valid approach; however, it's the stress pathways in the brain and brain inflammation that are the true problem. The adrenal glands are simply cortisol factories, churning out adrenal hormones in response to orders from the brain. Chronic stress causes them to overproduce cortisol, bombarding the brain and body with stress hormones. They may become exhausted from overuse and fail to make enough cortisol. Then the body cannot muster the energy to respond to even mild stressors, such as a common virus or a bad day at the office, and fatigue sets in. Although the adrenal glands may indeed need support, the best thing to do is support brain function and slow down brain degeneration. This, in turn, will relieve the brain's over activation of the adrenal glands.

One of the first things to look at when addressing brain-based inflammation is how to improve brain endurance. Are you getting enough of the right nutrients for healthy brain function, such as omega 3s or methyl B-12? Is poor neurotransmitter activity a problem, such as low serotonin or GABA? Maybe your brain just needs more overall stimulation, such as less time in front of the television and more time outdoors walking, engaging in social activities, or working on intellectually stimulating projects. Do you have anemia or blood sugar imbalances?

One thing people dealing with major or unrelenting stress can do to calm down the influence of stress on the brain is to use phosphatidylserine. You can take it orally, but I prefer liposomal methods of phosphatidylserine delivered through the skin. Phosphatidylserine dampens the effects of IL-6 on the midbrain reticular formation.

Herbal adrenal adaptogens are also powerful support when chronic stress is a problem. Although I have the word adrenal in there, these herbs do not work on the adrenal glands, but instead on the stress pathways in the brain, particularly in the hippocampus. Panax ginseng extract, ashwagandha, Holy basil extract, Rhodiola rosea, and eleuthero extract are all powerful botanicals that impact brain chemistry and stress responses in a positive way.[18][19][20][21][22] You can use them individually, but they have a greater synergistic effect when used in combination.

Herbs and nutritional compounds that act directly on brain inflammation can offer profound support. Supporting brain inflammation should be considered especially if you have symptoms of brain fog or have systemic inflammation. If your entire body is inflamed, you will probably have aches and pains everywhere, and there is a good chance your brain is also inflamed. In Chapter Ten, I will discuss detailed strategies to dampen brain inflammation.

Chronic stress responses can cause constriction of blood vessels and lead to poor circulation of blood to the brain. Oxygenation to the brain, which can become compromised when chronic stress impairs the parasympathetic response and autonomic function, may also need to be boosted to tame the inflammation response. I will talk more about this in the next chapter on brain blood flow and circulation.

Strategies to reduce the stress response, dampen brain inflammation, and support blood flow to the brain, in conjunction with supporting brain health and brain activity, have the potential to halt the nosedive into escalating brain degeneration and restore healthy function. For those who knowingly lead very stressful lives but are not in a position to change things, taking these nutritional compounds can help buffer the effects of a stressful schedule, and thus help prevent brain inflammation and fatigue. Unfortunately, however, these compounds cannot make up for a poor diet, blood sugar imbalances, and food intolerances. A good diet is critical. They also cannot make up for a lifestyle or career that is creating excessive mental and emotional stress. Stress-inducing lifestyles need to be modified for best results.

• •

Anya presented with non-responding insomnia coupled with significant autoimmune reactions and a history of head injury. After evaluation, I discovered she was also experiencing bouts of memory loss and a disruption in her body's ability to properly respond to stressors. As these stressors increased inflammation, her insomnia worsened and her mental function plummeted.

After supporting her body's stress cycle and modulating the inflammatory cascades from her autoimmune reactions, Anya found she no longer stayed awake all night, and she began to get the healing benefits of sleep. She awoke with energy and no longer needed naps to function.

As her mental clarity returned, she took on a new more demanding and more gratifying job. Also, due to the improvements in her inflammatory status, Anya was able to work with her rheumatologist on reducing both the pain and the anti-inflammatory medications she took to control it.

Today she is nearly pain free and able to enjoy a life she once thought had passed her by years ago.

David Arthur, DC, FACFN, DACNB, BCIM, DCCN
Denver, Colorado
www.DrDavidArthur.com

• •

CHAPTER SUMMARY

• Nothing is more damaging to the brain than stress.

• The most common stressor for most Americans is a sugary, high-carb diet.

• Other common stressors that contribute to brain degeneration include smoking, food intolerances and food allergies, anemia, bacterial gut infections, gut parasites, autoimmune diseases, joint pain and inflammation, poor digestion, and many more. Any time your body must struggle to compensate for imbalances and poor function, it creates a physiological stress response. If these metabolic issues go on unattended long enough, the brain becomes the ultimate victim.

• Stress also impacts the brain's command over the autonomic nervous system, that part of our nervous system that regulates all the bodily functions that happen without conscious input.

• A healthy brain sends 90 percent of communication output through an area of the brainstem called the pontomedullary reticular formation (PMRF). This output stimulates the parasympathetic system, also known as the rest-and-digest system, which oversees autonomic function. It also dampens the body's sympathetic, or fight-or-flight, system. When brain function suffers or the brain degenerates, output through the PMRF decreases, inhibiting parasympathetic activity and failing to dampen sympathetic activity.

• Chronic stress decreases firing into the PMRF.

• The midbrain is rich in receptors for IL-6, an inflammatory immune messenger. Chronic stress and inflammation bombard these receptors and plasticize the brain for stress. In other words, chronic stress and inflammation make the brain highly efficient at responding to stress. This is one mechanism behind PTSD.

• To reduce the stress response in the midbrain strategies include reducing inflammation in the body and the brain and addressing adrenal pathways in the brain. Several nutritional compounds are useful tools.

CHAPTER SEVEN

BRAIN CIRCULATION AND OXYGEN

SYMPTOMS OF POOR CIRCULATION AND BLOOD FLOW TO THE BRAIN

- Low brain endurance and poor focus and concentration
- Must exercise or drink coffee to improve brain function
- Cold hands and feet
- Poor nail health or fungal growth on toes
- Must wear socks at night
- White nail beds instead of bright pink
- Cold tip of nose

• •

Samantha came into my office complaining of severe headaches, fatigue, depression, and insomnia and carrying a bag full of supplements. She had seen numerous health care practitioners over the past couple of years and had tried virtually every nutritional and herbal supplement that was suggested to her. When I met Samantha I noticed the yellowish smoker's tint to her teeth and the smell of tobacco on her clothes and hair. Her lips and toes were blue; her fingernails, complexion, and hair looked unhealthy; and her hands and feet were very cold to the touch. These were all symptoms of poor circulation due to smoking. She admitted she had been smoking a pack of cigarettes a day for the past three years. She began smoking to curb her appetite and keep her weight under control. Unfortunately, this left her in a constant state of low blood sugar during the day and compromised lung function.

I made it very clear to Samantha that she needed to significantly cut down on her smoking and begin eating small meals of vegetables and proteins frequently during the day to stabilize her blood glucose. Otherwise there was no point for me to work with her as her smoking and low blood sugar were causing her symptoms and were deal breakers to success. She agreed to cut down on her cigarette smoking and to stabilize her blood glucose levels. I supplemented her with natural compounds that have been shown to increase circulation and blood flow to the brain. She quickly experienced complete resolution of her headaches, fatigue, depression and insomnia and no further care was required.

I share Samantha's case with you because it demonstrates the importance of addressing the root problem. Samantha had been given countless numbers of supplements for each of her symptoms to no avail because smoking and low blood sugar had decreased circulation to her brain. Without healthy blood circulation the brain cannot function. Remember, circulation carries blood and your blood carries nutrients, hormones, neurotransmitters, glucose, and oxygen necessary for proper brain function.

Datis Kharrazian, DHSc, DC, MS

• •

One of the most vital nutrients for the brain is oxygen. If your brain becomes deprived of oxygen for more than five minutes, you will suffer permanent brain damage. You would think as long as you're breathing you're brain is getting sufficient oxygen. However, while it may be getting enough oxygen to survive, it may not be getting enough to function at its peak. As a matter of fact, vascular dementia is the second most common form of dementia after Alzheimer's disease and is due to poor blood flow to the brain.[1] Healthy blood vessels and proper circulation are critical for a healthy brain. Don't forget that your blood is carrying everything your brain needs to function: nutrients, hormones, neurotransmitters, and, most importantly, oxygen.

Unfortunately, many factors common today can lead to poor circulation and starve the brain of oxygenation. The most common perhaps is stress. Stress not only causes shallow breathing, but also keeps the body in a state of fight or flight when most of the body's supply of blood, and hence oxygen, is shunted to the limbs, the heart, and the lungs. Other factors include anemia, smoking, low blood pressure, high blood pressure, poor lung function, poor cardiovascular function, and any mechanism that impairs blood vessels, such as diabetes.

Oxygen is one of the vital ingredients neurons use to make energy. When a neuron is starved of oxygen it can't make enough energy to function properly and survive.

In studies on brain degeneration, one of the criteria as to whether brain function is improving or diminishing is the rate at which the brain is getting blood or oxygen. Although the research recognizes how profoundly important oxygen is to brain function, it is, nevertheless, often overlooked by the average alternative or conventional health care practitioner.

CIRCULATION AND OXYGEN

Whenever overall circulation or blood flow in the body is reduced, the tissues farthest away from your heart are hardest hit. These are the hands, feet, and the brain. Unfortunately, as the most vertical tissue, our brain does not have gravity pulling blood downward as do our hands and feet. If you can't get blood flow to your brain, you can't get oxygen to your brain. If you're suffering from symptoms of poor brain function you need to evaluate whether you have any signs and symptoms of poor circulation. Typically, if your circulation is poor to your hands and feet you can bet it is also poor to your brain.

If you have chronic toenail fungal growth, you have a telltale sign of poor circulation. Fungal nail growth on your toes almost always takes place from poor blood flow to your toes. Your blood is carrying immune cells that would normally ward off fungal growth. We all have fungal growth from covering our feet and sweating in our shoes all day, but healthy circulation to our toes allows our immune cells to keep the fungal growth at bay. Although you can kill some of the fungus with anti-fungal baths or creams, it is likely to keep returning due to poor circulation. In my practice, as soon as I see a patient with poor brain function I always look for signs of poor circulation.

Weak nails or nails with multiple white spots are another indication of poor circulation. Your blood supplies vital nutrients to your nails

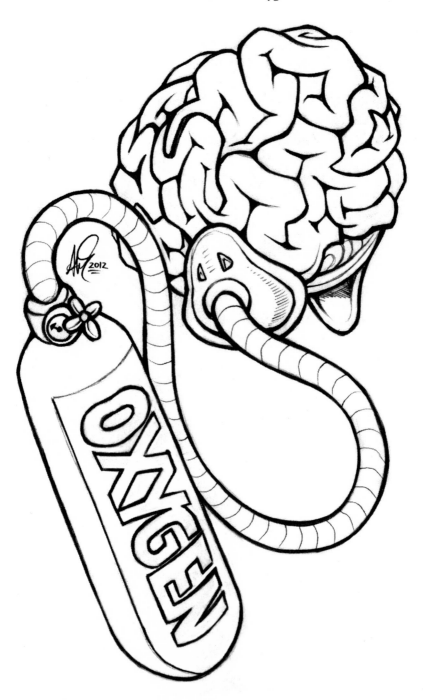

Factors such as anemia, hypothyroidism, smoking, low blood pressure, high blood pressure, and stress can restrict oxygen to the brain.

for healthy growth and repair. When your nails do not receive enough nutrients due to poor circulation, they cannot recover from the damages that occur from the normal trauma of banging your fingernails, which create white spots.

Another sign of poor circulation is poor capillary refill time: If you push on one of your fingernails, it should instantly return to its pink color once the pressure is taken off. In the case of poor circulation and blood flow, that pink color returns very slowly or—with even worse circulation—the fingernails were never pink to begin with.

Another way that I check for healthy circulation is by simply touching and comparing the temperature of my patient's fingertips and toes to their wrists and ankles. If they have poor circulation I would expect them to have colder fingertips than wrists, and colder toes than ankles. These patients usually need to wear socks all the time to keep their feet warm. They also tend to have cramping in their hands and feet from not being able to get oxygen and nutrients to those tissues.

At the end of this chapter I will review some strategies to help increase your circulation and get ideal blood flow to your tissues and your brain. There is no point in taking nutrients to support your brain if they cannot get to your brain due to poor circulation. The two most immediate and important functions to evaluate when brain function is poor are blood glucose imbalances and mechanisms that impair blood flow to the brain.

If you do not have ideal fuel or oxygen for your brain, your brain will not function well, and it will quickly degenerate.

BLOOD PRESSURE AND CIRCULATION

Both low and high blood pressure can impact the amount of oxygen delivered to your brain. If you have symptoms of poor brain circulation it is very important for you to check your blood pressure. Your blood pressure should be around 120/80. If the first or second number is higher or lower than 10 points, then your blood pressure is abnormal. The greater the amount of deviation from 120/80 the worse it is. Although most people focus on high blood pressure, low blood pressure is also an important concern and often overlooked.

LOW BLOOD PRESSURE

Let's first talk about low blood pressure, since it is completely neglected in the health care system. You need adequate pressure in your blood for healthy perfusion, or the ability of blood to be pushed into your tissues. If your blood pressure is low, let's say 90/65, there is not enough pressure for your blood, which carries oxygen and other vital nutrients, to be pushed into tissues such as your brain. You may not have increased risk for a stroke with low blood pressure, put you will have less than ideal brain function. Your brain is the most vertical part of your body, and you have lots of tiny blood vessels in your brain whose job it is to deliver blood to every neuron for ideal brain function. If your blood pressure is low the blood cannot get to these neurons very well. This reduces brain function and increases your risk for neurodegeneration.

If you have low blood pressure you need to get it up as close as you can to 120/80, as low blood pressure is not healthy. Don't confuse low blood pressure with low resting heart rate. Low resting heart rate is a good sign of health and not the same as low blood pressure. If your blood pressure is low you need to immediately start salting your food and even consume pinches of sea salt during the day to increase your blood pressure (people with Hashimoto's should avoid iodized salt for this purpose).

For patients with low blood pressure I also recommend an extract from licorice root called glycyrrhiza. This natural compound increases the hormone aldosterone, which helps you retain your sodium and can help raise low blood pressure. I personally prefer using a liposomal cream version with my patients, but you can use an oral licorice root extract. You will need to purchase a good automated blood pressure cuff and measure your blood pressure throughout the day and experiment with dosages. For most people, as soon as their blood pressure returns to normal levels they experience a dramatic increase in overall energy and brain function.

Many people can raise their blood pressure to normal by simply salting their food and supplementing with licorice root because their adrenal glands are not significantly impaired. Their bodies can make the necessary hormones, such as aldosterone, epinephrine, and norepinephrine. However, those with poor adrenal function may not be able to raise their blood pressure very well until their adrenal glands function better. Remember, the adrenal glands produce the necessary hormones to help raise and normalize your blood pressure if it is low.

The most common cause of functionally low blood pressure is a hypoglycemia lifestyle or depletion of the adrenal glands due to chronic stress, autoimmunity, or chronic infections. Chapter Five has suggestions regarding adrenal and blood glucose control if you have low blood sugar. The long-term hypoglycemia lifestyle of missing meals and having simple carbohydrates for meals depletes the adrenal glands. As a result they cannot produce sufficient hormones such as aldosterone to maintain healthy blood pressure and tissue perfusion.

HIGH BLOOD PRESSURE

High blood pressure is also a concern for vascular health of the brain. The increased risk of stroke from high blood pressure is directly related to how high your blood pressure is. The higher your blood pressure climbs above 120/80, the greater your risk for stroke. Additionally, high blood pressure narrows and damages your arteries, decreasing blood flow to your brain. The increased pressure can also break off a fatty deposit that then lodges into a tiny blood vessel in you brain, causing a clot called an "embolic stroke." Or the increased pressure can actually rupture the small artery in your brain, called a "hemorrhagic stroke." If you have a stroke, life as you know it will never be the same. You will almost always lose function that you will never get back, or you may die from the stroke.

If you have elevated blood pressure you must cut salt from your diet, exercise routinely, and reduce your stress. You can also take natural compounds such as magnesium and potassium to help bring your blood pressure down. Later in this chapter I also will discuss some strategies to increase circulation by modulating an enzyme called "nitric oxide synthase." These strategies may help you not only reduce your blood pressure, but also protect your blood vessels and improve your overall circulation. These mechanisms are all important to reduce your risk for stroke and improve blood flow to your brain.

In summary, if your brain isn't working well, you really need to look at your blood pressure. Both high and low blood pressure can impact blood flow to your brain. Low blood pressure leads to poor brain tissue perfusion in which your brain receives insufficient blood and oxygen.

High blood pressure can damage blood vessels and thicken arteries, reducing blood flow to the brain. Individuals with low blood pressure usually have the poorest blood flow to the brain, but the lowest risk for stroke. People with high blood pressure have a higher stroke risk, but generally it is long-term elevated blood pressure, which changes the structure of the arteries due to damage, that will restrict blood flow and oxygen to the brain. Either way, normalizing your blood pressure profoundly impacts the function and health of your brain.

ANEMIA

An obvious culprit in poor blood flow to the brain is anemia, a condition in which the red blood cells do not mature properly and become incapable of carrying and transporting oxygen to cells of your body. Anemia is a deal breaker for nutritional support of any kind since it literally starves the body and brain of oxygen. When cells are deprived of oxygen, basic functions that maintain, regenerate, and heal the body simply cannot operate adequately, if at all.

Anemia can be caused by a variety of factors. One common cause is pernicious anemia, an autoimmune disease in which the immune system attacks the intrinsic factor in the stomach, a substance necessary for the absorption of B-12. This form of anemia is often found in those with celiac disease, Hashimoto's disease, or other autoimmune diseases. B-12 anemia is due to low B-12, which is sometimes the case in vegetarian or vegan diets, or from poor absorption of B-12 from lack of stomach hydrochloric acid and digestive enzymes.

Other causes of anemia are iron deficiency, whether it's due to low iron in the diet or, more commonly, poor absorption of iron due to leaky gut or from excess blood loss. The breakdown of red blood cells can cause anemia, something I've seen in athletes who overtrain. Other possibilities include uterine fibroids, internal bleeding, chronic disease, liver disease, and genetic disorders.

If you have anemia you will typically be very tired all the time and suffer from depression and lack of motivation. You may notice you're pale and your heart rate may be increased. This is due to the body's attempts to compensate for the red blood cells inability to carry sufficient oxygen by pumping your blood faster. The only real way to know you have anemia is through blood test called a complete blood count (CBC).

The CBC can determine whether you have anemia and what type of anemia it is. If you have anemia, it is almost clinically impossible to improve your brain function until your red blood cells can carry oxygen efficiently to your brain.

STRESS AND OXYGENATION

In the previous chapter I explained how stress can become self-perpetuating in the brain. As the brain degenerates it loses the ability to stimulate the rest-and-digest parasympathetic system and dampen the sympathetic stress response. Stress also sensitizes the midbrain, which plasticizes the brain to become more efficient at stress so you get stressed out too easily. This in turn promotes brain degeneration, which further increases stress, and perpetuates the cycle of stress and degeneration.

Stress also inhibits the flow of oxygen to the brain. One of the fallouts of stress is that it decreases the supply of oxygen to all the organs, including the brain. When the body is in this fight-or-flight mode, blood and oxygen are shunted to areas of the body that will help it either run from the proverbial angry bison or stop and face it with quick reflexes and a good spear throw. When the body is frequently in some degree of sympathetic stress, the brain gets kicked toward the bottom of the to-do list for oxygen supply. As a result, brain inflammation sets in and can be very hard to calm down. The result is a spiral into worsening brain degeneration in what can become a vicious cycle.

NITRIC OXIDE AND YOUR BRAIN

Nitric oxide is a chemical-signaling molecule in the body involved with communication in the nervous, immune, and vascular systems. It was proclaimed the "Molecule of the Year" in 1992 by *Science* magazine because it is essential for normal function of the brain, arteries, and immune system, to name a few.[2] However, nitric oxide has both positive and negative influences on the brain, depending on the form of nitric oxide expressed.

Nitric oxide can be expressed in three different forms, also called enzymes or synthases:

- Inducible NOS (iNOS): pro-inflammatory and produces harmful free radical actions that promote brain degeneration
- Endothelial NOS (eNOS): dilates blood vessels, improves glucose uptake, and activates energy in the brain[3]
- Neuronal NOS (nNOS): used to optimize brain focus

To put it simply, nNOS and eNOS support ideal brain health, whereas iNOS promotes neurodegeneration. Ideal nitric oxide expression for healthy brain function would require greater eNOS and nNOS activity and suppressed iNOS activity.[4] In the next section I will discuss several natural compounds that can promote the beneficial forms of nitric oxide for better brain function and vascular health, and potentially reduce inflammatory mechanisms that have been linked to brain degeneration.

However, before I discuss those natural compounds, let's first talk about how lifestyle can impact the nitric oxide isomers. The single most important nitric oxide isomer for you to activate is eNOS, especially if you have poor circulation, abnormal blood pressure (high or low), or poor blood vessel health.

eNOS is found in the blood vessel walls and is activated by exercise to increase blood flow. eNOS then causes blood vessels to dilate, which improves circulation and literally dissolves built-up plaque on the arterial walls. Its effects last long after you exercise, which is why many people find their brain functions better after exercise. People who have cold hands and feet also notice their circulation improves for hours after exercise. The more eNOS you release in any given week, month, or lifetime, the better it is for your circulation, cardiovascular health, and brain health.

HOW TO RELEASE ENOS FOR BETTER BRAIN HEALTH

This means you must exercise if you have poor circulation. But not all types of exercise work the same in raising eNOS. You must really increase your heart rate to create the best environment for eNOS release. If you are trying to raise your eNOS levels you cannot be the person who casually walks on a treadmill at the gym while watching TV. You have to get your heart rate up, and I mean really up. The harder and longer you push yourself, the greater the eNOS response. But please do not exceed your limits, hurt yourself, or fatigue your adrenals by overtraining. Also, if you have any adverse symptoms with exertion, you must stop and make sure your heart is healthy enough to handle vigorous exercise.

If you are physically capable of pushing yourself to raise eNOS, then consider high-intensity exercises that really raise your heart rate, such as jump roping, jumping jacks, squat jumps, sprinting, rebounding (jumping on a trampoline), or any other type of high-intensity aerobic exercise. Just when you feel you can't go on, push yourself a little more. The type of exercise will vary depending on your physical fitness, weight, joint health, etc., but the key is to find a way to boost your heart rate safely. You may want to investigate some HIIT (high-intensity interval training) protocols to boost eNOS. Also known as sprint intervals, HIIT workouts alternate between intense bursts of activity and short periods of less-intense activity or complete rest.

For my patients with high or low blood pressure, poor circulation, or lack of brain oxygen, I recommend they do high-intensity exercise for five to 10 minutes after waking up in the morning to raise their heart rate as high as they can. This strategy has nothing to do with burning calories or losing weight. It is used instead to kickstart eNOS and blood flow to the brain. I also find taking compounds that directly stimulate eNOS before or after the exercise will produce much longer and greater impacts of eNOS from the quick workout. Let's talk about those compounds next.

Again, please exercise good judgment when doing exercise so as not to do more harm than good. Sprinting around the block or doing squat jumps may be perfectly appropriate for one person, while just increasing the walking pace may be enough for another.

NUTRITIONAL STRATEGIES FOR BRAIN CIRCULATION AND OXYGEN

For poor brain oxygenation I use a combination of botanical compounds: feverfew extract, butcher's broom extract, ginkgo biloba, huperzine, and vinpocetine. These compounds have been shown to dilate the cerebral arteries, support circulation in and blood flow to the brain, provide antioxidants that protect brain blood vessels, protect neurons when brain oxygen is low, and improve blood viscosity (how thick or thin blood is). Although they have been shown to dilate cerebral arteries, they do not increase blood pressure; in fact they can do the opposite.

They also work if you have low blood pressure. They may be helpful in preventing plaque build-up in the arteries and preventing the destruction of blood vessels that can potentially lead to stroke. Vinpocetine in particular has been shown to increase dilation of the cerebral arteries, improve blood viscosity, and protect the neurons in the brain with an antioxidant effect. Studies have shown its use after a head injury increases blood flow to the site of the injury to speed and enhance repair. I will summarize the most important compounds in order of importance.

Vinpocetine

Vinpocetine has been widely used for the support of vascular disorders in the brain. It improves blood flow in the cerebral vessels[5] and induces dilation of the cerebral artery.[6] It has been found to improve blood viscosity in vascular brain-related disorders.[7] A literature review of vinpocetine in the treatment of cerebrovascular disease concluded that vinpocetine has the ability to improve the blood flow and metabolism of affected areas of the brain and improves the quality of life in chronic cerebrovascular patients.[8]

Vinpocetine also is classified as a selective cyclic GMP phosphodiesterase (PDE) inhibitor, which means it modulates eNOS, the beneficial form of nitric oxide, and vascular tone.[9 10 11 12] By increasing eNOS activity, PDE inhibitors such as vinpocetine increase blood delivery to the hands, feet, and brain thanks to dilation of blood vessels.

In addition to activating eNOS, vinpocetine also influences the neurotransmitter acetylcholine, which will be discussed later in this book. Acetylcholine activity is critical not only for learning and memory, but also for ideal eNOS receptor site activity.[13 14 15]

Ginkgo biloba

Ginkgo biloba has been shown to promote blood flow, protect against restricted and low oxygen in the brain, affect energy metabolism in neurons, and enhance free-radical scavenger activity.[16] Although ginkgo biloba increases blood flow to the brain, it does not increase blood pressure. On the contrary, it appears to have an anti-hypertensive effect.[17] [18] It has also been demonstrated to protect against brain injury caused by hypoxia (lack of oxygen).[19] Not only has ginkgo biloba repeatedly shown its potential to increase blood flow to the brain, but also studies have confirmed its effect in enhancing brain activity.

ATP (Adenosine 5'-triphosphate)

ATP is the fuel source for all biochemical reactions. ATP can be found inside the cell (intracellular) or outside the cell (extracellular). Research has clearly demonstrated that supplementation with ATP increases extracellular and intracellular ATP.[20 21 22] Extracellular ATP has been found to activate the beneficial forms of nitric oxide, eNOS and nNOS.[23 24 25 26] More importantly, ATP does not activate iNOS, the pro-inflammatory form of nitric oxide, and has even demonstrated that it suppresses iNOS activity.[27 28 29] Together these effects are ideal for dampening inflammation, tissue destruction, and for balancing immune activity.

Huperzine A

Huperzine A is powerful compound for expressing the ideal forms of nitric oxide because it enhances acetylcholine activity necessary for eNOS and nNOS while inhibiting iNOS.[30 31 32] Not only does huperzine A inhibit iNOS, but it also suppresses the immune cytokines released during exercise that stimulate iNOS.[33 34 35 36]

Xanthinol niacinate

Xanthinol niacinate has very powerful vascular enhancing properties, improving blood flow to the hands, feet, and brain, and has demonstrated properties that increase eNOS.[37 38] A study on humans comparing the effects of a placebo and xanthinol niacinate found xanthinol niacinate significantly increased exercise tolerance (the capacity for enduring exercise) between one and nine hours after ingestion.[39] Clinical research has found xanthinol niacinate has antioxidant properties that may decrease iNOS activities. Several research studies have found it improves microcirculation and aids in healing.[40 41 42 43]

Alpha-Glycerylphosphorylcholine (Alpha GPC)

Alpha GPC is a compound isolated from lecithin. It is very well absorbed by the gastrointestinal tract and is used for the synthesis of acetylcholine. Alpha GPC has been shown to increase acetylcholine in the body,[44][45] which in turn promotes vascular dilation through eNOS and synaptic activity through nNOS.[46][47][48][49][50][51]

L-acetyl carnitine

L-acetyl carnitine is an amino acid compound that has a structure similar to acetylcholine. Research has shown that L-acetyl carnitine is effective in improving cognition and has the potential to delay the progression of Alzheimer's. Nitric oxide is activated by acetylcholine receptor activation.

Butcher's broom (Ruscus aculeatus)

Butcher's broom strengthens blood vessels, reduces capillary fragility, and helps maintain circulation.[52][53][54]

Feverfew

Feverfew has been used for decades as a safe and effective way to manage migraines[55][56][57][58][59][60] and has been shown to have many beneficial effects on the vascular system, including inhibition of inflammation of the brain's vascular system.[61]

USING COMPOUNDS TO SUPPORT BRAIN OXYGENATION

These herbs are so supportive and protective of the brain that I personally use them regularly. I find they are easier to take if compounded together into a liquid, especially before exercise or on an empty stomach. However, you do not have to use a liquid source.

Even people with great brain function and no signs of brain degeneration may notice an immediate improvement of focus and brain function taking these compounds, such as more alertness and less brain fatigue. Some people find them life changing. It's as if suddenly someone turned on the lights and colors become brighter and crisper, concentration and focus improves, brain fog lifts, or intellect sharpens. These are effects most people notice as blood flow to the brain increases. Many people also notice these types of changes after exercise since exercise increases blood flow to the brain.

For people who have suffered head injuries or strokes, these botanicals should be strongly considered (assuming there are no conflicts with medications). Athletes may find they improve athletic ability by enhancing focus and concentration—it's one approach I take with my patients who are professional athletes.

As with all nutritional compounds for the brain, dose depends on the degree of degeneration of the brain. You can start with minimum amounts and keep dosing up until you feel an effect. Then take some more to see whether you feel even more improvement. Adjust to your dose to the amount at which you last noticed a benefit.

CHAPTER SUMMARY

• One of the most vital nutrients for the brain is oxygen. If your brain becomes deprived of oxygen for more than five minutes, you will suffer permanent brain damage. You would think as long as you're breathing you're brain is getting sufficient oxygen. However, while it may be getting enough oxygen to survive, it may not be getting enough to function at its peak.

• Oxygen is one of the vital ingredients neurons use to make energy. When a neuron is starved of oxygen it can't make enough energy to function properly and survive.

• Many factors common today can lead to poor circulation and starve the brain of oxygenation. The most common perhaps is stress. Stress not only causes shallow breathing, but also keeps the body in a state of fight or flight when most of the body's supply of blood, and hence oxygen, is shunted to the limbs, the heart, and the lungs. Other factors include anemia, smoking, low blood pressure, high blood pressure, poor lung function, poor cardiovascular function, and any mechanism that impairs blood vessels, such as diabetes.

• Cold hands and feet, chronic nail fungus, poor capillary refill time, weak nails, and white spots on fingernails are symptoms of poor circulation that could be robbing your brain of oxygen.

• Low blood pressure causes poor blood flow to the brain. Low blood pressure is often a sign of adrenal fatigue, chronic stress, autoimmunity, or chronic infection. Using glycyrrhiza and adding salt to the diet are two strategies for raising low blood pressure, with a target of 120/80.

• High blood pressure narrows and damages your arteries, decreasing blood flow to your brain. The higher your blood pressure climbs above 120/80, the greater your risk for stroke. If you have high blood pressure you must cut salt from your diet, exercise routinely, and reduce your stress. You can also take natural compounds such as magnesium and potassium to help bring your blood pressure down.

• An obvious culprit in poor blood flow to the brain is anemia. There are many types of anemia, including iron-deficiency anemia, B-12 anemia, autoimmune pernicious anemia, or anemia caused by breakdown of red blood cells. A CBC can determine whether you have anemia and what type of anemia it is. It is almost clinically impossible to improve brain function until anemia is resolved.

• Stress inhibits the flow of oxygen to the brain. When the body is frequently in some degree of sympathetic stress, the brain gets kicked toward the bottom of the to-do list for oxygen supply. As a result, brain inflammation sets in and can be very hard to calm down. The result is a spiral into worsening brain degeneration in what can become a vicious cycle.

• Nitric oxide is a molecule essential for normal function of the brain, arteries, and immune system, to name a few.[2] However, nitric oxide has both positive and negative influences on the brain, depending on the form of nitric oxide expressed. Endothelial nitric oxide, or eNOS, is found in the blood vessel walls. Vigorous exercise activates eNOS, which improves circulation and dissolves built-up plaque on the arterial walls. Its effects last long after you exercise, which is why many people find their brain functions better after exercise. Certain nutritional compounds can also boost eNOS.

• For poor brain oxygenation I use a combination of botanical compounds: feverfew extract, butcher's broom extract, ginkgo biloba, huperzine, and vinpocetine. These compounds have been shown to dilate the cerebral arteries, support circulation in and blood flow to the brain, provide antioxidants that protect brain blood vessels, protect neurons when brain oxygen is low, and improve blood viscosity (how thick or thin blood is). Although they have been shown to dilate cerebral arteries, they do not increase blood pressure; in fact they can do the opposite.

Chapter Eight

GLUTEN SENSITIVITY AND BEYOND

GLUTEN SENSITIVITY SYMPTOMS

- Consuming grains makes you tired and makes it difficult to focus
- Consuming grains makes you bloated
- You feel better when you avoid breads and grains
- You have reactions to grain products

* *

Peggy, 12, suffered from chronic migraines, episodes of vomiting, gastric ulcers, joint pain, and bowel irregularities. It's not surprising she also did poorly in school. Her mother told me she had struggled with some type of health condition her entire life. She was a colicky baby, had chronic ear infections, developed asthma, and went through a period of having seizures that she outgrew. She had seen more doctors by the age of 12 than most adults have seen in their entire life, enduring countless blood tests, imaging studies, and medical evaluations by a multitude of specialists. She had also taken various medications over the years for her symptoms.

Peggy's mother read my thyroid book and incorporated some of the recommendations, which helped Peggy feel much better. This convinced Peggy's mother I was the only health care practitioner who could help her daughter, and they flew across the country for a consultation.

When I first saw Peggy it was obvious she was not growing appropriately. Although she was 12 she looked years younger. Peggy was sweet and behaved as if being in a doctor's office was normal. It's always sad to see a young child display so much experience visiting a doctor's office.

Peggy's mother had been diagnosed with hypothyroidism more than 20 years ago, but after she read my book she asked her doctor to test her for autoimmune Hashimoto's hypothyroidism. The test came back positive and she followed the many strategies in the thyroid book, including adopting a gluten-free diet. For the first time in years she felt energetic and was able to lose weight. Naturally, she was concerned her daughter might also have Hashimoto's or some other autoimmune disorder, and she asked me to look at Peggy's medical file.

Peggy's medical file was four inches thick and included numerous labs and medical tests. My initial concern was Peggy may have a gluten sensitivity or celiac disease. Her lab work showed she had been screened for celiac disease (an extreme form of dietary gluten sensitivity), and the results were negative. Peggy's mother put her daughter on a gluten-free diet for two weeks anyway, but it did not make a difference in her symptoms.

When I examined Peggy I found she had hyperreflexia, or overactive reflexes, in all of her limbs. When I tapped her knee, instead of her leg responding with a small kick her entire body jumped aggressively. She also had severe systemic hyperalgesia, or increased sensitivity to pain. When I stroked her skin anywhere on her body with a pinwheel she felt severe pain and withdrew. She also had severe sensitivity to high-pitched sound and to light. When I tested her eye reflexes with a pen light and her hearing with a tuning fork, she developed immediate head pain and nausea. These findings were not associated with a brain lesion or disease of the nervous system but rather with a metabolic or chemical imbalance that was impacting her brain and nervous system.

I ran a series of tests to evaluate her case, including a more comprehensive gluten sensitivity test, since many children of a parent with Hashimoto's are gluten intolerant. Gluten sensitivity is known to not only trigger autoimmunity, but also directly damage the nervous system. The tests her doctors ran were for classic celiac disease and were not thorough enough to rule out immune reactions to gluten. Additionally, going off gluten for two weeks is not enough for most people to see changes or improvements, especially if they have intestinal permeability or are still eating foods that cross react with gluten.

Peggy's results showed severe reactions to gluten, although not classic celiac disease. Instead, she had elevated antibodies to transglutaminase-6, which indicates an immune response from gluten against the nervous system. Classic celiac disease is associated with antibody elevations of transglutaminase-2, which indicates a reaction against the intestinal tract.

She also had reactions to milk and sesame, which are similar enough in their structure to gluten to create an immune response. Lastly, her labs also indicated intestinal permeability.

Based on her test results we started Peggy on a gluten-free, dairy-free, and sesame-free diet and a nutritional and lifestyle plan to address the intestinal permeability. Her response to the plan was completely life changing. She began to grow. The stomach aches, migraines, and joint pain disappeared. She began excelling in school for the first time.

When I talked to her mother during a follow-up consultation, she was crying and asked me why someone didn't diagnose her daughter properly years ago. I told her at least Peggy was properly diagnosed at age 12 and did not have to wait 30 years like her mother.

I share Peggy's story because she is one of many individuals with a gluten sensitivity who are overlooked by the health care system. Unfortunately, many doctors today are not trained to identify gluten sensitivity and are still stuck on outdated and limited models of celiac disease diagnosis. These models have been thoroughly debated in the scientific literature today and recent research has made it very clear the criteria for diagnosing celiac disease are very limited.

If your brain is not working or if you have a neurological disease, you must be properly tested for the entire spectrum of gluten sensitivity and not just for the limited markers for celiac disease. In this chapter I will teach you all of the key concepts.

Datis Kharrazian, DHSc, DC, MS

● ●

No food is a more powerful trigger of neurological issues and autoimmunity than gluten, the protein found in wheat. The average American eats wheat at every meal and we're seeing dramatic increases in gluten sensitivity today.

The term gluten comes from the Latin word for "glue" and it's the glue-like quality that gives wheat products an elastic, chewy texture. Gluten is found in wheat, spelt, barley, rye, kamut, triticale, and malts. Oats are often contaminated with gluten because they are grown in rotation with wheat or processed in the same facilities as wheat.

We define a gluten sensitivity as an exaggerated immune response to gluten that leads to inflammation throughout the body and potentially to an autoimmune reaction, in which the immune system attacks and destroys body or brain tissue.

Celiac disease is a severe reaction to gluten that causes autoimmune destruction of the gastrointestinal tract. I will distinguish between gluten sensitivity and celiac disease further, but they are both an abnormal immune response to gluten.

Gluten sensitivity and gluten-free diets have become very popular today. Many grocery stores have gluten-free sections, and they take up a large part of the aisle in health food stores. The numbers of gluten-free books, blogs, and online products has exploded. But is this really just a health fad, or the result of more awareness and diagnoses? Or are we seeing an actual increase in gluten sensitivity and celiac disease today? Although awareness has certainly grown, research shows the increase is *not* the result of increased detection clinically. Instead, the rates of gluten sensitivity have actually risen dramatically.[1]

A breakthrough study published in *Gastroenterology* in 2009 clearly identified a sharp rise in gluten sensitivity in the United States. Researchers compared blood samples collected between 1948 and 1954 of 9,000 healthy young adults to 13,000 gender-matched subjects in 2009. Their investigation found the prevalence of celiac disease increased dramatically during the past 50 years, from 1 in 700 to 1 in 100.[2] Also, this study only evaluated celiac disease and not the less severe but more common form of an immune reaction to gluten, gluten sensitivity. If researchers had looked for gluten sensitivity as well, I have no doubt the numbers would have been even more dramatic.

If you feel like your brain is not working, you must rule out a sensitivity to gluten. Also, the word gluten is technically a misnomer, as the word *gliadin* more specifically describes the portion of wheat that triggers an immune reaction. But since gluten is most commonly used, I will use both terms in this chapter.

* *

Unknowingly, I have been dealing with celiac disease for most of my life. I was finally diagnosed in 2000 after spending 18 years searching for answers to my medical symptoms. During those 18 years my symptoms steadily increased and worsened. Since my diagnosis, I have been on a gluten-free diet, and many of my symptoms have begun to disappear or have lessened in severity.

Twice in two years a restaurant accidentally served me food containing gluten. The first time I became very ill and contacted my medical doctor for assistance in clearing up the symptoms. I was referred to an endocrinologist because I seemed to be suffering from thyroid symptoms. After finally getting an appointment (which took three months), I received no assistance. I was told my blood test levels were not high enough for treatment and to come back in six months to be retested. I couldn't imagine waiting six more months feeling as ill as I did.

A friend mentioned Dr. Turnpaugh had helped her with her Hashimoto's hypothyroidism autoimmune disease. I couldn't comprehend that a chiropractor could help me, but I called Dr. Turnpaugh because conventional medicine had failed me. Dr. Turnpaugh ran all of the necessary blood work, and I was told I was close to adrenal failure. Taking the supplements he suggested, I have defeated the thyroid problem.

The second time I was exposed to gluten, I developed severe neurological symptoms. I was on vacation and called my medical doctor. As before, I was prescribed prednisone but had no improvement after three weeks. So I called Dr. Turnpaugh and within just two days of taking supplements for gluten exposure and neurological symptoms I felt much better.

Dr. Turnpaugh also introduced me to a lab that diagnoses other food sensitivities. We are now trying to reduce the inflammation that goes along with having celiac disease and intolerances to these other foods. From now on Dr. Turnpaugh will be the first person I call if have another gluten exposure or any neurological symptoms.

Laura W., patient of Dr. Turnpaugh
Chris Turnpaugh, DC, DABCN
Mechanicsburg, Pennsylvania
www.drchristurnpaugh.com

● ●

WHAT HAPPENED TO GLUTEN?

The gluten you eat today is not the same gluten you ate as a child, or your parents or grandparents ate. Although not technically genetically modified, gluten has nevertheless been significantly hybridized and deamidated over the years, processes that have rendered it inflammatory to humans.[3][4][5] Unlike genetic modification, which inserts or deletes genes, hybridization creates a new protein by combining different strains of wheat. This can alter a protein sequence by as much as 5 percent, making it quite different from the original source. Many people feel the hybridization of wheat has created a "new wheat," one that appears more prone to trigger immune reactions, especially in the brain and nervous system.

Deamidation, which is used extensively in the food processing industry, has also made gluten more immune reactive. Deamidation uses acids or enzymes to make gluten water soluble (it is normally only soluble in alcohol) so it mixes more easily with other foods.

Although deamidation makes wheat easier to use, it has also been shown to create a severe immune response in people. A double-blinded, placebo-controlled study found subjects did not react to native wheat flour but reacted severely to deamidated wheat. The researchers concluded deamidation of wheat generates new substances that activate the immune system.[6] Another study published in the *European Journal of Inflammation* concluded deamidated gluten is a new food compound and may be the major cause of hidden inflammatory responses to foods.[7]

The hybridization and deamidation of wheat appear to play a role not only in the sharp increases of gluten sensitivity and celiac disease, but also in inflammation, degeneration, and even autoimmunity of the brain and nervous system.

A 36-year-old single mother of four came to our office complaining of fatigue, anxiety, insomnia, heart palpitations, and occasional tremors. Her test results showed antibodies caused by a gluten intolerance were attacking her brain, nerve tissue, and intestinal tract. She was deficient in acetylcholine and vitamin D and had adrenal fatigue.

We immediately put her on a gluten-free diet. We gave her emulsified resveratrol and turmeric to help block inflammatory pathways. We also gave her a vitamin D complex and nutrients to support the HPA axis and acetylcholine activity. Within two weeks of this protocol she showed drastic improvement, and after six months, her symptoms had all but disappeared.

Joshua Redd, DC

Salt Lake City, Utah

www.drjoshuaredd.com

GLUTEN IS MORE A BRAIN ISSUE THAN A GUT ISSUE

The Dutch pediatrician Willem-Karel Dicke first identified gluten sensitivity in 1950 and termed it "celiac disease." In the 1960s, gastroenterologists identified patterns of destruction characteristic of celiac disease by studying intestinal tissue biopsies. Researchers later found certain gene types called HLA-DQ2 and HLA-DQ8 were associated with an increased risk of celiac disease. Researchers also found specific antibodies associated with celiac disease, such as gliadin and transglutaminase antibodies, which can be measured in the blood.

Over time they developed criteria for diagnosing celiac disease. The basic understanding for years and still held by many today is that only a few people with certain gene types are susceptible to celiac disease and that the destruction caused by gluten is limited to the intestinal tract.

However, studies today challenge these long-held concepts. First, the HLA-DQ2 and HLA-DQ8 celiac genotypes are very limited and cannot be used as sole determinants of gluten sensitivity or celiac disease.[8] Many people who do not have the genotypes still have severe reactions to gluten. Second, many people with gluten sensitivity have silent celiac disease, meaning their symptoms are not intestinal. Instead,

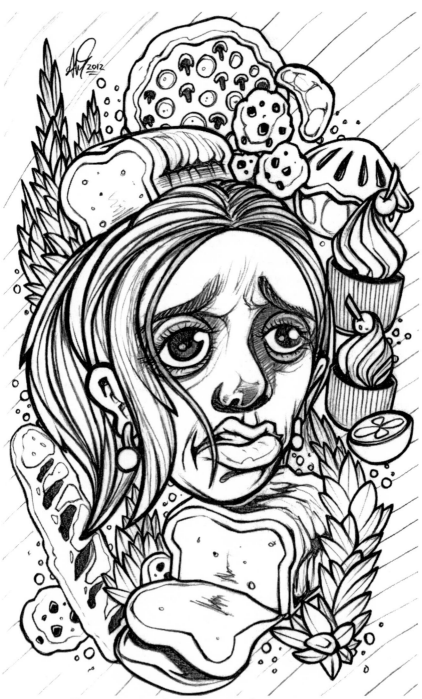

Gluten sensitivity destroys brain and nervous tissue more than any other tissue, including that of the gut.

they experience reactions to gluten in the brain, thyroid, joints, skin, or other tissues,[9] which are referred to as "extraintestinal manifestations." Finally, the most common area of non-intestinal manifestation of gluten sensitivity is the brain and nervous system.[10]

In fact, one study of patients who manifested gluten sensitivity in the brain found only a third of them also suffered from gastrointestinal disorders.[11] Another study in the journal *Neurology* showed that out of 10 participants with headaches, abnormalities in how they walked, and elevated anti-gliadin antibodies (gluten sensitivity), seven demonstrated complete resolution of symptoms on a gluten-free diet. The interesting part of this study was six out of the 10 subjects had no intestinal complaints.[12]

According to a recent paper titled *The Gluten Syndrome: A Neurological Disease*, research shows gluten sensitivity not associated with celiac disease or gut damage can nevertheless solely and directly harm the brain and nervous system, leading to a number of different neurological problems.[13] In other words, we are now learning gluten sensitivity destroys the brain and nervous tissue more than any other tissue in the body, including that of the gastrointestinal tract.[14]

So what does all of this mean to you? If your brain is not working, a sensitivity to gluten could be causing an immune assault on your brain. This will lead to brain inflammation and increase the risk for an autoimmune attack on brain tissue.

Despite the research, many physicians do not understand celiac disease, much less the concepts of gluten sensitivity, silent gluten sensitivity, or extraintestinal manifestations of gluten sensitivity. Your average gastroenterologist is still stuck on the outdated HLA-DQ and intestinal biopsy model for celiac diagnosis and unaware most gluten reactions do not cause gut damage or symptoms. Your average neurologist, on the other hand, has no idea a gluten sensitivity can cause any type of neurological disease.

If you have a neurological disorder or your brain is not working, you need to be tested for gluten sensitivity and not just celiac disease, which I will discuss later in this chapter. But before we go into testing, let me share with you some of the research related to the impact of gluten on the brain.

A psychotherapist referred a young high school teacher to me. He had been on disability for more than six months, suffering from severe depression and anxiety since he had been a high school student himself. He was receiving electro-shock treatments and had recently been hospitalized for depression.

From the time he was a teenager, he was in a number of in-patient and out-patient mental health programs and had been through trials of multiple medications. He also made several suicide attempts, his most recent being six months prior to our initial appointment.

He'd had brain scans done at the Amen Clinic and had undertaken some nutritional support recommended by that clinic, but he remained depressed and continued to have thoughts of suicide. In his last suicide attempt, he crashed into a telephone pole, lost consciousness, and was hospitalized with serious injuries for six weeks. Afterward, he was wheelchair bound for six months.

The client's wife joined him at his appointment and said she was willing to do whatever it took to help him. Throughout his nutrition program she prepared his meals, made certain he maintained his supplement regimen, and provided active emotional support.

He was on four medications for depression, anxiety, and bipolar disorder. Amazingly, he worked out every day and looked very fit. He was already supplementing with adrenal support, electrolytes, and very low doses of 5-HTP, along with fish oil, vitamin D, amino acids, and a multiple vitamin. He had begun to notice a slight improvement in his mood taking the 5-HTP.

I don't normally recommend neurotransmitter support when my clients are on medication, but this seemed to work for him. Most of our first interview was done with his wife, as he barely spoke to me and had a difficult time answering my questions. Frankly, I didn't know if I would be successful with him or not.

I recommended a comprehensive blood panel, an adrenal panel, and a male hormone panel. His blood test results indicated he was positive for an autoimmune thyroid, low B-6, and high liver enzymes. His adrenal panel indicated a circadian rhythm shift where his energy was very low for the first part of the day and *increased by evening time. This matched his mood and energy pattern exactly.*

Even though he had already eliminated gluten and his diet appeared well balanced and healthy, my first dietary recommendation was to eliminate all grains, legumes, dairy, and caffeine. From my experience, a low-antigenic food elimination program works well for those with autoimmune issues and especially for those with serious mood disorders; depression can be the result of inflammation. We increased his 5-HTP to three times a day, added gut restoration and digestive support, DHA, B-12, B-6, nitric oxide, and glutathione support.

For the first month he remained suicidal but noticed slight improvement in both digestion and mood. After we received results from a cross-reactive foods test for those foods that are most biochemically similar to gluten, I adjusted his diet. He was sensitive to most foods on the test, except rice and oats. This indicated he needed to continue with his gut restoration nutrients for another six months or more. We added more brain support for acetylcholine and to increase blood flow to the brain.

The increase of 5-HTP improved his mood somewhat, but I reasoned that acetylcholine support would increase the firing rate of the brain and therefore increase brain arousal enough to increase the viability of his medications and overall brain function. In addition, since the hippocampus (which regulates the adrenal response) is rich in acetylcholine receptors, adding acetylcholine support should help improve circadian rhythm function.

Within four months of beginning this regimen he was back to teaching and able to sleep through the night without medication. He continues to take his other medications as directed by his psychiatrist. He has elected to stay on the adjusted diet and the supplemental support, as he is no longer suffering from depression or anxiety and is enjoying his life with his wife and children.

Linda Clark, MA, CN
Fair Oaks, California
www.uwanutrition.com

* *

WHY GLUTEN IS SO HARMFUL TO THE NERVOUS SYSTEM

There has been an explosion of research on gluten and its impact on the nervous system in recent years; the timing of the hybridization and deamidation of grains and the onset of gluten-related diseases has aroused much suspicion about the safety of "new wheat."

Practitioners around the country are continually astonished by the profound therapeutic effect of a strict gluten-free diet on neurological disorders (the key word is "strict"). Studies have found associations between gluten sensitivity and disorders in every major part of the nervous system, including the brain, the spinal cord, and the nerves that extend into the arms and feet.

Gluten sensitivity has been shown to be a significant trigger in psychiatric disorders,[15] movement disorders,[16] sensory ganglionapathy,[17] ataxia,[18] general neurological impairment,[19] neuromyelitis,[20] multiple sclerosis,[21] neuropathy,[22] myoclonus,[23] apraxia,[24] myopathy,[25] neuro-muscular disease,[26] multiple systems atrophy,[27] cerebellar disease,[28] migraines,[29] hearing loss,[30] cognitive impairment,[31] dementia,[32] restless leg syndrome,[33] and disorders in virtually almost every part of the nervous system evaluated.

The immune system mistakes nervous tissue for gluten

Three main mechanisms appear to cause gluten to assault the nervous system. The first is related to cross-reactivity, a concept in immunology in which the immune system mistakes one protein for another—it appears the protein structure of gluten is similar to protein structures in the nervous system. When you are sensitive to gluten the immune system produces gluten antibodies to tag it for destruction. However, because gluten is similar in structure to nervous tissue, the immune system may accidentally produce antibodies to nervous tissue whenever you eat gluten. In this case, a gluten sensitivity may create an autoim-mune attack against the brain or other parts of the nervous system thanks to cross-reactivity.

One can easily test this concept with a test called ELISA, placing the blood of a person with gluten sensitivity into a dish of various neuro-logical tissues and then inspecting the dish for an immune response. A person should not have an immune response to tissues in the body, only to foreign invaders such as bacteria and other pathogens. An immune response to self-tissue is called autoimmunity.

Researchers have found gluten cross-reactivity leading to autoimmunity with synapsin,[34] a family of proteins located on neurons that help regulate neurotransmitter release; the brain's cerebellum, which can cause issues with balance, vertigo, or motor control; and an enzyme found in the brain called glutamic acid decarboxylase (GAD), which may cause symptoms related to anxiety.[35][36]

Gluten triggers nervous system transglutaminase autoimmunity

Another devastating mechanism gluten can trigger is an immune response against transglutaminase. Transglutaminases are enzymes that help bind proteins together and are also involved in the digestion of wheat. When looking at autoimmunity triggered by gluten, several transglutaminase enzymes concern us.

Transglutaminase-2 (TG2) is found in the intestinal lining, and TG2 antibodies have long been regarded as a laboratory marker for celiac disease. Celiac disease is an autoimmune disease in which the immune system destroys TG2 in the intestinal lining, thus causing damage, inflammation, and poor absorption of nutrients. Basically, when inflammation damages the gut lining, transglutaminases are found in the debris field. The body reacts to them and tags them with antibodies.

Transglutaminase-3 (TG3) is found in the skin, and a gluten-triggered autoimmune reaction to TG3 may lead to a skin disorder known as dermatitis herpetiformis, which presents as itchy red blisters frequently found on the knees, elbows, buttocks, and back, although they can appear elsewhere on the body.

When it comes to brain health, we want to be aware of the more recently discovered transglutaminase-6 (TG6), which is found throughout the central nervous system. Gluten can trigger immune reactivity to TG6, leading to autoimmune destruction of brain and nervous tissue.[37][38]

Also, transglutaminase is used by the food processing industry to tenderize meat and as a meat glue to hold processed meats together in distinct shapes. People with positive transglutaminase antibodies may react to this food additive.

Gluten can cause a leaky blood-brain barrier

The third mechanism is that immune reactions to gluten can break down the blood-brain barrier, the thin lining that protects the brain, and lead to what is called "leaky brain." A healthy blood-brain barrier prevents pathogens from getting into the brain but allows in necessary compounds, such as precursors for neurotransmitters. A leaky brain can allow in pathogens that increase the risk of autoimmune reactions in the brain and nervous system.[39][40] I describe this more in Chapter Nine.

* *

Christina, 28, remembers having symptoms of obsessive-compulsive disorder (OCD) as early as high school. She noticed she engaged in the same bizarre counting and tapping rituals as a classmate who had been diagnosed with OCD. In college, when stress ran really high, she said her OCD got "really weird."

For instance, handicapped signs painted into the asphalt of parking lots scared her, and she was unable to walk on them for fear something bad would happen. Before going through certain entry ways, she would have to perform complex counting and tapping exercises a set number of times. If she made a mistake, she had to start over before walking through the doorway. As exhausting as these rituals were, ignoring them was worse—she developed panic attacks and couldn't breathe.

Later in life her OCD served her in her job as a choreographer, dance teacher, and stylist for modeling agencies. "My OCD is what helped me to push ahead, as I was exceedingly particular and thorough," says Christina, who worked long hours dedicating herself to her job. However, she grew concerned when her OCD was also making her late for work.

"Before I could leave for work in the morning, everything in my house had to be perfect," Christina says. "There could not be a single dish out, not one speck of dust, nothing on the bathroom counter, or nothing out of place. The bed had to be perfectly made. I would rather be late to work than leave something out of place, or I felt something bad would happen to me."

She coped with the imposition of the disorder well into her 20s before finally seeking help.

It wasn't her OCD that drove her to seek professional help but rather a long list of other health issues: Bouts of crushing fatigue to where "I could barely lift a fork," says Christina. She also had trouble focusing, and a digestive system so sensitive that eating always caused bloating, stomach cramps, and a general ill feeling.

She woke every morning with aches and pains and had such severe hypoglycemia (low blood sugar) that if she didn't eat breakfast immediately upon waking she would end up on her hands and knees with severe nausea. Her hormones were "out of whack," she says, and she suffered two miscarriages in her attempts to get pregnant. She had chronic sinus infections and caught every bug that came around.

And yet repeated tests at her doctor's office showed she was in good health. "I felt isolated and emotional," she says. "Nobody believed me that I wasn't well. They all though I was a hypochondriac."

When she began seeing me, one of the first things I uncovered was a gluten intolerance. "I would have never known had he not told me," Christina says. "My medical doctor ran a blood test and I tested negative for celiac disease . However, around this time my brother tested positive for celiac disease, and since it's genetic, I knew there was a high probability I had it too."

I also found her hormones estrogen and testosterone were too high, and that she suffered from an overgrowth of candida, a naturally occurring yeast in the body that, when it becomes excessive, can cause myriad breakdowns in health. I also worked with her on her diet, as she wasn't eating regularly and was eating a diet high in sugar and starchy foods. "It's amazing how easily you can get a day's worth of sugar in one snack," says Christina.

Christina says working with me over the months hasn't been easy. In fact, it's been almost a full-time job changing her diet and lifestyle, but she has been rewarded 10 times over. "This has opened my eyes to how I have to be an advocate for my own health," she says. "I had to make my health a priority and stick with it. It's hard, but there's an enlightenment that happens. You see how the ways you care for yourself affect the quality of your life."

Christina's OCD is managed to the point that she actually lost a sweater recently, a first for someone who used to check things "five billion times," she says. Although she's still naturally tidy, she can go to work leaving a few dishes in the sink, the bed unmade, and even a few piles of mess here and there without having a panic attack She can now check the locks visually, instead of having to lock and unlock them numerous times. She no longer performs her counting rituals, unless she ends up in an unusually stressed state, or is in a new situation, such as traveling out of state. She's still in the process of improving her health.

"I'm so much better it's incredible," she says. "I'm calmer and more relaxed now. I know my limits and don't burn myself out and crash with exhaustion like I used to. The nice thing is I have more energy so now I can help my husband with things in his life, whereas he was always the one helping me before. He's especially happy because I'm not always hounding him to clean up."

Blake Ambridge, DC, DCANB
Santa Rosa, California
www.backtohealthsr.com

UNDERSTANDING GLUTEN TESTING

Different types of testing for gluten sensitivity exist, including genetic testing, intestinal biopsy evaluation, and antibody testing. As we have discussed, an immune reaction to gluten does not have to involve either the gut or specific genotypes, as many people develop neurological disorders instead. Therefore, it is not necessary to perform an intestinal biopsy or gene testing to evaluate gluten sensitivity.

A blood, saliva, or stool test that screens for immune antibodies to gluten are the established methods for identifying gluten sensitivity. Stool testing for gluten sensitivity has little evidence in the literature, so I do not use it or endorse it at this point. Most doctors screen for gluten sensitivity using blood tests, but saliva tests have shown great promise in terms of their reliability.[41 42 43]

Blood testing for gluten sensitivity involves placing samples of your blood in a dish of gluten proteins and seeing whether antibodies develop, an indication gluten activates your immune cells and you have gluten sensitivity.

⦁ ⦁

Darlene noticed her 75-year-old husband was changing drastically. His short-term memory was failing, and for the last couple of years he began to suffer from terrible brain fog after eating. He would be himself in the morning, then within two hours of eating breakfast and taking his blood pressure medication, he acted almost as if he were drunk.

"His head would droop, his eyes grew heavy and went to half-mast, and his hands would curl sideways and he couldn't open them," Darlene says. "He would also mumble instead of being able to speak clearly. Our doctor put him on a gluten-free and dairy-free diet and he immediately became much better," she says.

She said his symptoms of brain fog also get quite bad when he is under a lot of stress and anxiety. "Sometimes if he gets really anxious, he looks almost like he is going into anaphylactic shock," Darlene says. "He gets so pale and foggy-headed he can't even communicate."

They have learned that a gluten- and dairy-free diet and addressing his anxiety are important first steps in managing the inflammation causing his brain fog, and they are looking into whether he might be reacting to any fillers in his blood pressure medication.

Blake Ambridge, DC, DCANB
Santa Rosa, California
www.backtohealthsr.com

⦁ ⦁

The problems and solutions with gluten sensitivity testing

Testing for a gluten sensitivity is much more complex than most people and the standard health care model realize. This is because people can react to a number of different portions of the gluten protein. Most labs only test for antibodies to a portion of gluten called "alpha gliadin," which, thanks to current research, we now know is extremely limited and produces many clinically negative results.[44][45] If you have symptoms that suggest a gluten sensitivity but your gluten test came back negative, you may want to get tested again with a more thorough evaluation using the information below.

Gliadin

Gluten is made of a sticky portion called "glutenin" and a protein portion called "gliadin." Gliadin is further broken down into alpha, omega, and gamma gliadians. As I mentioned before, most labs only test for alpha gliadin antibodies, which is most commonly associated with celiac disease. Even worse, they do not report this limitation in test results. The reports usually state "gliadin" antibody, but do not specify it is *alpha* gliadin. The result often comes back negative, doctors tell patients they can eat gluten, and patient health further deteriorates. When the patient finally tests for the other branches of gluten, the results show severe gluten sensitivity. I have seen this happen many times.

Glutenin

Glutenin, the sticky portion, makes up 47 percent of the total protein content of wheat and is responsible for the strength and elasticity of wheat dough. Most labs do not test for glutenin sensitivity because it was believed glutenin is not immune reactive. However, this has been disproven.[46] Many people have severe reactions to glutenin but show normal results on the basic gliadin antibody test.

Deamidated gluten

As I mentioned earlier, deamidation is an acid or enzymatic treatment used by the food processing industry to make wheat water soluble so it mixes easily with other foods, and deamidated gliadin has been shown to trigger a severe immune response in people.[47] Many people will never test positive on a conventional gliadin antibody test, but will have profound immune reactions to deamidated gliadin. If you suffer from impaired brain function, testing for deamidated gluten is critical.

• •

A 63-year-old woman came to my office with a Mayo Clinic diagnosis of "relapsing multiple sclerosis." She complained of a weak immune system, fatigue, brain fog, an inability to find the right words, constipation, eczema, sugar cravings, thinning hair, and extreme short-term memory loss. The directions on how to get to my office confused her, she was unable to count backwards from 100 by sevens, and the consultation ran over by an hour because her speech was slow and she continually interrupted my intake questions by going off on tangents unrelated to her medical history.

MRIs of her brain indicated multiple sclerosis. Year-old blood tests revealed low white blood cells (poor immunity), B-12 anemia, and low triglycerides. She was taking interferon treatments as well as neurotransmitter and adrenal supplements recommended to her based on a urinary neurotransmitter test. Despite these measures, she was not improving.

While waiting for test results to come back I placed her on an anti-inflammatory diet and gentle gut cleanse. She stopped all other supplements and took only vitamin D, omega 3 essential fatty acids, methyl B-12, and nutritional compounds to support her digestion and liver detoxification. After the cleanse, her energy levels were coming up and her constipation was gone.

Advanced blood testing revealed autoimmune Hashimoto's thyroid disease, high homocysteine levels, and a weak, imbalanced immune system. Stool and saliva testing showed celiac disease, an autoimmune gluten intolerance, and a dairy intolerance. I then instructed her how to care for her immune system to minimize autoimmune thyroid attacks and placed her on a permanent diet eliminating dairy, gluten, and corn.

At this point I added nutritional support for her digestive system and adrenal health, and to calm inflammation in the brain and improve blood flow. I also added DHA and compounds to support acetylcholine, the learning and memory neurotransmitter. Within two weeks her brain fog lifted. After two months she declared she felt human again and her brain function was getting back to how it used to be. She wasn't worried about "going crazy" like her mother had done, and her family loved her recovery.

I was able to congratulate her for showing up on time for her appointments and keeping her consult within the time parameters. Seven months after the initial consultation she continued to see improvements, was taking her nutritional support, and assured me she would never go back to her brain-inflaming, autoimmune-provoking diet of gluten, dairy, and corn.

Kari Vernon, DC
Scottsdale, Arizona
www.karismaforlife.com

At this point, I hope you can see how gluten antibody testing conducted by most labs today captures only a small part of the picture, leading to many improper diagnoses and the continuation of patient suffering. A test should screen for an immune reaction to the alpha, omega, and gamma branches of gliadin as well as glutenin and deamidated gluten.

Lectins

This may seem like more than enough for which to test, but a couple of other components of wheat have been identified as immune reactive. Many people who react to wheat do not react to the gluten portion of wheat. Instead they react to the *lectin* portion. Lectins are substances that bind sugars and carbohydrates together. In wheat they are called wheat germ agglutinin (WGA).

The highest concentration of WGA is found in whole wheat or sprouted wheat, popular among health enthusiasts. WGA can pass through the blood-brain barrier and attach to the myelin sheath, the protective coating on nerves. This can inhibit nerve growth factor, a chemical critical for neuron growth and health.[48] Many people never test positive for gluten antibodies but have a WGA sensitivity. For these people eating lectins may cause a severe inflammatory response and destroy neurons.

Opioids

Lastly, people may react to gluten opioids, which is different than a reaction to gliadin, glutenin, or WGA.[49] [50] An immune response to opioids takes place in the nervous system and can be measured by antibodies to *gluteomorphin* and *prodynorphin*. Gluteomorphin is an opioid peptide formed during the digestion of gluten. Prodynorphin is an opioid that is the basic building block of endorphins.

If a person has elevated antibodies to these compounds gluten may cause a neurological reaction. The most difficult thing about an opioid sensitivity is that going gluten-free can cause severe withdrawal symptoms, including depression, mood swings, or abnormal bowel activity. It is similar to withdrawal from opioid drugs such as heroin. If this occurs the person must hang in there for a couple of weeks on a strict gluten-free diet and deal with the withdrawal symptoms until they've kicked the gluten addiction.

• •

Wanda, 60, was in her mid-50s and working as a teacher for troubled teens when her short-term memory started rapidly declining. It got so bad that she had trouble finding her way home on familiar routes and finding her car in parking lots, and it affected her performance at work to the point she had to retire early. She also withdrew socially, afraid of embarrassing herself.

Her husband Dave took her to the University of San Diego, and testing showed radical short-term memory loss, some long-term memory loss, and anxiety. Scans of her brain showed lesions throughout her frontal lobe, the area of the brain responsible for cognitive function.

Both avid health enthusiasts, Dave counted 35 different alternative health modalities they tried in an effort to halt her declining memory and restore her cognitive function; they had already decided against pharmaceutical approaches. After several years and many dead ends, an acquaintance mentioned Dr. Kharrazian, and they made an appointment with me.

They found a gluten-free diet to be one of the cornerstones of Wanda's recovery, as she was diagnosed with celiac disease. She immediately had to give up her two pieces of toast in the morning, a standard breakfast she had been eating for years, as well as all other forms of gluten in her diet.

"We noticed a difference in her cognitive abilities right away once she got on a gluten-free diet," says her husband Dave. "She has greater mental clarity and less anxiety. It's clear that gluten and her celiac condition are what caused the damage to her brain."

After six months on a gluten-free diet and incorporating other brain-healthy nutritional compounds and techniques, Wanda is able to drive again and enjoy more of a social life, having recovered much of her mental function. She still struggles some with memory and may have lost some of her memory permanently, but the couple has noticed dramatic improvements in her condition.

"When this happens to someone you love, it's devastating," says Dave. "She is able to get out more and be with her friends, without

fear of repeating herself or saying something wrong. Trying to cover for that was extremely stressful for her."

Wanda feels she has been given a second chance, and tears come to her eyes when she talks about the progress she's made. "This is the best thing that has ever happened to me," she says. "I'm so grateful because I wasn't in very good shape."

Blake Ambridge, DC, DCANB

Santa Rosa, California

www.backtohealthsr.com

• •

Transglutaminase

The last issue to cover with gluten sensitivity testing is transglutaminase, which I introduced earlier. Positive transglutaminase antibodies indicate gluten triggers autoimmunity.

There are three major transglutaminases: TG2, TG3, and TG6.

- TG2 is found in the intestinal tract and elevated TG2 antibodies indicates villous atrophy (destruction of the tiny finger-like projections in the small intestine that absorb food) and destruction of the intestinal lining.[51]

- TG3 is found in the skin and is associated with skin outbreaks triggered by gluten, such as dermatitis herpetiformis.[52]

- TG6 is found in the nervous system and is associated with neurological destruction triggered by gluten.[53]

The problem with labs today is they test only for antibodies to TG2, the intestinal transglutaminase, which indicates an autoimmune reaction in the gut. They also list the test results as "transglutaminase" and never specify it is only TG2. If you have neurological issues possibly stemming from gluten, you also need to evaluate TG6.

Also, it's important to test additionally for transglutaminase *bound* to gliadin or the test may miss transglutaminase antibodies, possibly resulting in a clinically negative result. Most labs only test for transglutaminase not bound to gliadin.

You can now see how flawed and limited gluten testing is today and why so many people continue to suffer despite a negative celiac test.

The most common tests my patients have done before they come to my office are an isolated alpha gliadin and TG2. As you now know, this is not nearly enough information, as many people have severe immune reactions to other types of gluten or may produce antibodies to a different transglutaminase enzyme.

• •

Roberta is an executive working in a high-stress environment that requires constant travel. After she was moved to an office that had mold growing in it her health plummeted. By the time she got to me she had persistent, profound fatigue, migraine headaches, and hypoglycemia, and she had been through so many sinus infections and courses of antibiotics that she lost count.

She often took antibiotics for six weeks at a time and often ran a low-grade fever. Though she didn't list anxiety as one of her symptoms, she was practically jumping out of her skin as she described her unbearably stressful job, which was made worse by the fact that she barely had enough energy to work.

Roberta's lab work suggested a previously undiagnosed autoimmune disorder and a gluten intolerance. A salivary adrenal panel revealed that Roberta's cortisol level actually went up at night, rather than being highest in the morning and low at night as they should be. This indicated her stressful life was causing poor function in her hippocampus, the area of the brain responsible for regulating the day-night cycling of cortisol. Unfortunately, the hippocampus is also the seat of short-term memory. A loss of normal cortisol rhythm can be an early indication of dementia, so this finding concerned me greatly.

I asked Roberta to completely avoid gluten. Based on her own observation that dairy tended to upset her digestion, I asked her to avoid all milk products as well. I gave her adaptogenic herbs to support her adrenal function and nutrients to repair her gut barrier system.

By the following week Roberta's migraines were improving and her energy level was going up. As the weeks went by her migraines completely disappeared, as did her sinus problems, chronic fever, and fatigue.

Roberta avoids gluten and dairy and maintains her protocol to keep her autoimmune response from flaring up. Her job is still stressful, but because her body is now in balance, she no longer pays a physical price for being in that environment. Though she described it as miraculous, I told her it's just a matter of knowing the physiology.

Samuel F. Yanuck, DC, FACFN, FIAMA
Chapel Hill, North Carolina
www.yanuckcenter.com

● ●

In summary, a complete gluten antibody screen should include:

- alpha gliadin
- omega gliadin
- gamma gliadin
- deamidated gliadin
- wheat germ agglutinin (WGA)
- gluteomorphin
- prodynorphin
- transglutaminase-2 (TG2)
- transglutaminase-3 (TG3)
- transglutaminase-6 (TG6)

This is the panel I use for my patients, and it has revealed countless misdiagnosed issues of gluten sensitivity. This panel is only available through Cyrex Labs (cyrexlabs.com), and it is called the Wheat/Gluten Proteome Sensitivity and Autoimmunity Panel.

If the test shows you are gluten sensitive you should avoid gluten at all costs. If you have positive reactions to any of the transglutaminases, it means you have an autoimmune reaction and should consider further screening for antibodies to neurological tissue if you suffer from brain decline. I discuss this in detail in Chapter Eleven.

● ●

My patient Derek, age seven, was suffering tremendously from mental, emotional, and dermatological symptoms. He could not bend certain joints because the eczema was so bad it caused loss of elasticity in his skin. He itched terribly and scratched so much he pulled pieces of flesh off. He also had terrible issues with stealing food. He snuck out of the house to steal food out of the trash and behaved in ways that were viewed as psychotic. Nobody understood his behavior. He had been on multiple antipsychotic medications typically prescribed for schizophrenia.

I ran some labs on Derek, and found he was profoundly reacting to multiple foods and various components of certain foods. He had profound gluteomorphin reactions that caused intense cravings and compelled him to steal foods. He had reactions to all transglutaminases—TG2, TG3, and TG6—which explained the extreme neurological symptoms and terrible skin reactions.

After eliminating all dairy and gluten from his diet, Derek was able to get off the medications. His skin is now healthy and normal, and he no longer steals food or behaves erratically. Just simple food elimination and a gut repair program changed this kid's life forever.

Joel Brandon Brock, FNP-C, DC, Nurse Practitioner
Rockwall, Texas
www.rockwallpediatrics.com/

● ●

GOING GLUTEN FREE

Going gluten free may seem difficult at first, especially if you regularly eat fast food and processed food. However, if you already eat a whole foods diet, it's not that difficult. Many gluten-free resources are available today, some of which are listed on my web site.

Sources of Gluten
- Wheat
- Barley
- Rye
- Spelt
- Kamut
- Oats (except from a gluten-free oat farm)

Foods suspected to cross-react with gluten (the immune system recognizes them as gluten)
- Casein (milk protein)
- Corn
- Oats (including gluten-free)
- Some brands of instant coffee

Hidden sources of gluten
- Modified food starch
- Food emulsifiers
- Food stabilizers
- Artificial food coloring
- Malt extract
- Dextrins
- Clarifying agents in some red wines

Commonly overlooked sources of gluten
- Processed condiments (ketchup, mustard, salad dressing)
- Deli meats
- Beer
- Soy sauce
- Imitation crab meat
- Shampoos

Transglutaminase is an enzyme used in the food industry to tenderize poor quality meat for cheap food or fast foods. It is not typically found in meats in grocery store meat departments or normal steakhouses. The food industry also uses transglutaminase to form meat into perfect shapes. Have you ever seen chicken nuggets that all look the same? If so, they probably used transglutaminase. If you have an immune response to transglutaminase, you may have an immune cross-reactive response to food industry transglutaminase and notice symptoms of inflammation if you eat it.

Going gluten free can be as simple as avoiding processed and fast foods, eating a diet of meats, vegetables, fruits, and using gluten-free condiments. If you have a confirmed gluten sensitivity and feel going gluten free is too difficult, it is time for you to put this book down and realize your brain has no chance, as you will continue to get worse.

You should also know there is no such thing as being "90 percent gluten free" or "pretty good," or "almost gluten-free." It is like saying you are 90 percent pregnant. You either are or you are not. If you are emotionally attached to gluten, you need to get over it and get serious to protect the health of your brain.

Getting serious means learning how to incorporate a gluten-free diet and gluten-free products into your lifestyle. It means when you eat out you cannot always trust the server or the chef, and you must stick to meat and vegetable dishes without heavy or processed sauces. It also means you must be patient and committed if family members give you a hard time at holiday gatherings. It can be challenging until you find your safe snacks, meals, and restaurants, and you often may need to prepare food in advance to bring along instead of eating out. Once you figure out your new routine, it becomes easier and easier. As you become established in your gluten-free lifestyle, you will get to the point where you don't even miss it.

Most people who react to gluten notice a change in their well-being within a week of adopting a gluten-free diet, though some will take longer. It may take several weeks or even months for the immune response to gluten to calm down, which is why cheating or small exposures can sabotage the entire program. "Just a bite" triggers a domino-effect immune response that can last for long periods of time, so please be strict.

• •

Like most people, Anna, 40, wasn't aware she was suffering from gradually deteriorating brain health. Instead it was her rapid and unexplainable decline in dental health that drove her to seek care from a natural health care practitioner. She had gone her entire life with healthy teeth and gums when suddenly she started getting multiple cavities and had to undergo several root canals and seven gum grafts, all despite her best efforts at good dental hygiene and a sugar-free diet. When her gums began to bleed constantly it was the last straw for Anna.

"My periods were also getting closer and closer together," says Anna. "My mom had these same issues when she was my age and had a hysterectomy. My grandmother had the same issues and ended up with Alzheimer's. My mom had hypothyroidism her whole life, and my grandmother had thyroid cancer. All the women in my family had marched to a place I didn't want to go."

Though her dental and hormonal issues most vexed her, Anna also acknowledged she was finding it increasingly difficult to multitask and her memory was getting worse. After doing an exam and ordering blood work, I was able to identify a variety of issues taxing Anna's health, including an intolerance to gluten and dairy.

After three months on a gluten-free diet and some nutritional support, Anna's symptoms cleared up. However, the importance of her new diet didn't sink in until she ate gluten during her vacation, and all her symptoms returned swiftly and severely.

"My gums started bleeding again and my periods got out of sync again," she says. "I had been constipated my whole life until I got on the gluten-free, dairy-free diet, and when I ate gluten on my vacation, I became really constipated—everything just stopped. I brought some geometry problems to work on for fun (Anna is a math tutor and enjoys math), and after eating gluten, I completely lost my interest and motivation in it."

In fact it wasn't until she went gluten- and dairy-free that Anna realized how much her previous diet had been affecting her brain health. Her perpetual brain fog lifted and her stress levels lowered.

"When I look back I feel like I had a screen pulled down over my brain, like I never came out of a dream state," says Anna. "On the new diet it's gone and I'm more awake, energetic, and alert, and able to process information better. I have also noticed I handle stress a lot better and can deal with little frustrations more easily, which helps with my overall concentration."

Joni Labbe, DC, CCN, DCCN
San Diego, California
www.brain-dr.com

WHEN GOING GLUTEN FREE IS NOT ENOUGH

Unfortunately, going gluten free alone may not be enough to manage declining brain function, autoimmunity, or inflammation. This is because proteins in other foods can cross-react with gluten. Cross-reactivity means the proteins in certain foods are similar enough to those in gluten to trigger a reaction.[54] Foods known to commonly cross-react with gluten include casein (the dairy protein), yeast, oats, sesame, and some brands of instant coffee.

The food that most commonly cross-reacts with gluten is casein. This is not to be confused with a lactose intolerance. Lactose is the sugar portion of milk whereas casein is the protein. Lactose intolerance is a condition in which some people lack the enzymes to digest milk sugars. It is not the same as an immune response to casein.

One study found 50 percent of patients with gluten sensitivity experienced only partial remission of symptoms on a gluten-free diet because they had a cross-reactivity to milk.[55] I have personally witnessed countless cases of individuals who needed to give up both gluten and dairy for a positive health response. Also, it's important to test for different antibodies to milk protein or you may miss a dairy sensitivity. These include alpha-casein, beta-casein, casomorphin, and milk butyrophilin.

The other common cross-reactive foods—oats, yeast, sesame, and some brands of instant coffee—can also be an issue. If your symptoms are not improving on a gluten-free diet you may need to get tested for these cross-reactive foods or simply avoid them completely.

The other main issue with going on a gluten-free diet is many people begin eating more of other grains, such as corn, rice, or quinoa, and develop sensitivities to those grains. This happens all the time with gluten-sensitive people. If you are gluten sensitive and have been on a strict gluten-free diet with minimal results, you may be sensitive to other grains.

● ●

Carmen sought my advice for fibromyalgia. She had also been diagnosed with Hashimoto's hypothyroidism, neuropathy, and constipation.

Testing revealed issues with her gall bladder, iron levels, blood sugar, and adrenal glands. Further testing also revealed positive transglutaminase antibodies against the intestines and sensitivities to gluten, dairy, soy, yeast, and eggs.

I instructed her to begin an anti-inflammatory diet eliminating these foods and gave her nutritional compounds for gallbladder, thyroid, adrenal, and gut support as well as vitamin D and essential fatty acids. Within a few days her constipation was relieved and she was off of her stool softeners.

Next we started functional neurological rehabilitation to further support brain function. Her pain in her legs was gone within three weeks and she slept better.

Carmen now has her life back and is off all medications.

Lonnie Herman, DC
Plantation, Florida
www.browardpaincenter.com

• •

Cyrex Labs offers a panel that checks for the foods that most commonly cross-react with gluten. It also screens for common sensitivities to other grains and non-gluten foods and is called the Gluten-Associated Sensitivity and Cross Reactive Foods Array 4.

Foods tested on the Cyrex Array 4 food sensitivity panel
(an [X] indicates a food that commonly cross-reacts with gluten; a [*] indicates the food is often contaminated with wheat during the processing of the food)

[X] Rye, barley, spelt, Polish wheat

[X] Cow's milk

[X] Alpha-casein and beta-casein (milk proteins)

[X] Casomorphin (peptide created during digestion of milk protein that produces an opioid effect in the nervous system)

[X] Milk butyrophilin (a protein in milk fat)

[X] Whey protein

[X] Milk chocolate

[X,*] Oats

[*] Some brands of prepackaged, preground, and instant coffee are contaminated with gluten

[X] Yeast

Sesame

Buckwheat

Sorghum

[X] Millet

Hemp

Amaranth

Quinoa

Tapioca

Teff

Soy

Egg

[X] Corn

[X] Rice

Potato

I have found this panel makes it easy to quickly identify which cross-reactive and gluten-free foods must be avoided on a gluten-free diet. If you do not have access to the testing, then follow a diet eliminating the entire list of grains, which is beneficial anyway if you have intestinal permeability, or leaky gut.

How to get the most out of your food sensitivity panel

To get the most out of your Cyrex food sensitivity panel, or any food sensitivity panel, it's important to know some immune basics.

A food sensitivity panel screens for antibodies (Cyrex measures IgA and IgG) to foods, and these antibodies take time to develop.

Antibodies are proteins the immune system makes to tag an antigen, or harmful invader. Once an antibody tags an antigen, the immune system knows to destroy and remove it. This immune reaction is very useful in the case of a virus. However, if it is happening against a food you eat at almost every meal it can cause inflammation, immune imbalances, and raise your risk of developing or worsening autoimmune disease.

In the event of a sensitivity, it takes about one month after eating a particular food for positive antibodies to show up on a test. If you have not consumed a food in the last three to four months, it most likely will not produce positive antibodies, even though you may be sensitive to it. For example, someone could be sensitive to teff, but because they rarely eat it, it may not show up as positive on the test.

What it means when all your results are below the reference range

Sometimes results show a person did not test positive for any foods and all the results are below the lab's reference range. This is not necessarily a green light to eat whatever you want. When all the results are below the reference range it can mean your immune system is suppressed and not able to produce enough antibodies for a positive test result.

One cause for this is steroid use, which suppresses antibody production. Another cause is the person's immune system is simply fatigued and under functioning. Testing for total IgA and IgG antibodies can verify whether this is the case.

General strategies to improve overall health—including an autoimmune diet, gut repair, and blood sugar balancing—can help restore antibody production for more accurate results on a retest. This mechanism explains why patients with an autoimmune disease, such as Hashimoto's hypothyroidism, see their antibody levels temporarily spike when they begin restoring their health, even though symptoms may improve.

However, if many of the values are below reference range but you still test positive to one or more foods, then immune suppression does not apply to you; the immune system is not selective about suppression.

What to do with your test results

You got your test results back, now what? You need to immediately eliminate the foods that showed positive on the test. Foods that are cross-reactive with gluten should be permanently avoided, particularly if you also tested positive for transglutaminase antibodies. If you tested negative for transglutaminase antibodies it's possible you may be able to eat these foods again after repairing leaky gut, but it depends on the individual.

The remaining foods are foods to which you have developed a sensitivity. Upon restoring gut health and reducing your overall immune load, it's possible you also may be able to eat these foods again in the future.

Many people with gluten sensitivity and gastrointestinal inflammation develop a leaky gut. As discussed in Chapter Nine, you can test for leaky gut using a panel from Cyrex Labs called the Intestinal Antigenic Permeability Panel. The dietary restrictions to repair leaky gut, which are discussed in the next chapter, include the removal of gluten, dairy, and all grains. Results can be profound.

Although these dietary changes can seem severe at first, they are the foundation to lowering overall inflammation and taming autoimmune reactions. Many people find that as their health improves they actually begin to love their new way of eating and how good it makes them feel.

Strategies for accidental gluten exposures

Despite your best intentions, there may be times when you are accidentally exposed to gluten. Many people with gluten sensitivity don't realize how awful gluten makes them feel until they have been off it for a while and then are exposed to it accidentally. It makes them realize how significantly gluten impacts their system.

Some have more adverse reactions than others. I have a patient with an inner ear autoimmune disorder called Meniere's disease. If she accidentally ingests gluten she develops dizziness and ringing in her ear. She can literally take a bite of a food with gluten and immediately develop symptoms that last for several days. Some people will notice mild abdominal bloating and brain fog. Others may have a subtle mental slowness or headaches. Everyone will be different.

⬤ ⬤

I have seen great results with many inflammatory conditions such as multiple sclerosis (MS). I recently had a patient diagnosed with MS come into my office. Her MRI showed multiple lesions in the brain and she had neurological symptoms. She complained of incontinence, brain fog, balance problems, numbness, and tingling. She was offered multiple drug therapies to counteract the effects from MS.

A comprehensive exam showed she had abnormal eye movements, she could not feel vibration on the left side of her body, and she had multiple balance issues. It was evident she was dealing with inflammation that led to her signs and symptoms of MS.

Her treatment plan consisted of an anti-inflammatory diet to reduce any food allergies and evaluate the impact gluten had on her immune system. I gave her neurological rehabilitative exercises to improve her balance, coordination, and perception.

We determined gluten was the major source of inflammation flaring her symptoms. She also found sugar, dyes, and preservatives impacted her health. After we removed inflammatory foods from her diet and supported proper brain function, she began feeling better.

A follow-up MRI six months later showed many lesions had resolved and only a few remained. Her neurological signs and symptoms were reduced and she stated improvement in her over-all life, affecting her life personally and professionally. She was able to continue writing a paper that later advanced her within her career.

Shane Steadman, DC, DACNB, DCBCN
Englewood, Colorado
www.integratedhealthdenver.com

● ●

If you have a gluten sensitivity and are exposed to gluten, several natural enzymes and compounds can reduce the adverse reaction and help you recover faster. These natural compounds help degrade the gluten protein to reduce the intensity and duration of the immune response.

DPP-IV

The first supplement is a digestive enzyme called DPP-IV. It helps digest gliadin and casein and regulate the immune response.[56][57] Research shows supplementing with DPP-IV is therapeutic for gluten sensitive people; the naturally occurring DPP-IV enzyme is less active in people with celiac disease and malabsorption.[58][59][60] Also, the effects of DPP-IV activity, gluten exposure, and inflammation have been shown to play a role in autism.[61][62]

Brush border enzymes

Brush border enzymes are digestive enzymes located in the intestinal microvilli and include amylase, cellulase, invertase, and lactase. Intestinal damage and leaky gut can destroy the microvilli and brush border enzyme activity. I do not recommend bromelain or pancreatic enzymes if you have positive transglutaminase antibodies and villous atrophy causing bloating after eating, anemia, weight loss, and other symptoms of malabsorption. These enzymes can "digest" the villi and make you feel worse. Plant-based enzymes are safer in the case of damaged guts.

Flavonoids

For people with gluten sensitivity and celiac disease, gluten promotes severe intestinal inflammation.[63] The flavonoids (colorful plant compounds) listed below can help dampen inflammation from gluten exposure.[64][65] I prefer using a combination of all of them. Please note: If you are gluten sensitive these are *not* to be used as an excuse to eat gluten; they are to dampen the consequences of minor exposures. There is no predetermined dose so you will need to experiment with doses that work best for you. These are not drugs, so you do not need to worry about overdosing.

- Lycopene
- Apigenin
- Quercetin
- Luteolin

Lycopene and quercetin have been shown to prevent immune activation from gluten.[66] Apigenin inhibits gut microflora from triggering inflammation.[67][68] Quercetin has been shown to work against intestinal histamine secretion in response to an antigen.[69] Luteolin inhibits LPS-induced inflammation in the gut lining.[70][71][72][73]

Together DPP-IV and these flavonoids can help dampen gut inflammation in the event of an accidental gluten exposure. You may find you need to take large amounts after an exposure, or take smaller amounts frequently to dampen inflammation and relieve symptoms.

● ●

Beth lives in Santa Rosa, California and is 63. She suffered from depression so severely for so many years that she was seriously contemplating suicide. She remembers the depression starting as early as her 30s but getting especially bad in her early 50s. She took four different medications for her depression, none of which helped much.

As the depression worsened, I began to take classes from Dr. Kharrazian. After learning about the effects of gluten on brain function, I had Beth tested for gluten intolerance and learned she had celiac disease. She immediately started on a gluten-free diet and was amazed to find her depression and suicidality lifted after just two weeks. If she cheated, however, the depression would return a few days later.

"When I decided I was going to cheat and eat something with gluten in it, I always paid for it," Beth said. "The depression and suicidal feelings would return. Now I am very strict."

Beth says she feels so much better than she remembers feeling in a long time, and no longer battles her weight. "I feel a lot better about myself," Beth says. "I'm more patient with my grandchildren and happier with my family. I used to be on edge all the time and always yelling at the grandkids, but now it's just not an issue. I'm calmer, more relaxed, and not hating the world. I wish I had been that way with my own kids."

Beth is on just one medication now instead of four and says she feels badly for people who are on so many medications with no relief, when a simple diet change might be all they need. "It takes a lot of willpower to give up something you shouldn't eat," says Beth. "But I have a whole different life now."

Blake Ambridge, DC, DCANB
Santa Rosa, California
www.backtohealthsr.com

• •

CHAPTER SUMMARY

• No single dietary protein is a more potent trigger of neurological dysfunction and neurological autoimmunity than gluten, the protein found in wheat. We're seeing dramatic increases in the number of people sensitive to gluten in the United States. Research shows gluten sensitivity has risen sharply in the last 50 years.

• The gluten you eat today is not the same grain it once was. Gluten has been significant hybridized and deamidated over the years.

Hybridization has created a "new wheat" that appears to trigger immune reactions, especially in the brain and nervous system. Deamidation, which is used by the food processing industry to make wheat water soluble, has been shown to cause a severe inflammatory process in people.

• The criteria for diagnosing celiac disease and gluten sensitivity are either outdated or incomplete. HLA-DQ2 and HLA-DQ8 celiac genotypes are very limited and cannot be used as sole determinants of gluten sensitivity or celiac disease. Many people who do not have the genotypes still have severe reactions to gluten. Second, many people with gluten sensitivity have silent celiac disease, meaning they do not manifest intestinal symptoms. Instead, the immune reaction to gluten is experienced in other tissues, such as the brain, thyroid, joints, or skin. Lastly, the most common area of non-intestinal manifestation of gluten sensitivity is the brain and nervous system.

• Despite the research, many physicians do not even understand celiac disease, much less such concepts such as non-celiac gluten sensitivity, silent gluten sensitivity, or extraintestinal manifestations of gluten sensitivity. Your average gastroenterologist is typically not aware of gluten reactions that do not cause intestinal destruction. Your average neurologist has no idea a gluten sensitivity can cause any type of neurological disease.

• Studies have found associations between gluten sensitivity and disorders in every major part of the nervous system, including the brain, the spinal cord, and the peripheral nerves that extend into the arms and feet. Countless practitioners all over the country and I are continually astonished by what a profound therapeutic effect a strict gluten-free diet has on all types of neurological disorders.

• Three main mechanisms appear to cause gluten to assault the nervous system. The first is that the immune system mistakes nervous tissue for gluten. Eating gluten may trigger an autoimmune attack against brain or nerve tissue. Another mechanism is that gluten can trigger immune reactivity to transglutaminase-6, leading to autoimmune destruction of neurons in a reaction similar to celiac disease. Lastly, immune reactions to gluten can also break down the blood-brain barrier, the thin lining that protects the brain, and lead to what is called "leaky brain."

• Gluten is made of a sticky portion called glutenin and a protein portion called gliadin. Gliadin is further broken down into alpha, omega, and gamma fractions. However, most labs only run an isolated alpha gliadin test. This means most people receive incomplete gluten sensitivity testing and may not be diagnosed properly.

• A complete gluten antibody screen should include:
  • alpha gliadin
  • omega gliadin
  • gamma gliadin
  • deamidated gliadin
  • wheat germ agglutinin
  • gluteomorphin
  • prodynorphin
  • TG2
  • TG3
  • TG6

• Going gluten free alone may not be enough to manage declining brain function, autoimmunity, or inflammation. This is because proteins in other foods can cross-react with gluten. Cross-reactivity means the proteins in certain foods are similar enough to those in gluten to trigger a reaction.

• If you have a gluten sensitivity and are exposed to gluten, several natural enzymes and compounds can reduce the adverse reaction and help you recover faster. These natural compounds help degrade the gluten protein to reduce the intensity and duration of the immune response. They include the enzyme DPP-IV and the flavonoids lycopene, apigenin, quercetin, luteolin.

• If you have a confirmed gluten sensitivity and feel going gluten free is too difficult, it is time for you to put this book down and realize your brain has no chance and you will continue to get worse.

CHAPTER NINE

THE GUT-BRAIN AXIS

SYMPTOMS OF AN IMPAIRED GUT-BRAIN AXIS

- Difficulty digesting foods
- Constipation or irregular bowel movements
- Increased bloating and gas
- Distention after meals
- Intolerance to food types such as proteins, starches, and/or fats
- Frequent abdominal discomfort after eating

• •

Sarah, 56, was a naturopathic doctor who had been suffering from chronic gastrointestinal disorders for more than 20 years. She had helped countless patients for various digestive conditions, but she couldn't help herself. She came into my office with two grocery bags full of supplements and a box filled with various laboratory tests.

Her labs indicated she had recurring yeast and bacteria overgrowths and multiple food sensitivities. She had treated various parasitic infections with medications and herbs many times over the years, none of which made a substantial impact on her health. She had taken every supplement known in natural medicine to support her gastrointestinal tract. Many of them helped her digest her food and maintain regular bowel movements, but she was dependent on them for regular daily function.

Her diet was impeccable. She only ate organic foods and even had a small farm at her house for various vegetables, herbs, and spices. She never ate processed foods and rarely ate out. She said she needed to follow such a strict diet in order to function.

Her health began declining during the last year of her doctoral program 20 years ago. She had been under significant stress and also in a car accident that caused her to lose consciousness. She was taken to the hospital, told everything was fine, and released the same day. She said it took several weeks to feel stable after the accident, but she had never really been the same since.

Sarah had significant abdominal bloating and eczema all over her body. When I checked her pupil responses with light she immediately became nauseous and developed a headache. This finding and several others indicated her brain was not healthy.

I ordered several laboratory tests that indicated she had severe immune reactions to wheat germ agglutinin, the lectin portion of wheat, as well as antibodies to glutenin, a protein portion of wheat (I discussed both of these in the previous chapter). Standard tests screen for alpha gliadin only and not these other parts of wheat. This explains why Sarah's previous tests for gluten sensitivity came back negative.

She also had antibodies to her cerebellum and intestinal trans-glutaminase, which shows up in those with celiac disease. In other words, she was suffering from autoimmune reactions to gastrointestinal and brain tissue and a compromised gut-brain axis, which is the communication loop between the gut and the brain.

It became obvious Sarah needed to address her disrupted gut-brain axis. I had her immediately go off all grain products and I placed her on an intestinal permeability repair program. I also found many of her nutritional supplements used wheat as a filler, which is typical of some whole-food supplements. We implemented many of the strategies that will be covered in this chapter to re-establish integrity of the vagus nerve (which coordinates communication between the brain and the gut), support her autoimmunity, and improve her brain health with neurotransmitter support.

I took her off most supplements except the ones she depended on, focusing instead on nutritional support for her autoimmunity

and brain health. After several weeks she experienced dramatic changes in her digestive function for the first time in 20 years.
Datis Kharrazian, DHSc, DC, MS

• •

Sarah's case is a great example of how impaired brain function can affect the digestive system. Sarah's case is not unique. I have seen numerous patients from all over the world with chronic gastrointestinal complaints similar to Sarah's. If you suffer from poor brain function and chronic gastrointestinal complaints, you may need to learn how to address the intimate relationship between the gut and the brain, called the gut-brain axis.

The gastrointestinal tract consists of a long tube of muscle, nerves, intestinal bacteria, and an immune system. Collectively these different components are known as the "gut" (not to be confused with the term "gut" to describe belly fat). The communication between the brain and the gastrointestinal tract is known as the gut-brain axis and is bi-directional, meaning communication travels in both directions. If your brain is not working and you have chronic digestive symptoms, you may have an impaired gut-brain axis.[1][2][3]

Most people and even physicians are surprised to hear the brain and the gut communicate with each other. Conventional medicine separates the body into independent systems and doctors are trained to view the nervous system as separate from the gastrointestinal system, with the two having nothing to do with each other. Pick up any physiology book and you will see a chapter for every system, but no chapter explaining the intimate relationships between each of them.

Even worse, the standard health care model has created a medical specialty and drugs for each system. If you have constipation you take a laxative, if you have indigestion you take an antacid, if you have depression you take an antidepressant, and so on. It's no surprise the health care system is failing people despite billions of dollars and countless medications. The compartmentalized model of physiology is outdated and linear.

Fortunately, the world of science and research has exploded with insights into how these various systems interact with each other. Many journals and scientific symposiums have clearly established the interconnected web that is basic human physiology. For example, a recent review paper published in the journal *National Review of Gastroenterology and Hepatology* shows irritable bowel syndrome to be a result of disturbed neural function along the gut-brain axis.[4]

In this chapter I will simplify information about the gut-brain axis and review how you can support this system.

THE BRAIN'S ROLE IN THE GUT-BRAIN AXIS

The brain plays a major role in gastrointestinal function, including controlling the movement of food through the intestines (motility), releasing digestive enzymes to chemically break down food, and regulating blood flow that carries vital nutrients and chemicals to support gut health and repair. There is no question poor brain function can compromise gut health. This happens to many people and may even be happening to you.

One of the earliest signs of a poorly functioning brain is poor digestion. I am not referring to full-blown neurological or gastrointestinal disease, but rather to general poor brain function—poor memory, inability to find words, or difficulty learning new things—leading to an increasing difficulty digesting foods, constant episodes of bloating and gas, or alternating constipation and diarrhea. The health care model today overlooks these symptoms because they are not associated with disease, or it blames them on aging.

Gut-brain axis basics

Let's start with the basics of how everything works. Your brain constantly receives messages called "presynaptic inputs" and it constantly sends messages called "postsynaptic outputs." These inputs include visual stimulation from your eyes, touch sensation from your skin, sound from your ears, gravitational input to your joints and muscles, tastes from your tongue, and smells from your nose. These presynaptic inputs activate your brain, causing neurons to fire. The constant stimulation of neurons keeps them healthy and strong, just as physical exercise keeps your muscles healthy and strong. Your brain processes these presynaptic inputs and then sends messages to various parts of your nervous system, which is called "postsynaptic excitation."

Two major postsynaptic pathways make up the brain's total output. The first is the motor system, which is used to move your muscles. This accounts for only 10 percent of your brain's output and is volitional, which means you have voluntarily control over it, such as moving your arms and legs.

The autonomic postsynaptic pathways account for 90 percent of your brain's output and involve no voluntary control. They activate areas of your brainstem associated with heart rate, respiration, digestion, and other functions that are non-voluntary. In essence, 90 percent of your brain's output influences the digestive system and other autonomic functions.

Why is this important? When the brain ages, degenerates, or otherwise becomes impaired, total output lowers, which decreases activation of the brainstem. As a result, the brainstem cannot sufficiently activate the gastrointestinal tract and digestive imbalances arise.

● ●

Many people have heard we only use 10 percent of our brains but this is not true. We use 100 percent of our brains. The rumor is a misinterpretation of the fact that we use only 10 percent of our brain for voluntary control. The other 90 percent of our brain directs the non-voluntary autonomic function used to breath, control blood circulation, control our heart, and digest our food. Therefore, we use 100 percent of our brain and every nerve cell counts if we want to maintain our health.

● ●

THE GUT'S NERVOUS SYSTEM

The digestive system has its own nervous system called the "enteric nervous system." The brain communicates with the enteric nervous system through a large, meandering nerve called the vagus nerve. The term *vagus* is Latin for "wandering," as the vagus nerve emerges from the brainstem and wanders to all the organs of the body, including those in the digestive tract. The vagus nerve carries information to and from the brain, happening somewhat like this: The brain activates the brainstem, the brainstem activates the vagus nerve, and the vagus nerve stimulates the enteric nervous system. The enteric nervous system then stimulates intestinal muscles to move food along, also known as motility.[5] I will talk later about how the gut communicates with the brain.

Lack of sufficient output through the brainstem can impair the vagus nerve, which may result in poor motility and constipation. Poor motility is a concern because it leads to fermentation in the gut and the overgrowth of intestinal bacteria and yeast. Any time a patient with a poorly functioning brain complains of chronic constipation, a dysfunction in the gut-brain axis must be considered.

As the brain degenerates a person loses digestive ability first, then bowel and bladder control. These are situations in which seniors need to wear diapers. It's as if they return to the beginning of life as a baby. A baby's brain and gut-brain axis are not fully developed at birth, which is why babies cannot control their bowel and bladder until digestive function develops. This explains the correlation between a child learning to crawl, walk, and talk and his ability to eat solid food.

We can see gut-brain axis dysfunctions in childhood developmental delays. For example, a child who has difficulty speaking and learning to walk likely still wears diapers because he or she has not yet developed bowel and bladder control. The child may also suffer from poor gastrointestinal motility and constipation.[6]

As the gut-brain axis loses its efficiency the vagus nerve also loses the ability to activate the release of stomach hydrochloric acid (HCl) to digest proteins. People with low HCl may notice they can no longer digest high-protein foods such as meats and eggs without feeling like they have a brick in their stomach. Or they develop symptoms of burning from the undigested proteins putrefying in the stomach and creating an acidic environment. Many of these people are diagnosed with acid reflux as a consequence of poor gut-brain axis.

Enzymes secreted by the pancreas[7] digest fiber and starches, while the gallbladder releases bile to digest fats. If these systems falter due to poor gut-brain function, one may develop an inability to digest fiber-rich or fatty foods. This can also lead to gallstones. Of course there may be other factors to consider, but it's important to know brain degeneration can lead to poor digestion and malnutrition.

LEAKY GUT

An impaired vagus nerve also leads to the development of intestinal permeability, more commonly known as "leaky gut." In the lining of the small intestine cells join together to create what is called a "tight junction." These tight junctions form an impermeable barrier to protect the sterile bloodstream from the contents of the gut. A healthy gut breaks food down into low molecular weight particles small enough to cross the tight junctions. Signaling proteins open and close the tight junctions as necessary to regulate the transport of nutrients into the bloodstream.

Leaky gut happens when these tight junctions weaken and allow large, improperly digested proteins, bacteria, fungus, and other pathogens to cross the intestinal wall. As these proteins pass through the leaky gut they inflame the intestinal wall and cause a buildup of mucus. The mucus prevents the low molecular weight nutrients from crossing but does not keep out the larger, heavier undigested proteins. The consequence is both leaky gut and malabsorption (poor absorption of nutrients).

Researchers identified this mechanism using a test called the "mannitol and lactulose challenge." Mannitol is a small molecular weight sugar (monosaccharide) particle similar to the size of nutrients. Lactulose is a large molecular weight sugar (disaccharide) similar in size to undigested proteins.

The study involves ingesting both sugars and collecting a urine sample six hours later. In an individual with healthy digestion and no leaky gut, only the small-weight compounds are measurable in the urine. In a person with leaky gut the small-weight compounds are not found in the urine because a buildup of mucus prevented their absorption, but the urine does contain the large-weight compounds. This indicates a leaky gut with poor nutrient absorption.[8]

Also, because pathogens don't belong in the bloodstream they alert the immune system to attack and destroy. When a person has leaky gut this immune activation is constant, which may lead to inflammation causing pain, food sensitivities, rashes, brain health issues, and other imbalances. Because inflammation contributes to leaky gut, it becomes a self-perpetuating vicious cycle between the two.[9]

Poor brain health, brain trauma, or brain degeneration play a role in leaky gut by decreasing activation of the vagus nerve. This lack of activation inhibits blood flow to the intestines, which prevents the intestinal wall from functioning and regenerating normally. Combined with the other consequences of impaired vagal function—low HCl, poor enzyme release, poor motility, and yeast and bacteria over-growths—leaky gut develops.[10][11]

IDENTIFYING AN IMPAIRED VAGUS NERVE AND GUT-BRAIN AXIS

In a clinical setting we can identify an impaired vagus nerve and gut-brain axis through examination. For instance, since the vagus is responsible for bowel motility, a practitioner should be able to hear rumbling in the abdomen with a stethoscope. When the gut-brain axis is impaired, it is common to hear very little rumbling.

The vagus nerve is responsible for raising the uvula, the tissue in the back of your throat that looks like a punching bag. When you visit your doctor and say "ahh" he or she is looking for it to rise. When the vagus is not working well the uvula does not rise much.

The gag reflex is also not very responsive. When exam findings show these functions are poor in a person with chronic digestive problems and a poor brain function, it indicates a strong possibility the gut-brain axis is not working well.

It is not uncommon for doctors to ignore the gut-brain axis in patients with chronic gut complaints. Interventions such as enzymes, probiotics, and other digestive aids may improve digestive health, but the clinical focus should also support brain health to improve the gut-brain axis.

IMPROVING YOUR VAGUS NERVE

Like muscles, neurons need constant stimulation to be healthy. If you break your arm and wear a cast, the muscles shrink within a few weeks from reduced activity. Neurons are no different. Without activation they lose function. Remember, 90 percent of the brain's output goes through the brainstem. If a poorly functioning brain does not stimulate the vagus nerve, the result is reduced activation of the gastrointestinal tract.

In functional neurology, a discipline introduced by Dr. Ted Carrick, practitioners rehabilitate the vagus nerve through exercises that make it stronger. Brain pathways can be strengthened just like muscles.

For example, a person with weak biceps can make them stronger doing bicep curls, which develops proteins in the muscles to build strength. Functional neurology brain rehabilitation is no different. As you stimulate weak neurons they develop more proteins to become stronger. This is called the development of positive plasticity and can be done with any part of the brain. If you have a poorly functioning gut-brain axis and vagus nerve, neurological exercises can increase the plasticity and function of the vagus pathway.

Vagal exercises are easy to perform at home. I commonly prescribe the exercises below to my patients who have poor vagal tone and gut-brain axis failure.

Gargling

The first exercise is to gargle with water several times a day. The vagus nerve activates the muscles in the back of the throat that allow you to gargle. Gargling contracts these muscles, which activates the vagus nerve and stimulates the gastrointestinal tract.

Drink several large glasses of water per day and gargle each sip until you finish the glass of water. You should gargle long enough and deep enough to make it a bit challenging. A two-second light gargle may be equivalent to using a 2-pound dumbbell to strengthen your arm versus a 10-pound dumbbell. It will not work unless it is more challenging. Do this exercise for several weeks to help strengthen the vagal pathways.

Sing loudly

I also encourage my patients to sing as loudly as they can when they are in their car or at home. This works the muscles in the back of the throat to activate the vagus. This exercise may become a nuisance for family members, but I still recommend it.

Gag

I also have patients purchase a box of tongue blades so they can stimulate their gag reflex throughout the day. Do not to jab the back of your throat with the tongue blade and hurt yourself, just lay the tongue blade on the back of your tongue and push down to activate a gag reflex.

Gag reflexes are like doing push-ups for the vagus while gargling and singing loudly are like doing sprints. It will take some time using these exercises to strengthen vagal tone and the gut-brain axis. You need to perform them for several weeks to produce change, just as you would with weight training. You cannot go to the gym for just a few days and expect your muscles to grow. Nor can you perform these exercises for a couple of days and expect to see profound change, although it does produce change very quickly for some.

Coffee enemas

In patients with brain degeneration who are having significant difficulty with regular bowel movements, I encourage them to perform daily coffee enemas. Distending the intestines with an enema activates the vagus. The caffeine in the coffee stimulates intestinal motility by acting on cholinergic receptors. This allows the patient to relieve bowel contents, which is very important for overall health.

Many people notice bowel function improves over time and they can begin weaning off the enemas. This is because the enemas help develop positive plastic change in their vagal system pathways. Unfortunately, some people have such rapid brain degeneration that it outpaces the ability to gain positive changes. In this case the coffee enema is used to prevent impacted bowels.

A coffee enema is very easy to do. First you need to purchase an enema bag with an anal insert tube and a lubricant such as KY Jelly. Then make organic coffee and cool it to room temperature. (Do not use instant coffee as many brands are contaminated with gluten.) The next step is to fill the enema bag with coffee and lubricate the anal tip of the tube. You will then need to lie on your right side. It is best to perform this in the bathtub in case you spill anything. Then insert the tube into your anus and raise the bag with your hand so it is higher than your head. The higher you raise the bag the faster the bag will empty.

Once the coffee has drained from the bag into your intestines try to hold the contents in your bowel for five to 10 minutes. You will have urges to have a bowel movement, but hold the contents as long as you can. The coffee will stimulate the cholinergic receptors in your intestines and activate motility as well as stimulate your vagal system to develop plasticity. The cholinergic stimulation from coffee will also cause your gallbladder to contract, helping release liver metabolism end-products into your bowel for elimination.

If you do not have significant constipation but your gut-brain axis is compromised, it is still a good idea to build vagal tone (along with gargling, singling loudly, or performing gag reflexes on yourself). Loss of vagal tone is almost always secondary to poor brain function. Strategies to improve overall brain function are absolutely critical and will be examined throughout this book.

* *

Larry, 58, was a retired pediatrician. He was referred to my office by a friend of the family because he was suffering from chronic gastrointestinal complaints. He had had three fecalith obstructive surgeries. A fecalith is a stone of fecal material formed in the gastrointestinal tract due to lack of motility. All his surgeries and complaints were on his left side. He had come into my office to see what alternative approaches and natural compounds could offer him.

He had found that whenever he took fiber supplements for a few weeks he developed fecaliths. During the intake exam, it was obvious Larry's mental speed and memory were compromised. Larry's wife had to constantly interject to finish his thoughts.

When I examined Larry I heard very few bowel sounds and he had no gag reflex. These findings and his history indicated his chronic gastrointestinal issues and motility failure were from impaired brain inputs to the vagus and gastrointestinal tract. It also explained why taking fiber resulted in fecaliths. Because he didn't have the neurological input to move the fiber, it developed into a stone. Larry also presented with early signs of dementia and failure of his acetylcholine system.

I gave Larry gargling exercises to strengthen his vagus and supported his acetylcholine system. He noticed improvements in his digestion, but unfortunately I was not able to work with him on his early signs of dementia. He and his wife felt that was just normal aging and were satisfied with addressing Larry's digestive complaints. I have not seen Larry in years and think about him every now and then.

Datis Kharrazian, DHSc, DC, MS

* *

BRAIN DEGENERATION IS GUT DEGENERATION

As I have explained, when the brain loses function it reduces output to the vagus nerve, which leads to decreased gut function. But there are deeper concerns. Like the brain, the gastrointestinal tract has a nervous system that includes neurons, neurotransmitters, and electrical signals. Called the enteric nervous system, it is sometimes referred to as the "second brain."

Researchers have concluded mechanisms that degenerate neurons in the brain also degenerate neurons in the enteric nervous system.[12] We now know that many neurodegenerative diseases of the brain also indicate neurodegenerative disease in the gastrointestinal tract. Sometimes chronic gut problems are the first sign of brain degeneration.

As a matter of fact, Parkinson's disease has been found to cause degeneration in the gut before the brain.[13] Chronic constipation occurs years before a Parkinson's disease patient ever develops tremors. If your gastrointestinal symptoms are chronic and progressing, your brain is not working and you really need to take your imbalance seriously. It may not be Parkinson's disease, but it certainly suggests potential early neurodegeneration leading to failure of the gut-brain axis.

THE GUT'S ROLE IN THE AXIS

Up until now we have looked at how brain dysfunction can impair gut function, but now we will look at how the gut impacts the brain. At the end of the chapter I will summarize the vicious cycles of gut-brain axis disorders and provide suggestions for help.

The relationship between the brain and the gut is an exciting area of research today. It appears the gastrointestinal tract contains chemical messengers—peptides and hormones—that profoundly impact brain health. These gut peptides include substance P, neurotensin, galanin, cholecystokinin, various cytokines (immune messengers), and many other peptides.[14]

Gut peptides influence the brain's immune system and its neurotransmitter pathways. I will talk more about neurotransmitters later in the book, but neurotransmitters are brain chemicals that relay information between neurons and profoundly affect brain function, mood, personality, and more.

Studies have linked gut peptides to depression, mood disorders, schizophrenia, Parkinson's disease, and memory loss.[15] One amazing discovery showed the gut peptide ghrelin circulates from the gut into the brain's hippocampus, where it enhances memory and learning.[16]

Neurotensin has a close relationship with the dopamine system of the brain (dopamine enhances feelings of pleasure and reward) and plays a role in psychiatric and neurological disorders.[17] Cholecystokinin also functions as a neurotransmitter and plays a role in regulating both the digestive system and the brain.[18]

We know multiple communication pathways travel back and forth between the gut and the brain and that gut health affects brain function.[19] Perhaps you have noticed a particular food significantly affects your mood. For example, have you ever eaten something that made you bloated and then you became irritable and angry afterwards? Your mood swing developed right along with your digestive symptoms. This is an example of how a chemical introduced to your gastrointestinal environment immediately impacted your brain chemistry.

Gut flora and the brain

Researchers have also discovered our gut flora, the several pounds of bacterial organisms we carry in our intestines, affects brain chemistry. Healthy gut flora serve many beneficial roles. However, poor diets, stress, excess sugars and carbs, repeated antibiotic use, and other factors tip the balance of gut flora so that harmful bacteria outweigh the beneficial.

Newer studies implicate gut flora in mood disorders such as depression and in various psychiatric disorders.[20][21] Has taking antibiotics for several days ever changed your brain function or mood? It is quite possible the antibiotics could have imbalanced your gastrointestinal flora and thus your gut-brain neurochemistry.

Leaky gut and the brain

Leaky gut has also been shown to play a role in severe depression by allowing harmful bacteria into the bloodstream. These bacteria carry in their membranes lipopolysaccharides (LPS), large molecules that trigger inflammation. LPS inflame the gut wall and, once in the bloodstream, cause inflammation throughout the body, which can ultimately change brain chemistry and cause depression.

This mechanism is called the "cytokine model of depression" because it is associated with inflammation instead of neurotransmitter deficiencies (for which antidepressants or amino acids may relieve symptoms). Leaky gut increases production of inflammatory cytokines, which activate the brain's immune system, creating brain inflammation and degeneration. This alters how well neurons function and communicate, which can result in such disorders as severe depression.[22]

The scientific literature has numerous papers beyond the small selection I referenced that clearly illustrate the profound impacts of the gut on the brain. This may come as no surprise to anyone who has eaten foods that immediately altered their mood, personality, focus, or concentration.

If your brain is not working, you need to address not only the health of your brain but also the health of your gut. Gastrointestinal health means you have daily, regular bowel movements and don't regularly suffer from bloating, pain, burning, or other gastrointestinal symptoms. If you are constipated, have constant bloating, feel like you are not digesting your food, or have developed several food intolerances, your digestive system may need a tune-up.

• •

A patient told me her fiancé Mark had just been diagnosed with multiple sclerosis (MS). His MRI showed the characteristic plaque formations associated with the condition, and he was getting progressively worse every week.

Mark came into my office with muscle weakness and a limp. He had episodes of blurriness and double vision, and was unable to perceive sensations such as temperature and light touch in different areas of his body. His laboratory tests showed high levels of myelin antibodies, indicating his immune system was attacking his nervous system. He was depressed and very scared about what was going on.

Mark ate the standard American diet loaded with fast food, partially hydrogenated fats, processed foods, and sugar. His diet was almost completely deprived of good fats, or essential fatty acids. I placed Mark on a diet that completely restricted partially hydrogenated fats, fried foods, and inflammatory foods and had him take various forms of essential fatty acids. Within a couple of months

he noticed his MS was not progressing anymore and within six months all of his findings were either dramatically improved or gone. As soon as he felt better Mark would go back to his old ways of eating, and the symptoms would return in a few days. Mark's case is a great example of how a gut on fire is a brain on fire.
Datis Kharrazian, DHSc, DC, MS

• •

GUT ON FIRE EQUALS BRAIN ON FIRE

Poor gut health can do more than cause depression. A study published in the *Lancet* found subjects with inflammatory bowel disease developed white-matter lesions in the brain, as identified by MRI, with almost the same frequency as patients with multiple sclerosis (a disease of brain myelin destruction). Forty-two percent of patients with Crohn's disease and 46 percent of patients with ulcerative colitis had white matter lesions in their brain.[23] Several other studies have shown the same results.[24][25][26]

It is interesting to watch this mechanism at work in people. When the gut and the brain are "on fire" people don't experience pain. This is because neither the brain nor the mucosal lining of the intestinal walls have pain fibers. Instead of pain you might see bloating followed by brain fog—intestinal inflammation causes gut distention while brain inflammation slows the transmission of information from one neuron to another, resulting in brain fog.

For example, a person who is dairy-intolerant may notice her belly becomes distended when she eats dairy, she cannot find the right words when speaking, and she loses her ability to focus and concentrate. Food sensitivities, leaky gut, and gut flora imbalances can cause these inflammatory responses.

LEAKY GUT AND SYSTEMIC INFLAMMATION

When the digestive tract becomes inflamed, the normally tight junctions weaken and allow undigested foods, toxins, and bacteria into the bloodstream. As these compounds pass through the tight junctions they trigger the intestinal immune system, releasing inflammatory cytokines, or immune messenger cells.

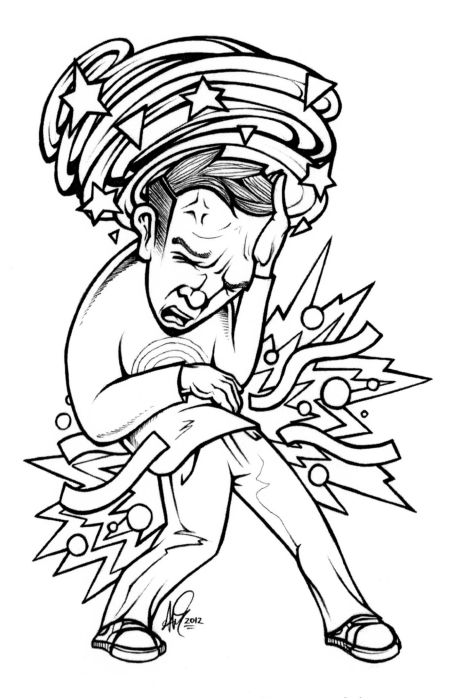

Inflammation in the gut can cause inflammation in the brain.
Symptoms include bloating and brain fog.

These cytokines make their way into the bloodstream, where they cause inflammation throughout the body (systemic inflammation), including in the brain, joints, heart, skin, blood vessels, and other tissues. This explains why systemic inflammation can manifest in so many different ways.

Once the intestinal mucosa is damaged, the gastrointestinal tract is unable to produce the enzymes necessary to properly digest food. This leads to malnutrition, further intestinal inflammation, further permeability, and the development of food sensitivities, bacteria overgrowths, yeast overgrowths, and poor intestinal immune health. In essence, leaky gut syndrome impacts a vast network of mechanisms, which all feed back into creating more leaky gut.[27] It is not uncommon for these individuals to suffer from chronic leaky gut for years or decades.

LEAKY GUT AND AUTOIMMUNITY

Research shows leaky gut can lead to autoimmune attacks in the brain.[28] This is because the chronic inflammation leaky gut causes makes the immune system overzealous, always on red alert. An overzealous immune system begins to have trouble distinguishing between real intruders, such as bacteria or undigested foods, and the body's own tissue. This creates a situation in which the immune system may erroneously tag body tissue, such as the thyroid gland, brain tissue, or pancreatic cells, for attack, thus creating an autoimmune reaction.[29][30][31][32]

In summary, systemic inflammation caused by leaky gut can impair brain health, degrade the blood-brain barrier, alter neurochemicals in the gastrointestinal tract (which then impact brain chemistry), inflame the brain, and trigger autoimmune reactions. If your brain is not working and you have symptoms of leaky gut, the concepts in this chapter can be very important for you.

SYMPTOMS OF A LEAKY GUT

How do you know if you have leaky gut? You may have mild to moderate gastrointestinal symptoms, such as such as bloating, gas, abnormal bowel movements, systemic inflammation, and food sensitivities. You may also have developed reactions to foods that include skin rashes, headaches, abdominal pain, joint pain, body aches, swelling, or bloating.

If leaky gut is inflaming the brain, this may cause depression or brain fog, thanks to decreased nerve conduction. Systemic inflammation from leaky gut can impact energy levels and cause fatigue, poor muscle endurance, or poor recovery from injuries. Or perhaps the inflammation is perpetuating pain from a previous injury and you have trouble healing.

It's also important to know many people with leaky gut have no intestinal or inflammatory symptoms, especially if they already eat a healthy, non-inflammatory diet. Therefore, leaky gut should always be considered for anyone with brain fog, persistent depression, chronic systemic inflammation, or any autoimmune condition—even if you don't have digestive symptoms.

MECHANISMS THAT CAUSE LEAKY GUT

Because leaky gut and inflammation may be responsible for numerous disorders, patients experience profound changes in brain function when they follow an anti-inflammatory diet.[33] [34] One of the most common things they report is improved mental clarity and cognition.

Before I discuss what to do about leaky gut, we need to know more specifically what causes it so you can identify the best strategies to improve your gut and brain health.

• •

I never thought at 25 I would have health problems. I was tired, anxious, and depressed and the symptoms seemed to have worsened in just a few short years. I didn't have the energy to be productive at home or at work, my mind was not crisp and clear like I knew it should be, and anything that required mental focus made everything worse. My medical doctor had all but given up on me, and I really didn't want to go back to her and get another prescription that either worked for only a short period or not at all.

I visited several alternative doctors and they all promised me they knew what was wrong and could fix it. I took vitamins, did detoxes, and did some things I don't even know what they were for, but I was desperate and would do anything. I jumped from doctor to doctor hoping to find an answer, any answer, but always coming up empty. I started giving up myself.

I finally found Dr. Steven Noseworthy in Tampa. The first thing he did that put me at ease was to say that he didn't know what the problem was, but he knew what tests to do to figure it out. That was different. After some blood tests and a stool sample he explained I had a blood-sugar problem and a gut infection.

He told me the brain is extremely sensitive to anything that causes poor energy production (such as a blood sugar imbalance) and that recent medical research shows depression often stems from inflammation. In my case my gut infection was affecting my brain. He helped me understand how my bad eating habits were destroying my health and that you don't have to live in the Third World to pick up a parasite.

We changed my diet and I learned to eat the right foods and to eat on a more regular basis. He recommended nutritional support for my brain, my blood sugar, and a protocol of special herbs to kill the gut infection and help repair the gut lining. As my blood sugar stabilized and my gut came under control, the fog lifted and I had the energy I needed to be a good mom and run my small business again. I was far less anxious and, for the first time in years, had a sense of hope that I could be healthy again. Thank you Dr. N!

a patient of Dr. Noseworthy
Steven A. Noseworthy DC, DACNB, DCCN
Tampa, Florida
www.DrNoseworthy.com

● ●

Diet and leaky gut

We can't discuss intestinal health without first addressing diet and lifestyle. If you eat the standard American diet (SAD) high in fast foods, processed foods, gluten, and dairy with little consumption of fresh fish, raw nuts and seeds, and vegetables, you are at risk for developing leaky gut. Basically, an inflammatory diet promotes leaky gut.

One of the most inflammatory foods, as discussed in the last chapter, is gluten. Clear evidence links gluten with intestinal inflammation and leaky gut.[35] Other inflammatory foods include dairy, processed foods, and fried foods. If you eat these foods daily you are basically on a pro-inflammatory diet that encourages leaky gut. If you have gluten sensitivity or celiac disease, it is almost certain you have leaky gut, unless it is ruled out with proper testing.

Excess alcohol consumption may also cause leaky gut. It is difficult to define excess. If you drink several drinks at one sitting more than once a week you probably drink too much. Excess alcohol produces acetaldehyde and reactive oxygen species, both of which induce intestinal leakiness.[36]

Chronic stress and leaky gut

Chronic stress is a major risk factor for developing leaky gut. The constant release of stress hormones suppresses immunity and inhibits blood flow and oxygenation of the intestines, leading to intestinal permeability.[37] Always being on deadline or always struggling with personal or financial concerns increases your risk for leaky gut, as does lack of sleep or physically overtraining. Unhealthy relationships, bad jobs, and other negative life situations can also influence stress.

Other factors

Several other mechanisms not directly related to diet and lifestyle may also promote leaky gut. Intestinal inflammation from infections (parasite, bacterial, or viral) may break down the proteins that keep the intestinal junctions tight.[38] The use of antibiotics and other medications can lead to intestinal permeability. Deficiencies in hormones such as testosterone, estradiol, progesterone, or thyroid may promote intestinal inflammation and reduce intestinal regeneration, leading to permeability.[39][40][41][42] Glycosylated end products from high blood sugar associated with diabetes may destroy the intestinal tight junction proteins.[43][44] Lastly, autoimmune diseases increase cytokines that activate a pro-inflammatory enzyme called inducible nitric oxide synthase (iNOS). iNOS destroys the proteins holding the tight junctions together, leading to intestinal permeability.[45][46]

In my experience the most common cause of intestinal permeability is a sensitivity to gluten and casein, or some other food intolerance. I find patients always underestimate their immune reactions to inflammatory foods and the effects of stress. However, several different factors typically promote leaky gut.

For patients who don't have much stress in their life and who maintain a healthy diet and lifestyle, the issue can be chronic gastrointestinal infections, such as from parasites. Parasite infections are more common than you may think, and you don't have to travel to a Third World country to develop one.

Also, don't forget the gut-brain axis—head trauma, progressed neuro-degeneration, or a brain not firing well into the vagus nerve can all cause leaky gut. Many times I have to wean a patient off inflammatory foods, support their gut nutritionally, place them on a strict leaky-gut diet, and improve their brain and vagal function to re-establish the gut-brain axis.

I will discuss management of leaky gut later in this chapter, but let's first look at laboratory testing for intestinal permeability.

LABORATORY ANALYSIS OF LEAKY GUT SYNDROME

To appreciate the best test for leaky gut you first need to understand what regulates the opening and closing of the tight junctions in the intestinal wall.

Our understanding of leaky gut and its relationship to autoimmune disease is based in large part on the discovery of zonulin. Zonulin is a protein that opens up the tight junctions of the intestinal wall, thus regulating how permeable the gut is.

Researchers first discovered zonulin while studying cholera. When given to animal subjects, zonulin created immediate intestinal permeability. This instigated further research into the leaky gut model. For people with celiac disease gluten triggers zonulin to open these junctions, thus promoting leaky gut. Zonulin also opens the junctions in the blood-brain barrier for those with celiac. But many researchers believe zonulin release is not specific to the celiac population. Some research shows gluten opens these junctions in *all* people. Occludin is another messenger protein that regulates intestinal permeability.[47] [48] [49]

Zonulin and occludin antibodies

As the gut becomes inflamed and breaks down during leaky gut, the immune system makes antibodies to zonulin and occludin. One way to evaluate leaky gut is to test for elevated zonulin-occludin antibodies. Because the blood-brain barrier also has zonulin and occludin, positive antibodies could indicate a leaky blood-brain barrier as well.

Actomyosin antibodies

Actomyosin antibodies are another indication of intestinal destruction. Actomyosin is a complex of proteins that makes up muscle fibers and contributes to muscular contractions. Antibodies to actomyosin signal a breakdown of the membrane lining the digestive tract and hence leaky gut. Actomyosin antibodies indicate gut damage is severe enough to break through the cells, not just open the spaces between cells. This type of damage takes longer to repair.

LPS antibodies

We also look at antibodies to LPS, the compound in the membranes of harmful bacteria that trigger inflammation. Immune cells in the mucosal lining do not interact with LPS unless the walls are breached due to leaky gut. Upon exposure, the immune system produces antibodies to LPS, another marker we can measure to identify leaky gut. LPS antibodies also signify gut flora dysbiosis, or the overgrowth of harmful bacteria in the digestive tract. When we see LPS antibodies in the bloodstream we know it is causing inflammation throughout the body and may have breached the blood-brain barrier, causing inflammation in the brain.

Antibodies to zonulin, occludin, actomyosin, and LPS are measurable with a blood test, now understood to be the most accurate way to analyze the immune response to intestinal permeability.[50][51][52][53][54][55] Cyrex Labs (Cyrexlabs.com) offers this test, called the Intestinal Antigenic Permeability Panel. If you do not have access to the lab test, then you can just begin the protocols for intestinal permeability I discuss next. The only problem with not having the lab test done is you don't have confirmation that leaky gut is the cause of your symptoms, and you cannot confirm whether you have corrected the problem with a follow-up test.

UNWINDING LEAKY GUT

Unwinding leaky gut consists of following a restricted diet and tak nutritional compounds that help reduce intestinal inflammation and repair the intestinal membranes. It can be followed for as few as three days for a quick recovery after an accidental exposure to a food that causes an immune reaction. More advanced cases may need to follow the program for as long as 90 days.

You will need to follow the diet religiously. I admit these gut-repair diets can be difficult and make you feel left out and deprived, especially in social situations. However, many people struggling with chronic autoimmune disease whose quality of life is seriously compromised have found it's a small price to pay for getting their health back.

Length of program

The length of the program can vary. The average leaky gut program will take 30 to 60 days. You will know it has been long enough when your symptoms resolve. However, if you have an autoimmune disease or celiac disease, staying on the diet and nutritional support long term provide the best outcome.

An autoimmune condition creates inflammation that affects the intestinal tight junction proteins. These people will struggle to varying degrees with intestinal permeability throughout their lives. There is no exact and predictable time frame for leaky gut support. You will have to follow the program for a length of time and then go off of it to evaluate how you feel. You will know if you need to go back on the program based on how you feel. If you do not have obvious symptoms, the only way you can be certain is with lab testing before and after the program.

- Average leaky gut: 30 days
- Moderate leaky gut: 60 days
- Severe leaky gut: 60–90 days
- Autoimmune disease or celiac disease: ongoing for life as needed

THE INTESTINAL PERMEABILITY PROGRAM

Eat regularly and do not allow yourself to become overly hungry—stabilizing blood sugar is a primary aim to avoid the stress of low blood sugar. For more resources supporting this diet, visit my web site.

Foods to avoid

- ALL sugars and sweeteners, even honey or agave
- High-glycemic fruits: watermelon, mango, pineapple, raisins, grapes, canned fruits, dried fruits, etc.
- Tomatoes, potatoes, and mushrooms
- Grains: wheat, oats, rice, barley, buckwheat, corn, quinoa, etc.
- Dairy: milk, cream, cheese, butter, whey, etc.
- Eggs or foods that contain eggs (such as mayonnaise)
- Soy: soy milk, soy sauce, tofu, tempeh, soy protein, etc.
- Alcohol
- Lectins—a major promoter of leaky gut—found in nuts, beans, soy, potatoes, tomato, eggplant, peppers, peanut oil, peanut butter and soy oil, among others
- Instant coffee: Many brands of instant coffee appear to be contaminated with gluten. It's important to eliminate it to be sure it's not an immune trigger.
- Processed foods
- Canned foods

Foods to eat

When confronted with this diet the first thing people ask is what *can* they eat. In fact you'll be eating the way people ate for most of human history—there's plenty of food that doesn't come from a factory or an industrialized farm.

- Most vegetables (except tomato, potatoes, and mushrooms): asparagus, spinach, lettuce, broccoli, beets, cauliflower, carrots, celery, artichokes, garlic, onions, zucchini, squash, rhubarb, cucumbers, turnips, and watercress, among others.

- Fermented foods: sauerkraut, kimchi, pickled ginger, fermented cucumbers, coconut yogurt, kombucha, etc. You will probably need to make your own or buy one of the few brands that are genuinely fermented and free of sugars or additives.

- Meats: fish, chicken, beef, lamb, organ meats, etc. Best choices are grass-fed and pastured meats from a local farm. Second best is organic. Avoid factory-farmed meats that contain antibiotics and hormones. For a source of good meat near you, contact your local Weston A. Price chapter leader or farmer's market.

- Low-glycemic fruits: apricots, plums, apple, peach, pear, cherries and berries, to name a few.

- Coconut: coconut oil, coconut butter, coconut milk, coconut cream

- Herbal teas

- Olives and olive oil

WHY NO GRAINS OR LEGUMES?

People with intestinal permeability often have difficulty digesting grains, starchy vegetables, legumes, and most sweeteners. A diet that eliminates these types of foods, called a monosaccharide (single sugar) diet, is more commonly known today as the Gut and Psychology Syndrome (GAPS) diet, or the Specific Carbohydrate Diet (SCD). (However, these diets allow foods not on the anti-inflammatory diet.) It is based on consuming a diet free of foods that contain disaccharides or polysaccharides, the more complex sugars and carbohydrates found in all grains, most beans, and most sweeteners. These complex sugars feed harmful bacteria in the small intestine that prevent its repair or proper function.

Grains and legumes are also high in lectins. Lectins have been shown to degrade the intestinal barrier,[56] and once in the bloodstream they may bind to insulin and leptin receptors (leptin acts in concert with insulin to control appetite). Some believe lectins may desensitize these receptors, thus contributing to insulin resistance and leptin resistance.[57]

The research is convincing, but more convincing is the experience of someone with chronic leaky gut issues who has transitioned into a grain- and legume-free diet. Many report a remarkable turn-around in their health. As with everything, this is individual. For some a gluten- and corn-free diet is enough. For others, however, especially those grappling with autoimmunity, a diet that removes grains, legumes, all sweeteners (including natural ones), and starchy vegetables (such as potatoes) can produce a significant improvement in health. More importantly, it is something you can do yourself without visiting a doctor.

Fortunately, ample support exists on the internet today. There are online "tribes" for many variations of this diet. They include Paleo, primal, GAPS, SCD, and probably some other variations I haven't heard of yet. Many, many people have adapted some version of this diet and are happy to help and support others.

I don't like to give hard and fast rules as to what to eat or how many grams of carbs to eat beyond the guidelines in this chapter. Your health and your symptoms are the best feedback—getting trapped in dogma or group-think can sabotage your ability to monitor your body and how it responds to the foods you eat. I do like people to pay attention to their blood sugar symptoms and markers and keep blood sugar stable, often a good basic guideline with which to start.

• •

Brenda was referred to my office suffering from fear and anxiety. She also complained of brain fog, which she described as having a blank feeling in her head when it came to searching for words and memories, and the sense that her overall mental function was in decline.

An assessment determined Brenda had poor GABA activity and a high level of brain inflammation. We also discovered a strong connection between her irritable bowel disorder and flare-ups of brain fog and the anxiety. In other words, when her bowel trouble worsened so did her mental function.

Within one week of support for brain and gut inflammation, Brenda was a different person. She reported no more inner tension, her anxiety was under control, and her mood swings stabilized. In

*addition, her gut pain was gone and she enjoyed weight loss and
a boost in energy.*
   David Arthur, DC, FACFN, DACNB, BCIM, DCCN
   Denver, Colorado
   www.DrDavidArthur.com

* *

NUTRIENTS TO HELP REPAIR THE INTESTINAL LINING

The emphasis of the anti-inflammatory diet is on reducing intestinal inflammation and repairing the intestinal membranes. The literature shows a variety of botanicals and nutritional compounds restore and maintain the intestinal lining. They support tissue during intestinal inflammation or discomfort, help regulate the enteric nervous system and motility, and support the secretion of digestive enzymes.

These nutrients can be taken therapeutically for anywhere from a few days to a few months, depending on the severity of the gut permeability. The time each person should be on a gut-repair diet and protocol depends on the individual and his or her circumstances. There isn't a time period set in stone; it depends on when you start to see symptoms diminish and disappear. A person with severe issues may need to adapt it for months or longer.

L-glutamine

L-glutamine is the preferred fuel source for the cells of the small intestine and has been shown to support the regeneration and repair of the intestinal lining. It has been shown to increase the number of cells in the small intestine and the number of villi on those cells, as well as the height of the villi. Studies have shown L-glutamine reduced permeability of the lining that accompanies leaky gut patterns that promote intestinal inflammation and the development of delayed food intolerances.[58 59 60 61 62 63 64 65 66 67 68 69 70 71 72 73 74 75 76 77 78 79]

Deglycyrrhizinated licorice

Deglycyrrhizinated licorice is a popular and substantially studied natural compound with flavonoids that helps repair the gastric and intestinal lining. Many different mechanisms have been shown with regard to its restorative properties, including stimulation and differentiation of glandular cells, protective mucus formation, protective mucus secretion, increased intestinal blood flow, and growth and regeneration of intestinal lining cells.[80 81 82 83 84 85 86 87 88 89 90 91 92 93 94 95 96 97 98 99]

Aloe leaf extract

Aloe leaf extract contains natural phytochemicals and powerful antioxidant properties that reduce intestinal inflammation, soothe the intestines, aid in intestinal wound healing, and have an anti-ulcer effect. It also appears to have antifungal properties, support cholinergic intestinal motility, and reduce intestinal pain and discomfort.[100 101 102 103 104 105 106 107 108 109]

Tillandsia

Tillandsia, also known as Spanish moss, has historically been used for intestinal irritation and allergies. Research on the plant has identified rich sources of flavonoids and other phytochemicals that provide antimicrobial activity and free radical scavenging properties.[110 111 112 113 114 115]

Marshmallow extract

Marshmallow extract has high content of mucilage that can sooth and help heal compromised intestinal barrier tissue. It is also rich in antioxidants that can support healing of tissue. It is has properties that inhibit hyaluronidase, the enzyme involved in the break down of hyaluronic acid, which promotes intestinal tissue destruction.[116 117 118]

Methylsulfonylmethane (MSM)

Methylsulfonylmethane is a rich source of natural sulfur that acts as a substrate for the antioxidant defense systems as well as support for substrates for hepatic phase II sulfation pathways. It has antifungal and anti-inflammatory properties that help support the compromised liver-gut axis.[119 120 121 122]

Gamma oryzanol

Gamma oryzanol is a mixture of plant sterols and ferulic acid esters from rice. It has been demonstrated to be a powerful antioxidant. Numerous papers have shown its effectiveness for gastrointestinal complaints, ulcers, irritable bowel syndrome, and non-specific gastrointestinal conditions. It has also been shown to modulate and support the enteric nervous system in its ability to activate intestinal motility and secrete digestive enzymes.[123 124 125 126 127 128 129 130]

Slippery elm bark

Slippery elm bark is very high in natural mucilage and helpful in soothing inflamed intestinal cells. It reduces contact of inflammatory proteins with the intestinal mucosa, thereby enhancing recovery from intestinal barrier compromise and inflammation.[131 132 133 134]

German chamomile

The chief constituent of German chamomile has been identified as esters of angelica root and tiglic acid, together with amyl and isobutyl alcohols. These constituents have been shown to enhance wound healing time and modulate prostaglandins and nitric oxide activity to provide gastric and intestinal protection.[135 136 137 138 139 140 141 142 143]

Marigold flower extract

Marigold flower extract constituents include saponins, carotenoids, flavonoids, mucilage, bitter principle, phytosterols, polysaccharides, and resin. It has been used historically for varied gastrointestinal complaints. It provides substrates for digestive enzyme production, reduces inflammation, and provides antibacterial activity.[144 145 146 147 148 149 150]

PROBIOTICS AND LEAKY GUT

If a probiotic must be refrigerated its integrity in the warm, acidic environment of the stomach is questionable. Therefore, I prefer shelf-stable strains that can withstand stomach acid so they survive intact to inoculate the upper and lower intestines.

I go for probiotics that reduce intestinal ammonia, improve intestinal pH, increase short-chain fatty acids, and improve the balance of healthy bacteria in the intestines. The strains below appear to combat toxins, candida, and bacterial infection, as well as nourish intestinal cells.

I also find arabinogalactan, a compound made up of protein and sugar, helpful for immune support. In addition to being a food supply for friendly bacteria, it also has been shown to stimulate and modulate the function of immune cells.

Saccharomyces boulardii

Saccharomyces boulardii is a non-pathogenic yeast and is resistant to stomach acid, bile, and pancreatic juices so it can tolerate varying pH levels of the intestines, unlike common probiotics, and inoculate the upper and lower gastrointestinal tracts effectively. Additionally, antibiotics have no impact on these organisms so the two can be taken together without contraindications. There are more than 200 papers published on the benefits of this probiotic. Numerous randomized, double-blinded placebo-controlled studies have shown Saccharomyces boulardii's efficacy for diarrhea, irritable bowel syndrome, intestinal infection, and inflammatory bowel conditions.[151 152 153 154 155 156 157 158 159 160 161 162 163 164]

Lactobacillus sporogenes

Lactobacillus sporogenes is a gram-positive, spore-forming, lactic-acid producing bacillus. It has the ability to pass through the stomach in its spore form and multiply rapidly in the intestines. The mechanism of action is thought to help replenish the quantity of desirable obligate microorganisms. At the same time it provides antagonizing effects on pathogenic microorganisms.[165 166 167 168 169 170 171]

DDS-1 Lactobacilli acidophilus

The DDS-1 Lactobacilli acidophilus strain has been investigated extensively and is considered the most stable bacterial probiotic resistant to adverse conditions such as heat, humidity, oxygen, and light. The DDS-1 strain produces natural antibiotic acidophilin and inhibits the growth of 23 toxin-producing microorganisms. It also produces enzymes to digest protein, fat, and lactase and produces B vitamins, folic acid and B-12. Lastly, it produces hydrogen peroxide to fight adverse bacterial and yeast overgrowth. Numerous papers have found it effective for diarrhea, intestinal bacteria and yeast overgrowths, and intestinal inflammation.[172 173 174 175 176 177 178 179 180 181 182 183 184 185 186 187 188 189 190 191]

Arabinogalactan

Arabinogalactan is a highly-branched polysaccharide that is non-digestible and resists breakdown by intestinal enzymes, so it can populate the large intestine and ferment into powerful supportive colonic bacteria. It has been shown to increase the production of healthy and beneficial microorganisms including short-chain fatty acids and beneficial microflora. It has also been shown to decrease the adverse generation of intestinal ammonia. Lastly, these compounds have been shown to demonstrate significant impacts in improving the integrity of the gastrointestinal immune system.[192 193 194 195 196 197 198 199 200 201 202 203 204 205 206]

ADVANCED LEAKY GUT SUPPORT

Many people with advanced gut problems have significant issues with candida overgrowth, fungus, bacterial infections, or parasites. In these cases, eradicating these organisms is necessary to calm the inflammation and allow the digestive lining to repair.

However, it's also necessary to tread gently in this territory. Too aggressive of a detox makes some people very ill with symptoms of nausea, vomiting, diarrhea, or other effects. Therefore, it's important to always start slowly and with small doses when taking gut detoxifying compounds.

Yeast and fungal overgrowth

Yeast and fungal overgrowths are well known for accompanying and contributing to leaky gut. Certain botanicals have been shown effective in combating these growths.

When used in combination the following botanicals have demonstrated broad-spectrum anti-fungus, anti-mold, and anti-ova properties. They inhibit the growth of molds, yeast, and fungus, and they help correct the unhealthy microbial environment produced by these microorganisms.

Undecylenic acid

Undecylenic acid is a natural 11-carbon monounsaturated fatty acid derived from castor oil that has been shown to be very powerful for mold, yeast, and fungus inhibition. It has demonstrated antifungal properties and helps support the healthy balance of the intestinal and vaginal flora as well as inhibit the morphogenesis of Candida albicans. Its mechanism of action is thought to be its ability to interfere with yeast, mold, and fungal fatty acid biosynthesis by disrupting the pH of the cell cytoplasm and preventing the development of the pathogenic organism into the active hyphae form.[207 208 209 210 211 212 213 214 215 216 217 218 219 220 221]

Caprylic acid

Caprylic acid is a medium chain fatty acid found naturally in coconut oil, palm oil, and butter fat, as well as in milk from humans, cows, and goats. It has been used as a natural antifungal and anti-yeast product for almost 50 years. The short length of its carbon chain allows it to easily penetrate the walls of fungus and yeast. Caprylic acid is thought to dissolve the cell membrane of yeast, causing changes in fluidity and permeability that leads to membrane disaggregation.[222 223 224 225 226 227 228]

Uva ursi

Uva ursi has been used medicinally since the second century. Its constituents include Arbutin, hydroquinone, and tannins. These constituents have been shown to have antimicrobial properties and also have astringent effects, helping to shrink and tighten mucus membranes and reduce inflammation. It has historically been used to support chronic diarrhea, urinary tract infections, and to reduce uric acid. Yeast organisms produce large amounts of uric acid by activating uric acid synthase and promoting inflammation.[229 230 231 232 233 234 235 236 237 238 239 240 241]

Cat's claw

Cat's claw has been used in Peruvian medicine for hundreds of years for a wide range of health problems. It is rich in a diverse set of alkaloids, glycosides, and proanthocyanidins that seem to enhance the gastro-intestinal immune system, dampen inflammation, and provide antimicrobial properties. Cat's claw may help prevent opportunistic growth of bacteria and yeast.[242 243 244 245 246 247 248 249 250]

Pau d'arco

Pau d'arco is a native to South America, where it has been used for hundreds of years to address a wide range of health problems. The chemical compounds in the plant include naphthoquinones, specifically lapachol and beta-lapachone. These constituents appear to have antifungal and antibacterial properties.[251 252 253 254 255]

Parasites and leaky gut

People can unknowingly host a variety of parasites, whether they are pinworms, roundworms or tapeworms, or something less obvious but just as destructive, such as single-celled protozoa: giardia, cryptosporidium, or amoebas.

The following botanicals work to provide natural support to help the body expel parasites, and have also been shown to demonstrate antioxidant properties that support anti-inflammatory mechanisms. When used together they also have an impact on pathogenic bacteria.

Wormwood extract

The active constituents of wormwood (*Arthemisia annua*) include absinthin, anabsinthin, and thujone. These constituents have been shown to have antiparasitic, antifungal, and antibacterial properties. Wormwood has also been shown to have antioxidant properties, increase digestive enzymes, and reduce intestinal discomfort. In addition to its antiparasitic properties, it has demonstrated therapeutic uses in the expulsion of parasitic worms and is classified as a vermifuge.[256][257][258][259][260][261][262][263][264][265][266][267][268][269]

Olive leaf extract

Olive leaf extract contains oleuropein phenolic compounds. These compounds have very powerful antioxidant, anti-inflammatory, and immune modulating properties. These activities have been shown to serve as a natural agent with antifungal, antimicrobial, antiviral, and antiparasitic properties. Various mechanisms have been discovered related to their anti-pathogenic effects, including inhibiting pathological organism reproduction, altering pathogenic organisms to build cell walls, altering protein production of pathogenic organisms necessary for replication, inhibiting assembly of pathogenic organisms at the cell membrane, interference of reverse transcriptase and protease production of the pathogen, and enhanced formation of the immune system cells to combat the pathogenic organism.[270][271][272][273][274][275][276][277][278][279][280][281][282][283][284][285]

Garlic extract

Garlic (*Allium sativum*) is a rich source of thiosulfinates and allicin. Garlic has been used for various medicinal purposes by many different cultures for thousands of years. The thiosulfinates' mechanisms of action have been extensively studied in vitro and in animal and human clinical trials for various conditions. It is very clear that it contains antiparasitic, antibacterial, and antifungal properties. Additionally, it does not appear to compromise the healthy gut bacteria despite its antiparasitic and antimicrobial effect.[286][287][288][289][290][291][292][293][294][295][296][297][298][299][300][301]

Black walnut extract

Black walnut (*Juglans nigra*) is rich in tannin, juglandin, juglone, and juglandic acid content. These constituents are known to have antiparasitic, antifungal, and antimicrobial activity. It has classically been used for its vermifuge properties of expelling tapeworms, pinworms, and ringworms. It is also very well known for its intestinal yeast overgrowth management.[302 303 304 305 306]

H. pylori and bacterial overgrowth

H. pylori is a naturally occurring bacterium that lives in the highly acidic environment of the stomach. Many people today experience an overgrowth of H. pylori, which researchers discovered to be the cause of stomach ulcers. An H. pylori infection can cause symptoms of bloating, nausea, or a burning pain in the stomach an hour or so after eating. It also can cause hypochlorhydria, or too little stomach acid, which impairs digestion and nutrient absorption and, paradoxically, causes symptoms of heartburn and acid reflux.

Imbalanced gut flora and bacterial infections are typically a problem with leaky gut.[307 308] As part of their intestinal permeability test, Cyrex Labs measures levels of LPS antibodies. Remember, LPS are in the cell walls of pathogenic bacteria and provoke an immune reaction. When higher than normal levels of LPS antibodies show up on the test, it indicates that bacterial overgrowth plays a role in leaky gut by triggering inflammation. Eradicating these bacteria is a helpful tool to restoring gut integrity.

The following botanicals have been shown to be effective in eradicating excess H. pylori and serve as good all-around antibacterial and antifungal substances. They have also been shown to support a healthy immune response in the gut, inhibit intestinal inflammation, serve as an intestinal antispasmodic, and support intestinal mucus membranes.

Berberine

Plants with high Berberis alkaloids have been used in both Chinese and Ayurvedic medicine for centuries. These plants appear to demonstrate significant antimicrobial activity against a variety of bacteria,[309 310 311 312] fungi,[313 314] protozoans,[315 316 317] helminths,[318] chlamydia,[319 320] and viruses.[321] Berberine has demonstrated the ability to inhibit the growth of giardia lamblia, trichomonas and entamoeba histolytica.[322] These plants also demonstrate anti-inflammatory properties such as inhibiting arachidonic acid-induced thromboxane A3 release, and the ability to activate macrophages.[323 324]

Yerba mansa

Yerba mansa is not related to the berberine-containing plants chemically or botanically, but it is used to treat similar conditions. The active compound in Yerba mansa is methyleugenol, an antispasmodic similar in chemical structure to compounds found in nutmeg, which is used to treat irritable stomach.[325] It also appears to have anti-inflammatory effects and is used to treat inflammation of the mucus membranes.[326] The plant has also been shown to have antifungal properties.[327]

Oregano extract

Oregano extract has been used for the management of gastrointestinal-related infections in natural medicine for hundreds of years. It appears to have properties that inhibit enteric parasites and has immunostimulatory effects on lymphocyte production.[328 329 330 331 332 333]

CHAPTER SUMMARY

• If you suffer from poor brain function and chronic gastrointestinal complaints you may need to learn how to appropriately address your gut-brain axis, the intimate relationship between the gut and the brain.

• Symptoms of an impaired gut-brain axis include:
  • Difficulty digesting foods
  • Constipation or irregular bowel movements
  • Increased bloating and gas
  • Distention after meals
  • Intolerance to food types such as proteins, starches, and/or fats
  • Frequent abdominal discomfort after eating

• One of the earliest signs of a poorly functioning brain is poor digestion.

• The digestive system has its own nervous system called the "enteric nervous system." The brain communicates with the enteric nervous system through a large, meandering nerve called the vagus nerve. Poor brain function impairs the vagus nerve, which may result in constipation and general poor digestive function. Any time a patient with a poorly functioning brain complains of chronic constipation, a dysfunction in the gut-brain axis must be considered.

• Studies have linked poor gut health to depression, mood disorders, schizophrenia, Parkinson's disease, and memory loss.

• Gut and brain inflammation don't cause pain because neither the brain nor the intestinal walls have pain fibers. Instead intestinal inflammation causes gut distention (bloating) while brain inflammation slows the transmission of information from one neuron to another, resulting in brain fog. Leaky gut syndrome impacts a vast network of mechanisms, which all feed back into creating more leaky gut.

• Leaky gut can also lead to autoimmune attacks in the brain. This is because the chronic inflammatory response leaky gut causes makes the immune system overzealous, always on red alert. An overzealous immune system constantly on the prowl for stuff to attack begins to have trouble distinguishing between real intruders, such as bacteria or undigested foods, and the body's own tissue. This creates a situation in which the immune system may erroneously tag body tissue, such as the thyroid gland, brain tissue, or pancreatic cells, for attack, thus creating an autoimmune reaction.

• Although brain degeneration can cause leaky gut, more often it is the result of such factors as poor diet, chronic stress, blood sugar imbalances, chronic inflammation, autoimmunity, antibiotic use, or hormone imbalances.

• Unwinding leaky gut consists of following a restricted diet and taking nutritional compounds that help reduce intestinal inflammation and repair the intestinal membranes. It can be followed for as few as three days for a quick recovery after an accidental exposure to a food that causes an immune reaction. More advanced cases may need to follow the program for as long as 90 days. People with autoimmune disease or other chronic conditions may find sticking to the diet as a way of life improves health.

• A variety of botanical compounds, nutrients, and probiotic strains have been shown to help repair leaky gut along with a leaky-gut diet.

Chapter Ten

BRAIN INFLAMMATION

One of the reasons your brain may not be working is because of inflammation in the brain, also referred to as "neuroinflammation." Do you have any of these symptoms?

SYMPTOMS OF NEUROINFLAMMATION

- Brain fog
- Unclear thoughts
- Low brain endurance
- Slow and varied mental speeds
- Loss of brain function after trauma
- Brain fatigue and poor mental focus after meals
- Brain fatigue promoted by systemic inflammation
- Brain fatigue promoted by chemicals, scents, and pollutants

• •

Michelle, 52, was a defense lawyer. Her work schedule was so stressful that at times she suffered from social isolation, frequent crying, and even emotional meltdowns. She had more responsibilities than her brain could handle. When she came into my office she started crying within minutes of telling me her story. She told me she had days where she could not think straight or find the words she was looking for. Entire days were a blur where she felt almost useless because her brain would not work. Afraid she might be developing Alzheimer's she visited a neurologist, who gave her a clean bill of health after a 10-minute visit.

When I examined Michelle it was clear she did not have Alzheimer's or a disease of the nervous system. Nevertheless, her brain was not functioning at its peak. Her diet was atrocious and void of antioxidants, she smoked cigarettes every day, and she drank way too much alcohol to cope with her stress. It was very apparent her stress load was out of control and her lifestyle full of inflammatory triggers.

After the examination and history I ordered a series of tests, but the results would not come back for a couple of weeks. She insisted she could not wait that long and needed help immediately. I placed her on a brain inflammation protocol of high doses of various flavonoids and antioxidants that have been shown in the literature to dampen brain inflammation by suppressing inflammatory activity of microglia, the brain's immune cells.

I told her to increase the dose every day to the point her brain fog went away. After a week of taking the supplements she found the dose that cleared her brain fog and allowed her to function again. Because her response to the supplements was positive, it indicated brain inflammation as a diagnostic mechanism. Although the supplements made her feel much better they were still a band-aid approach—her case required tackling the issues causing the brain inflammation.

Brain inflammation can destroy brain tissue just as chronic joint inflammation can destroy joint tissue, leading to joint deformity, stiffness, and pain. If your brain is not working well, you may be suffering from brain inflammation. This is serious because brain inflammation is associated with a significant risk for various degenerative brain diseases, including Alzheimer's. Even if you do not have brain inflammation, taking antioxidants and certain natural flavonoids can protect your brain similar to the way taking certain antioxidants can protect your heart.

In this chapter I will teach you how to recognize brain inflammation and what mechanisms promote it. I also will give you the list of compounds researchers have found help dampen brain inflammation and potentially protect your brain. The information in this chapter is so critical that I personally incorporate all of these strategies for myself and my family despite the absence of any

symptoms. If your brain is on fire you need to put the fire out before
you lose brain function.
    Datis Kharrazian, DHSc, DC, MS

● ●

In this chapter I am going to cover the concepts of inflammation, because it rapidly ages the brain. By learning ways to dampen brain inflammation you can preserve your brain health and slow the aging process, or even just boost mental function and overall well-being, which is useful at any age.

Inflammation in the body—chronic joint pain, infections, inflammatory bowel disease, or an unmanaged autoimmune condition—releases immune messengers called cytokines. These cytokines send messages across the blood-brain barrier that activate inflammation in the brain, which alters brain function and destroys brain tissue.[1][2][3][4][5][6][7] Likewise, inflammation or degeneration in the brain can activate the body's immune system and trigger systemic inflammation that results in such issues as joint pain, gut pain, skin disorders, or more.[8][9][10][11][12][13] In the literature this is referred to as "neurogenic inflammation."

For example, researchers are studying this model as a major cause of chronic depression, which in some cases is the result of brain inflammation decreasing the firing rate of neurons in the frontal lobe.[14][15][16] In these cases, people typically don't respond to antidepressants since the medications do not address the underlying inflammation.

● ●

Studies of brain lesions in animals have found relationships
between brain function and immune function. In these studies,
researchers measure the immune status prior to and after inducing
a brain lesion. They found that a brain injury can distort various
aspects of immune function, causing drops in white blood cells,
T-cell dysregulation, B-cell dysregulation and altered natural killer
cell function, and promoting leaky gut syndrome.[17][18][19][20][21][22]

● ●

It is always important to consider this inflammatory cytokine model of depression when someone complains of brain fog, chronic pain, swelling, and inflammation. Addressing the causes of inflammation and providing natural compounds to dampen neuroinflammation can produce very promising results.

While inflammation in the body can inflame the brain, poor brain health can inflame the body. Good brain function is critical for maintaining a healthy immune system that does not become overzealous or out of control. Many practitioners have seen a correlation between poor brain health and chronic inflammation or autoimmunity.

For example, a person who sustains a head injury suddenly develops an autoimmune disease. Or a problem in brain function sparks multiple food intolerances. When brain injury or impairment triggers an inflammatory response in the body it's known as a "brain-immune dysregulation disorder." This is an emerging field in neuroimmunology and researchers now understand the brain profoundly impacts the body's immune system. Compromised brain health can alter immune regulation and modulation (balancing) of inflammation throughout the entire body.

● ●

A 27-year-old woman came to me complaining of episodes of depression, mood fluctuations, and memory loss. She had suffered two wakeboarding accidents a couple of weeks apart in which her head impacted the water, rendering her unconscious. After she partially recovered from the first accident, she went wakeboarding again and had the second accident.

She experienced immediate loss of memory for several days after the second accident and felt very disconnected. Her symptoms continued to worsen to the point she began experiencing severe anxiety and panic attacks, and her doctor prescribed her an antidepressant. After taking the antidepressant, she experienced severe chest pains. Continued medical treatment of her condition consisted of trials of various medications.

After examining her I supported her condition nutritionally with compounds to reduce inflammation and increase oxygenation to the brain. She increased her dose of these compounds every four hours until the brain fog and mood instability dissipated.

An MRI scheduled the following day by her neurologist reported abnormalities in several areas. Her MD thought it might be multiple sclerosis and ordered a spinal tap.

The patient continued on the compounds for brain inflammation and oxygenation multiple times a day. After two weeks she attempted to reduce her dose and found her symptoms returned. Upon returning to the previous dosage the symptoms again dissipated. After three weeks at the original dosage, she reported she was able to sleep through the night.

Several months later she was able to reduce her dosages successfully. Her moods had stabilized and her memory was returning. Over the next four months she was able to reduce the dosages of the nutritional compounds significantly, so that she was taking a smaller amount only once a day.

Seven months after our first visit her neurologist performed a follow-up MRI and told her the abnormalities on her brain were either smaller or gone. After another four months I contacted the patient for a follow-up evaluation. She reported none of the previous symptoms and even said she was pregnant.

David Peterson, DC

St. Louis, Missouri

www.wellnessalternatives-stl.com

● ●

THE BRAIN'S IMMUNE SYSTEM

At the root of brain inflammation are microglia cells, the brain's immune soldiers. They determine whether your brain is inflamed and aging too quickly. Microglia cells have received attention only in the last 20 years or so. Prior to that they were considered merely to be glue that held the brain together; glia is the Latin word for glue.

Newer research, however, shows the complex interplay between microglia and hormones, cytokines, neurotransmitters, and other chemical messengers in the body and brain. There are 10 glia cells for every neuron in the brain, and if you weigh the brain, more than 50 percent of it is glia cells. In other words the brain is more glia cells than neurons.

Microglia cells are either in a resting state or an active state. In normal conditions the microglia perform many functions vital for healthy brain function. They dispose of dead neurons, beta amyloid plaque, the substance that predisposes one to Alzheimer's, and other cellular debris that may interfere with healthy communication between neurons. However, in a heightened state of activation, they create an overzealous inflammatory immune response that causes brain inflammation, or neuroinflammation.

Neuroinflammation leads to both immediate and long-term complications. Short-term consequences are that it immediately hinders the transmission speed and conductivity of neurons, which means neurons fire more slowly. This slows down brain function and creates symptoms of brain fog, slower mental speed, slower recall, and slower reflexes.

Another immediate consequence of neuroinflammation is that it shuts down energy production in the cells so that brain endurance plummets. This causes limited endurance for reading, driving, or mental tasks, and may also cause depression.

A longer term of consequence of chronic neuroinflammation is neuron death and the development of neurodegenerative disorders.

Many things can activate the microglia and inflame the brain, such as diabetes, high-carbohydrate diets, poor blood circulation in the brain, and inflammatory triggers from areas outside of the brain, including an inflamed gut or environmental pollutants. In the end it comes down to whether the brain's microglia cells have been activated. Luckily, there are things you can do about it.[23][24]

Mechanisms that increase the risk of activating brain microglia[25][26][27][28][29][30][31][32][33][34]

- Diabetes and high-carbohydrate diets lead to the production of glycosylated end products, which activate the microglia cells
- Lack of oxygen from poor circulation, lack of exercise, chronic stress response, heart failure, lung disorder, anemia
- Previous head trauma
- Autoimmune reaction to neurological tissue
- Dietary gluten for those who are gluten intolerant
- Low brain antioxidant status

- Alcohol and drug abuse
- Environmental pollutants
- Systemic inflammation
- Inflammatory bowel conditions
- Compromised blood-brain barrier

• •

I had suffered from extreme fatigue and depression for years and was diagnosed with Hashimoto's about 10 years ago. I felt better after being put on a natural thyroid hormone, and became pregnant with my first child. The fatigue and depression returned shortly after giving birth, which my doctor blamed on postpartum depression, although I also struggled with insomnia, weight gain, and constipation. A friend referred me to Dr. Geronimo and within a couple of months of working with him, I began to see marked improvements in my energy levels. It's been a rough battle, but I have lost more than 40 pounds and finally feel like I have my life back.

However, this story is about my daughter. It is an embarrassing story for my husband and me but I hope it will give others hope. When my daughter was around 18 months old she began exploring her private area. At first, I thought that it was normal childhood behavior and didn't think much of it, however, it evolved into an increasingly persistent coping mechanism. By the time she was three she would start rubbing herself when she had tantrums or became anxious, such as when she was around strangers or in a public area, and the behavior worsened when she started school. You can imagine the embarrassment this caused her teacher, other parents, and us.

We spent thousands of dollars on doctors, MRIs, and ultrasounds and my daughter was diagnosed with "persistent genital arousal disorder." The treatments they offered ranged from nerve blocks to surgery, procedures my husband and I decided we could not agree to.

I asked Dr. G if her behavior could have originated from a brain development issue since I was coping with Hashimoto's during pregnancy. He said it was possible since the mother's immune health affects brain development of the fetus. He had just started a functional neurology program and wanted to apply what he learned along with some nutritional approaches.

The first thing we did was remove gluten and dairy from her diet, which was not easy. He then put her on high doses of DHA and had me perform functional neurology eye movement and balance exercises with her. It took four to five months of much time and work, but my daughter's rubbing issues are about 90 percent less frequent, and she no longer does it in public.

She's in second grade now and has fewer tantrums, is less clumsy, and her reading and writing have improved. My parents insist she just grew out of it, but I know all the hard work with the diet, supplements, and brain exercises were crucial to her development. I don't know what I would have done without Dr. G's guidance and I cannot thank him enough.

A patient of Dr. Geronimo
Rommel Geronimo, DC
San Diego, California
www.fecsd.com

Microglia have no off switch

The body's immune system involves many different components, each playing a specific role in the immune response, whether it's to a virus or a splinter. Part of that response is a fine-tuned orchestration for turning *off* the immune response when necessary. Otherwise a splinter might continue to produce swelling and pus long after it has been removed.

Unfortunately, for all its miraculous wonder, the brain is quite simplistic when it comes to inflammation. Once microglia become overstimulated, they are like fierce little Chihuahuas with AK-47s. They startle at anything that comes by, firing off their machine gun in a 360-degree circle, including at healthy brain tissue.

When microglia are overactivated, neurons die. With no built-in off switch, the microglia can continue on their rampage for their entire lifespan, destroying healthy brain tissue and speeding brain degeneration in the process. That there are 10 microglia cells for every neuron doesn't help, nor does it help that they recruit other microglia cells during the inflammatory process.

Microglia activation induces a domino effect in which one microglia activates another and so on. These activated cells perpetuate an ongoing vicious cycle that can lead to chronic and persistent neuroinflammation that may last for weeks, months, or years.

As I discuss in Chapter Seventeen, healthy hormone levels dampen microglia activity, keeping their overactivity in check. Later in this chapter I'll introduce some natural compounds found in plants and spices that researchers have discovered are highly effective in dampening microglia.

Once again, it's important to point out that microglia cells are not all bad. The problem is they don't operate well in an environment that includes processed, genetically modified, and inflammatory foods, heavy metals, bacteria, environmental pollutants, or other harmful substances—all of which heighten their activation.

• •

At the age of 19 Daniel was in a severe car accident. He was flown by helicopter to a large trauma hospital, diagnosed with a shear brain injury, and remained in a coma for three months. Daniel left the hospital in a wheelchair he controlled with his mouth. His mother refused to accept this was his only option.

The first time I saw Daniel he could not walk, his speech was difficult to understand, and his memory was virtually nonexistent. Daniel could not move his right hand at all, and his left hand had severe dystonia, shaking uncontrollably whenever he moved it. He had double vision 50 percent of the time and his eyes moved uncontrollably.

We started a functional neurology rehab program with Daniel and soon realized there was hope. He still had brain function. Unfortunately, only two weeks later, Daniel's brain began fatiguing faster than it was recovering. It was at this point that I highly recommended we add a nutrition program to dampen inflammation and support brain function.

Almost overnight Daniel improved significantly. Over the next several months Daniel returned to college and ultimately resumed his studies in engineering. He walks independently, carries a full course load, and works more than 20 hours a week at an electron-

ics store. He has made miraculous improvements and achieved outcomes considered impossible by conventional medicine.

While he still limps and is unable to drive a car independently, Daniel is a long from way from living life in a wheelchair he operates with his mouth. To this day Daniel continues to support his brain health with nutrition. He confirms this choice as the single most important step in his recovery since leaving the hospital.

Chris Turnpaugh, DC, DABCN
Mechanicsburg, Pennsylvania
www.drchristurnpaugh.com

• •

Key concepts related to brain inflammation

- Your brain is saturated with immune cells called microglia cells.
- The microglia cells perform many important functions under normal conditions to help transmission between neurons, such as removal of dead neurons and plaques.
- In a heightened state of activation, microglia create a persistent, self-perpetuating state of neuroinflammation.
- Microglia cells can become activated and promote neuroinflammation in response to inflammatory diets, head trauma, lack of oxygen, diabetes, environmental toxins, autoimmunity, and systemic inflammation.
- Neuroinflammation decreases the speed of neuron responses and leads to symptoms such as brain fog and depression. Chronic neuroinflammation leads to neuron death and neurodegenerative changes.

THE BLOOD-BRAIN BARRIER AND NEUROINFLAMMATION

One of the biggest risks to overactivating the microglia is a leaky blood-brain barrier. The blood-brain barrier is a finely woven mesh of astroglia cells and blood vessels that surrounds and protects the brain. It is designed to allow only nano-sized particles in or out as needed and keep unhealthy things out.

However, like the gut, it can become damaged and "leaky," allowing dangerous intruders to slip in and potentially trigger the ultra-sensitive microglia. The blood-brain barrier is extremely vulnerable to various aspects of modern life, such as inflammation and high cortisol from chronic stress. The most common symptom of a leaky blood-brain barrier is brain fog or reduced brain function after exposure to environmental insults such as gasoline fumes, chemical cleaning products, or inflammatory foods.

The good news is that even though the blood-brain barrier degrades easily, it also has the potential to regenerate quickly. For instance, high stress degrades the blood-brain barrier, but normalizing stress can allow it to repair. This doesn't mean you have to quit your job and become a beach bum. Simply stabilizing your blood glucose and cortisol levels, reducing inflammatory triggers such as gluten, clearing up a gut infection or chronic virus, boosting your antioxidant system, and supporting anti-inflammatory mechanisms can help restore the blood-brain barrier and better protect your brain.

In addition to stress and systemic inflammation, other factors that degrade the blood-brain barrier are elevated homocysteine (homocysteine, measured by a simple blood test, is an inflammatory compound that elevates with B vitamin deficiency), alcohol, advanced glycosylated end products (these are free radicals made during diabetes and high blood glucose when glucose cannot enter the cells), and harmful free-radical compounds, such as pollutants or other compounds that trigger inflammation.

Causes for breakdown of the blood-brain barrier[35 36 37 38 39 40 41 42 43 44 45 46]

- Chronic stress
- Alcohol
- Elevated glucose and diabetes
- Chronic environmental toxic exposure
- Elevated homocysteine from B vitamin deficiency
- Poor diet and antioxidant status
- Systemic inflammation

The leaky blood-brain barrier challenge

The tight junctions of a healthy blood-brain barrier only allow nanoparticles, which are very tiny, to pass through while preventing the passage of antigens and environmental compounds.

GABA, a supplement popular for producing a calming, relaxing effect, exceeds the nanoparticle size and does not have a blood-brain barrier transport protein. Therefore, it technically cannot cross a healthy blood-brain barrier.[47][48][49] If you take GABA and notice it has an effect, then you probably have a leaky blood-brain barrier.

Take 800–1,000 mg of GABA and give yourself a two-to-three hour window to see whether it affects you. It is best to take GABA between 6 p.m. and 9 p.m., so you can sleep it off if it sedates you. If GABA causes relaxation, calming, and sedation, don't keep taking it regularly or you risk shutting your GABA receptor sites and a retest won't be accurate.

If the GABA causes anxiety, irritability, or panic this also indicates a permeable blood-brain barrier (for reasons explained in the neurotransmitter section). Eating some protein may help alleviate these symptoms.

Feeling no change after taking GABA is a good sign your blood-brain barrier is intact. GABA should produce no symptoms as GABA "bounces off" a healthy blood-brain barrier.

It's useful to do the GABA challenge periodically to see how various things might affect you. For instance, if you are gluten intolerant a GABA challenge can show you that eating gluten will cause leaky brain for a week or two (which can be restored simply by avoiding gluten).

If that's the case, then you know to be careful after an accidental exposure to gluten. This can mean making sure you get enough sleep, avoiding stressful situations, avoiding pesticides or pollutants, and being careful to avoid sugars, alcohol, and high-carbohydrate foods. All these steps will help reduce inflammation and the possible exposure of your brain to antigens that could trigger the microglia cells.

In addition to removing the triggers for leaky brain, certain nutritional compounds have been shown very useful in repairing the blood-brain barrier, which I will discuss later.

Why heavy-metal chelation can be dangerous if you have a leaky blood-brain barrier

In my thyroid book I discussed one reason doing chelation, a popular therapy that involves pulling heavy metals out of the body, can be dangerous. Some people may react to a heavy metal the way one reacts to peanuts or pollen, provoking an immune response. In other words, someone may have a "mercury immune sensitivity," which is more common than people realize. When that's the case, chelation triggers this sensitivity, which can be devastating to brain health. This sensitivity is common among children with autism and a reason why they may regress during chelation.

Chelation can also be dangerous in the event of a leaky blood-brain barrier. I would never expose a person to chelation if they failed the leaky-brain challenge. Chelation pulls toxic metals out of body tissues and into the bloodstream for removal. When the blood-brain barrier is compromised, these chelated toxic metals can move from the bloodstream into the brain. This sets off the microglia cells on their endless inflammatory rampage and accelerates brain degeneration.

There are exceptions: In some cases when a neurodegenerative disease is severe and progressed and one will obviously fail a GABA challenge, it is assumed these toxic metals have already reached the brain and removing them might be advantageous. However, for a relatively healthy person who isn't suspected of having heavy metal toxicity in the brain yet who failed the GABA challenge, chelation can unnecessarily expose the brain to heavy metals.

● ●

When I first saw eight-year-old Matthew in my waiting room, he was sitting next to his mother, grimacing in pain. She looked exhausted. Matthew had undergone two surgeries to address a bacterial infection in his brain and to place a shunt to relieve the pressure caused by the buildup of fluid. Though the procedures were successful, they left Matthew with a persistent, intense headache that got much worse when he lay down.

Though this is not uncommon after brain surgery, Matthew's pain had not gone away as expected. Months later, Matthew was still in constant pain, as well as exhausted and anxious. As I sat with his mother discussing his case, I watched Matthew try to lie down on my exam table because of his exhaustion, only to grimace again from the pain when he put his head down. He repeated this attempt several times, eventually crying with frustration. This was all too much for such a young boy. His mother said that he used to be polite, social, and comfortable with himself. He was now angry, irritable, and anxious all the time.

Inflammation makes it hard for cells to make energy. Because Matthew's brain was still inflamed, his brain cells couldn't make the energy they needed to function normally. This created his headaches and mood changes.

What's worse, Matthew loved sweets, which provided reliable pleasure for a boy in a lot of pain. Unfortunately, the blood sugar instability this created meant that his body wasn't making much GABA, the neurotransmitter the brain uses to keep itself calm. Matthew's sweets habit was making his anxiety worse.

Matthew's brain inflammation and lack of GABA meant he was unlikely to respond successfully to neurological rehabilitation. Therefore, changing his brain chemistry was the first priority. I gave Matthew nutritional compounds to reduce brain inflammation and improve brain cell metabolism. I also asked his mother to get him off sweets so he could make GABA, and off gluten and dairy to further reduce his inflammation.

When Matthew returned to my office it was clear his brain inflammation was resolving. He was alert, polite, and comfortable. His pain was fading, and he had transformed back into his former self.

Samuel F. Yanuck, DC, FACFN, FIAMA
Chapel Hill, North Carolina
www.yanuckcenter.com

● ●

TAMING MICROGLIA CELLS

Fortunately, there has been an explosion of research on microglia cells in the last 10 years, and this has allowed me to comb through a mountain of literature on ways to dampen brain inflammation and degeneration. A paper published in the 2009 *Journal of Current Opinion in Neurology* covered the key aspects of neurological research in the last 20 years, spotlighting the dampening of microglia as the target for neurodegenerative diseases such as Alzheimer's.

The pharmaceutical industry appears to be focused on developing drugs to shut down microglia cells, which would be therapeutic in Alzheimer's and Parkinson's diseases, head trauma, stroke, and other conditions that cause rapid inflammation and degeneration. However, the drugs' success has yet to match the performance of many natural compounds that have demonstrated in peer-reviewed literature excellent microglia-quenching abilities. They are flavonoids that include apigenin, baicalein, resveratrol, catechin, rutin, and curcumin. These flavonoids cross the blood-brain barrier and have powerful anti-inflammatory effects in the brain.

One might also want to use these flavonoids preventively, considering the many stressors we endure these days. I personally take a combination of all these flavonoids daily as a way to decrease brain-based inflammation because I know, like anyone else with a stressful lifestyle, that I have some degree of brain-based inflammation that I want to dampen. If you don't have a major inflammatory process happening, you may not notice their effects, but they can still be protective.

BRAIN FOG AND INFLAMMATION

The effects of these flavonoids can be profound for those suffering from brain fog, a condition in which it's hard to think clearly and one feels disconnected or fuzzy headed. Inflammation in the body, whether it's in the joints or on the skin, is often painful. However, the brain has no pain fibers, so brain inflammation doesn't hurt. It presents instead as brain fog.

Brain fog can be secondary to a food intolerance, lack of sleep, gut infections, hypothyroidism, extreme stress, autoimmunity, systemic inflammation, and other factors. Brain inflammation distorts healthy neurotransmission, leading to fuzzy and incomplete synapses and symptoms of brain fog. If your brain fog clears up with the flavonoids, that indicates brain inflammation is an issue. I find these flavonoids useful for patients with brain fog, depression, and slow mental speed associated with chronic pain, swelling, or autoimmunity.

Although these flavonoids can address brain inflammation, they do not necessarily address the underlying cause of inflammation. That should always be dealt with as well.

Sometimes these flavonoids are great to help unwind the self-perpetuating stress cycle I talked about in Chapter Six, where inflammation creates stress, which just creates more inflammation, such as sometimes happens after a stroke or head injury.

In addition to dampening neuroinflammation, these compounds have also been suggested as nutritional support for neurodegenerative conditions, such as brain trauma, stroke, peripheral neuropathy, and for overall brain antioxidant protection. I use them in my practice with all cases of head trauma and degenerative brain conditions.

I find using the flavonoids in combination creates a synergistic effect; however, the use of any of them in isolation is also effective. The biggest clinical issue with these flavonoids is using an amount large enough to dampen the neuroinflammation. Supporting neuroinflammation is not a simple, linear model in which a dosage can be based on a patient's body size or symptom severity. It is like asking how much water you need to put out a fire—it depends on the extent of the inflammation. It is not uncommon for a person with neuroinflammation to require several hundred to a couple of thousand milligrams of each of the compounds to dampen their inflammation. The biggest mistake clinicians and individuals make is they do not use doses significant enough to dampen neuroinflammation.

The best way to use these compounds is to start with a small dose and increase it slowly until the desired outcome is reached. The more symptomatic you are, the easier it will be to identify the correct dosage. For example, if you take 200 mg a day of curcumin and do not notice any impact on your inflammation-based depression, brain fog, or poor mental endurance, you may notice significant improvement at 2,000 mg a day.

In those who have no noticeable symptoms, there is no way to determine the correct dosage, but 100–500 mg of each flavonoid may be good as a preventive strategy. It is a brain-protection strategy I use for myself.

In addition to using flavonoids to dampen neuroinflammation, you also need to address pro-inflammatory factors in your diet and environment and neurological autoimmunity.

COMPOUNDS THAT DAMPEN MICROGLIA NEUROINFLAMMATION

- Apigenin
- Luteolin
- Baicalein
- Resveratrol
- Rutin
- Catechin
- Curcumin

Apigenin

Apigenin is a bioflavonoid found in parsley, artichoke, basil, and celery. It has very powerful neuroinflammation quenching and neuroprotective properties. Research has demonstrated the compound can modulate activation of the microglia cells during neuroinflammatory processes. Apigenin has demonstrated the ability to inhibit microglial proliferation. Apigenin has also demonstrated the ability to protect neuronal cells from artery occlusion that may occur after stroke.[50][51][52][53]

Luteolin

Luteolin is a bioflavonoid found in celery and green peppers and has been shown to block inflammatory responses in the brain by inhibiting microglia activation. Luteolin has been shown to inhibit several different microglial activating pathways and demonstrated the ability to protect neurons from inflammation-induced injury in research studies.[54][55][56][57]

Baicalein

Baicalein is a flavonoid that has been shown to exert anti-inflammatory and antioxidant properties on the brain microglia system.[58] It has a long history of safe administration to humans and has been found to easily cross the gastrointestinal tract and the blood-brain barrier by membrane permeability assays.[59] Baicalein has demonstrated neuroprotective properties to dopaminergic neurons implicated in the pathogenesis of Parkinson's disease.

Animal subjects given MPTP (a dopamine neurotoxin) in combination with Baicalein demonstrated decreased neuronal damage and microglia activation.[60 61 62 63] Baicalein has been reported to protect cortical neurons from beta-amyloid, the protein involved in Alzheimer's disease.[64] It has demonstrated to ameliorate inflammatory processes of diabetic retinopathy and have inhibitory activity against neuron loss in diabetic retinas.[65]

Baicalein has been found to protect neurons from decreased blood flow to the brain.[66 67] Traumatic brain injury triggers a complex series of inflammatory responses that contribute to secondary damage. Research has found that post-injury treatment with baicalein improved functional outcomes and reduced pro-inflammatory activity in traumatic brain injury.[68]

Resveratrol

Resveratrol, a flavonoid found in grapes and wine, has been reported to reduce the activation of microglia in numerous studies. Activated microglia produce excessive nitric oxide, which leads to neuronal inflammation. Resveratrol has demonstrated nitric oxide attenuating properties on microglia cells.[69 70] Resveratrol has potent antioxidant effects on oxidative stress activity derived from microglia cell activation.[71 72] Resveratrol reduces activated microglia cell activity and may reduce neuroinflammation.[73 74]

Resveratrol has demonstrated the ability to protect against microglia-dependant amyloid-beta toxicity through inhibiting NF-kappaB signaling and may provide a novel compound to be considered for Alzheimer's disease.[75] Research on resveratrol has found it inhibits LPS-induced nitric oxide and TNF-alpha production in microglia by blocking phosphorylation, and is suggested as potential support compound for neurodegenerative conditions.[76 77]

Rutin

Rutin, a citrus flavonoid found in plants, acts as a powerful antioxidant. It attaches to the iron ion Fe^{2+}, preventing it from binding to hydrogen peroxide and allowing it to become a free radical. Rutin has demonstrated the ability to quench lipid peroxidation.[78] It has demonstrated the ability to modulate microglia inflammatory mediators TNF-alpha and nitric oxide.[79] It has been found to protect against toxicant-induced hippocampal injury by suppression of microglia activation of inflammatory cytokines.[80]

Catechins

Catechins are polyphenolic antioxidant plant metabolites abundant in various tea leaves. They have been shown to protect microglia cells and neurons from DNA damage by oxidative stress by increasing their expression of DNA repair by the enzyme poly(ADP-ribose) polymerase and by translocation of NF-kappaB.[81 82]

Catechins have been reported to possess divalent metal chelating, antioxidant, and anti-inflammatory activities, to penetrate the brain barrier, and to protect neuronal death in a wide array of cellular and animal models of neurological disorders. They appear to have both an iron chelating and antioxidant effect.[83 84] One study demonstrated catechin is a potent inhibitor of microglia activation and thus is a useful candidate for alleviating microglia-mediated neuronal injury.[85]

Curcumin

Curcumin are antioxidant compounds found in the Indian curry spice of turmeric that have been found to modulate microglia neuroinflammation. Curcumin has demonstrated the ability to protect dopaminergic neurons against LPS-induced neurotoxicity in animal neuronal/glia culture.[86] Curcumin has been found to have neuroprotective effects by blocking the production of pro-inflammatory and cytotoxic mediators such as nitric oxide, TNF-alpha, IL-1 alpha, IL-6, and NF-kappaB by activated microglia.[87 88 89 90 91] Curcumin has been found to inhibit amyloid peptide-induced chemokine gene expression and may represent a potential therapeutic aid to ameliorate the inflammation and progression of Alzheimer's disease.[92]

My favorite example of the effect inflammation can have on the brain comes from working with a mother who had a herniated disc in her low back. She would come to the office with her small son, Conner, who showed signs of developmental delay, increased cranial size, and poor speech development. On her third visit I gathered up the nerve to ask her whether he was a big two-year-old or if he was delayed. She verified my suspicion, telling me that he was already in a state-run program for speech therapy.

She shared her frustration that the program was not going well, even with the meager goal of learning two new words a week. I explained how inflammation can be associated with developmental delay and that, if she would bring her child in, I might be able to help.

Being very Western-based medicine in her mindset, she declined. I asked her to purchase a glutathione cream that would be anti-inflammatory and perfect for use with children. Glutathione is a powerful antioxidant and anti-inflammatory compound. She declined. Ultimately, I gave her the cream at no charge and asked her to please apply it twice daily on her boy's belly to see if it made any positive change. She agreed.

On our next visit three days later she came in and immediately demanded to know what was in the cream. Her child had picked up 30 words over the weekend! I explained that although he had been learning the words taught in occupational therapy, the inflammation in his brain diminished his ability to vocalize them. I also explained the cream was not the solution. The real solution was to identify the source of the inflammation and stamp it out for good.

We ran a three-month gut rehab program on her son and continued with the cream for the duration of the program. Six months after she began applying the cream her son was dropped from the speech therapy program. The occupational therapist informed her he was truly exceptional and that no other case like his had ever been documented in their program.

Ben Anderson, DC
Austin, Texas
www.vanguardchiropractic.com

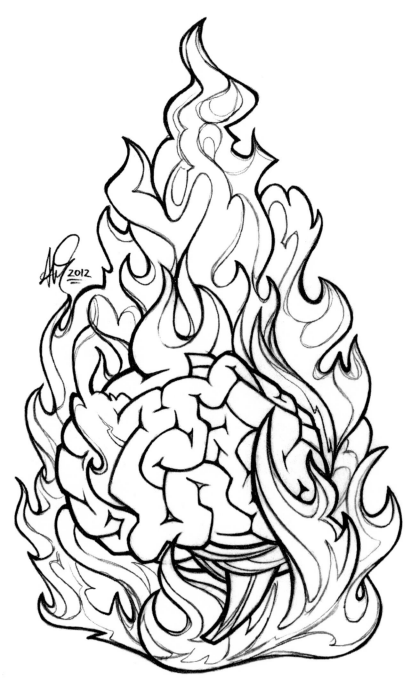

Brain inflammation can cause brain fog, slower mental speed, poor brain endurance, depression, and neurodegenerative disorders.

APPLYING THIS INFORMATION

- Evaluate the checklist of symptoms in the beginning of the chapter. If you have several of the symptoms, you should consider strategies to reduce neuroinflammation and improve your brain function.

- If you have symptoms of neuroinflammation, evaluate the list of mechanisms that activate microglia and may be a continuing cause of neuroinflammation.

- If you suspect your blood-brain barrier is breached take the GABA challenge.

- If you have symptoms of neuroinflammation or had a poor outcome with the GABA challenge, consider support with the natural flavonoids that dampen microglia.

• •

This patient came in for neck pain. When giving her history she off-handedly mentioned she had some minor numbness on the left side of her body. Upon physical examination I found she had diminished motor function on her entire left side. She also indicated she had an infected tooth. I explained that inflammation in her oral cavity could be negatively affecting her brain, manifesting as weakness and the numb feelings she noticed.

She had a root canal within the week. The day after the root canal, the numbness had completely resolved and never returned. Motor function was normal on her return visit to my office. The detrimental effect of long-term inflammation on her brain was resolved by removing the inflammatory insult in her jaw.

Ben Anderson, DC
Austin, Texas
www.vanguardchiropractic.com

• •

＊ ＊

Brian, 17, was first knocked unconscious at age 11. Like most contact sports, hockey carries an assumed risk of head injury. Brian believes he suffered at least 15 concussions while playing the sport he loved. He had been evaluated by multiple specialists, diagnosed with post- concussion syndrome, and told to rest. His mother, Paula, said, "It was after great frustration that we realized we must take things into our own hands and seek out our own resources. I will not accept my son's headaches and dizziness as normal."

Brian and Paula flew from Canada to Texas for an evaluation. He complained of vertigo, motion sickness, brain fog, feeling "off," difficulty concentrating, poor memory, fatigue, mood swings, agitation, relentless headaches, sensitivity to light, heartburn, and a weak immune system.

Over a three-day period I evaluated Brian with advanced diagnostic equipment that allowed me to quantify his balance disorder and abnormal eye movements. I was able to provide specific brain-based therapy to enhance the function of these areas.

However, the neurochemical component is commonly overlooked. A concussion is a mechanical insult that alters brain chemistry. It creates a chemical insult (inflammation) that must be handled by the immune system. This process, called "immunoexcitotoxicity," alters the function of pathways in the nervous system.

With an understanding of this critical component I asked Brian to modify his diet and incorporate nutritional products to help unwind brain inflammation and support brain health.

Shortly after returning to Canada, Brian reported his daily headaches and fatigue had resolved and his brain fog had lifted. Paula said, "His smile is more apparent, I see a glimpse of what my son used to look like! I feel our family has regained some hope and optimism."

Dr. Thomas Culleton, DC, DACNB, FACFN
Austin, Texas and New York, New York
www.CNWcenter.com

＊ ＊

CHAPTER SUMMARY

• One of the reasons your brain may not be working is because of inflammation in the brain, also referred to as "neuroinflammation."

• Inflammation in the body—chronic joint pain, infections, inflammatory bowel disease, or an unmanaged autoimmune condition—releases immune messengers called cytokines. These cytokines send messages across the blood-brain barrier that activate inflammation in the brain, which alters brain function and destroys brain tissue.

• Likewise, inflammation or degeneration in the brain can trigger systemic inflammation that results in such issues as joint pain, gut pain, skin disorders, or more. In the literature this is referred to as "neurogenic inflammation." Many practitioners have seen a correlation between poor brain health and chronic inflammation or autoimmunity.

• Brain inflammation is a major cause of chronic depression.

• At the root of brain inflammation are microglia cells, the brain's immune soldiers. They determine whether your brain is inflamed and aging too quickly. In normal conditions the microglia perform many functions vital for healthy brain function. However, if triggered by an antigen or injury, they create an overzealous inflammatory immune response that causes brain inflammation, or neuroinflammation.

• Neuroinflammation causes neurons to fire more slowly, which may cause brain fog, slower mental speed, slower recall, and slower reflexes. It also shuts down energy production in the cells so that brain endurance plummets. A longer-term consequence of chronic neuroinflammation is neuron death and the development of neurodegenerative disorders.

• Many things can activate the microglia and inflame the brain, such as diabetes, high-carbohydrate diets, poor blood circulation in the brain, and inflammation from areas outside of the brain, including an inflamed gut or environmental pollutants.

• Microglia have no built-in off switch. Once activated they promote inflammation for their entire lifespan, destroying healthy brain tissue and speeding brain degeneration.

• Microglia activation induces a domino effect in which one microglia activates another and so on. These activated cells perpetuate an ongoing vicious cycle that can lead to chronic and persistent neuroinflammation that may last for weeks, months, or years.

• One of the biggest risks to over activating the microglia is a leaky blood-brain barrier. The blood-brain barrier is a finely woven mesh that surrounds and protects the brain. As with the gut lining, it can be leaky and allow pathogens into the brain, which activate the microglia and cause inflammation.

• You can assess whether you have leaky brain with the leaky brain challenge using GABA. GABA, a supplement popular for producing a calming, relaxing effect, is too large to cross a healthy blood-brain barrier. If you take GABA and notice it has an effect, then you probably have a leaky blood-brain barrier.

• Chelation can be dangerous relates to a person with a leaky blood-brain barrier as it can allow chelated metals into the brain. This sets off the microglia cells on their endless inflammatory rampage and accelerates brain degeneration.

• A variety of dietary and lifestyle factors can tame brain inflammation. Stabilizing your blood glucose and cortisol levels, reducing inflammatory triggers such as gluten, clearing up a gut infection or chronic virus, boosting your antioxidant system, and supporting anti-inflammatory mechanisms can all help restore the blood-brain barrier and better protect your brain.

• Factors such as diabetes, high homocysteine, and regular alcohol consumption can cause brain inflammation.

• The flavonoids apigenin, baicalein, resveratrol, catechin, rutin, and curcumin cross the blood-brain barrier and have powerful anti-inflammatory effects in the brain. However, dietary and lifestyle factors should also be addressed.

Chapter Eleven
WHAT IS NEUROLOGICAL AUTOIMMUNITY?

SYMPTOMS AND SIGNS OF NEUROLOGICAL AUTOIMMUNITY

- Brain and neurological symptoms with a history or family history of autoimmune disease
- Brain and neurological symptoms at an early age not associated with age-related brain degeneration
- History of celiac disease or gluten sensitivity
- Brain and neurological symptoms and signs with a relapsing and remitting pattern associated with stress, poor sleep, or immune activation

＊＊＊＊＊＊＊＊＊＊＊＊＊＊＊＊＊＊＊＊＊＊＊＊＊＊＊＊

Kate, 62, began having almost weekly six-hour episodes of dizziness and uncontrollable vomiting when she was 50 years old. She went to various doctors and nobody knew what was causing the episodes. Out of desperation her physicians put her on steroids and antibiotics, but they did not help. She stopped going out or driving for fear of the episodes, becoming a prisoner in her own home. Her entire life and future changed.

After four years of suffering, Kate was finally diagnosed with a condition called Meniere's disease. It is a deteriorating disease of the inner ear that leads to hearing loss, dizziness, and ringing in the ear. She was forced to take an anti-anxiety medication daily to calm the dizziness.

Kate's condition continued to progress and eventually her doctor performed surgery, cutting her left inner ear nerve and inserting a shunt. It resulted in permanent deafness in her left ear but relieved some of her dizziness. Her doctor suggested future surgery in her right ear, but Kate was still struggling every day with vertigo, nausea, fear, digestive symptoms, emotional outbursts, significant fatigue, and a broken spirit.

Kate sat next to my wife on long airplane trip. They talked and Kate told my wife her story. My wife put her hand on Kate's shoulder and told her, "My husband can help you; he sees complex cases such as yours all the time. He will know what to do. Please call his office when you land."

My wife told me about Kate when she got home and made me promise to take her as a patient. Kate called and I was able to see her after several weeks. When she came into my office I could tell she was scared and really worried about how much worse her condition might become.

An examination made it clear Meniere's disease was impacting both inner ears and that her overall brain function was quite compromised. Just simple visual eye movements gave her vertigo and nausea, and her inner ear system was inappropriately stimulating her limbic system, which led to uncontrollable emotional responses. She could barely function during the day and had zero capacity to deal with any stress. Her hearing was continuously declining. She also had a few episodes of "drop attacks," in which the nerve in her inner ear spontaneously fired and pushed her straight to the ground, as if someone was pushing her forcefully.

I was worried about Kate because I could see how rapidly she had been declining. She had Meniere's disease but she also had a brain with very little endurance, which was why her brain had so little ability to compensate for her inner ear nerve disorder. I organized inner ear and brain exercises for her condition based on functional neurology rehabilitation, but her brain had no capacity to perform them without immediate fatigue. Her brain chemistry was severely challenged.

Kate's laboratory tests showed she had neurological autoimmunity to nerve proteins and to the protective sheath surrounding her nerves. She was also having severe episodes of hypoglycemia (low blood sugar), had no ability to digest food, and had developed significant intestinal and blood-brain barrier permeability as evidenced by high levels of occludin and zonulin antibodies. We also found Kate had laboratory markers for celiac disease.

Basically, her immune system was attacking her nervous system. Her neurons were not able to function because of the significant inflammation affecting her brain and nervous system. Her brain was deficient in fuel and she had a disrupted gut-brain axis. Anti-anxiety medication and surgery on her other inner ear nerve were not going to make these mechanisms go away.

We followed clinical strategies to modulate her autoimmunity with diet, lifestyle, and nutritional interventions. She followed a diet to stabilize her blood glucose levels, and we started correcting her gut-brain axis imbalances. Kate responded very quickly to her treatment plan; soon she no longer had any drop attacks or emotional swings. Her mood, energy, and balance all improved significantly.

I spoke with Kate on the phone a few weeks after we started treatment. I immediately noticed the strength in her voice and the sense of empowerment in her personality—she had transformed into a completely different person. Although her autoimmune condition is incurable, Kate is doing much better today. She is functioning at a very high level and has the ability to enjoy her life once again.

We figured out strategies to improve her brain function and to dampen the mechanisms that were destroying it. These strategies are not part of the standard health care model for patients with her condition. The only strategy the world's leading Meniere's clinic could give her was to surgically remove her inner ear nerves followed by lifelong therapy with anti-anxiety and anti-nausea medications.

Fortunately, we were able to dig a little deeper and look at her overall brain health with the goal of improving its function and health instead of just suppressing her symptoms or cutting out areas of dysfunction. Kate has something in common with most people with autoimmune neurological disorders—they are never given any strategies to manage the autoimmunity.

Datis Kharrazian, DHSc, DC, MS

● ●

The immune system is responsible for fending off common colds and killing bacteria when we cut our skin. Immune cells serve as our personal army of soldiers to protect us from opportunistic organisms such as bacteria, viruses, parasites, and other pathogens. However, people's immune systems are going haywire these days, with the rates of autoimmunity having exploded worldwide. In autoimmunity the immune system becomes dysfunctional and cannot distinguish body tissue from infectious organisms. As a result, it inappropriately attacks the tissue it was designed to protect as if it were a pathogen. In the world of immunology this is called "loss of self-tolerance."

The number of *known* cases of autoimmunity in the United States is staggering. One out of every nine women and one out every 12 men has an autoimmune disease in the United States today.[1] Statistics from the National Institute of Health (NIH) show 50 million diagnosed autoimmune cases in the United States and the prevalence is rising.[2] Compare this to 9 million cancer cases and 22 million cases of heart disease—there are more known cases of autoimmune diseases in the United States than cancer and heart disease combined.

However, the number of people suffering from autoimmunity is actually much greater because most people are not diagnosed. According to the American Autoimmune Related Diseases Association, doctors receive minimal education in autoimmune diseases and initial symptoms are difficult to diagnose, even by medical specialists.[3]

A common area of autoimmune attack is the brain and the nervous system. The attack can be against the brain, the spinal cord, or the peripheral nerves that carry information to our hands and feet. When the immune system attacks its own nervous system it is called "neuroautoimmunity." Such autoimmunity can involve any part of the nervous system and therefore create diverse symptoms, such as weakness, poor brain function, dizziness, burning sensations in the hands and feet, obsessive compulsive disorder, and more.

The main clue a person may be suffering from neuroautoimmunity is a history of another autoimmune disease. However, many patients don't know an autoimmune process is behind their symptoms, so let's first discuss autoimmune disease in general.

The most common autoimmune diseases today are hypothyroidism, celiac disease, pernicious anemia, ulcerative colitis, Crohn's disease, and rheumatoid arthritis. The majority of people with hypothyroidism have antibodies to their thyroid and thus an autoimmune disease called Hashimoto's. Celiac disease causes antibodies to the intestinal enzyme transglutaminase in response to dietary gluten, the protein found in wheat. Pernicious anemia is a B-12 anemia caused by antibodies against intrinsic factor, the transport protein for B-12. Ulcerative colitis and Crohn's disease are inflammatory bowel diseases that involve autoimmunity to the large intestine, and rheumatoid arthritis involves autoimmunity to joint cartilage.

If you feel your brain or nerves are not working properly and you or a genetically related family member has been diagnosed with any of these conditions, you may have neurological autoimmunity.

Another red flag for possible autoimmunity is neurological and brain dysfunction that appears early in life, before age related brain decline is more likely. This includes decline of brain function in adults under the age of 50 and autism in children.

In the immunology literature autism is considered an autoimmune disease that develops during pregnancy. This is evidenced by both the presence of antibodies to the fetus' brain in the mother's blood and elevated neurological antibodies in children with autism.[4] Autism and many childhood developmental delays are extreme examples of profound neurological autoimmunity in early life.[5]

Neurological symptoms in children and young adults who do not have autism are also a cause to be suspicious of neurological autoimmunity. These symptoms may include significant memory loss, worsening balance, memory lapses, vertigo, and obsessive compulsive disorder, all of which are possible signs of early autoimmunity.

THE STAGES OF AUTOIMMUNITY

Neuroautoimmunity and autoimmune reactions take place in stages.

1. Silent autoimmunity

The first stage of autoimmunity is called silent autoimmunity. This is the beginning of an autoimmune reaction in which the immune system is attacking body tissue, but does not result in any significant loss of tissue or even symptoms. We can identify silent autoimmunity through elevated tissue antibodies in the blood (such as to the thyroid gland or the cerebellum). However, the patient may not experience signs or symptoms at this stage because not enough tissue has been destroyed to produce noticeable changes.

2. Autoimmune reactivity

The second stage of autoimmunity is called autoimmune reactivity. In this stage the autoimmune reactions have progressed to the point that enough tissue has been destroyed so that signs, symptoms, or loss of function are noticeable. However, the condition is not so advanced as to be labeled an autoimmune disease.

3. Autoimmune disease

The last stage of autoimmunity is called autoimmune disease. At this point symptoms and loss of tissue are significant. The loss of tissue is also advanced enough to be identified with imaging studies and other tests, such as nerve conduction studies.

Stage 1: *Silent autoimmunity—Positive antibodies but no symptoms or loss of function*

Stage 2: *Autoimmune reactivity—Positive antibodies with symptoms and loss of function, but not complete destruction of the tissue associated with disease.*

Stage 3: *Autoimmune disease—Positive antibodies and significant symptoms with significant loss of function. Can be identified with imaging studies such as MRI, nerve conduction testing, etc.*

When autoimmunity sets in, a person first loses tolerance to his or her own body tissue. It then progresses to stages of early destruction that cause some symptoms but not significant enough to be labeled an autoimmune disease. Finally, the tissue destruction leads to significant tissue loss, creating noticeable symptoms and loss of function. At this stage the condition can be called autoimmune disease.

For example, let's say a person develops autoimmunity to myelin, the sheath that covers the nerve cells. In the very early stages a blood test for myelin basic protein antibodies will come back positive, but the person does not have noticeable symptoms or loss of function. This is the early silent stage. The medical world also calls this "benign autoimmunity," but it is not benign as the person is at a high risk for developing autoimmune disease.

If the autoimmunity progresses, the person develops subtle symptoms associated with myelin destruction, which reduces nerve communication from one nerve cell to another. Symptoms may include weakness in one of the extremities, a tingling sensation in the body, numbness in various muscles, or double vision (seeing two images in certain directions instead of one).

At this point a person does not have enough damage to produce an abnormal MRI—the destruction must affect 70 percent or more of the myelin sheaths to show up on an MRI. If the myelin loss is only at 40 percent, imaging is normal. A neurologist's examination findings may show subtle imbalances, but because the MRI is normal doctors cannot diagnose or offer support.

Finally, if the autoimmunity progresses to cause significant destruction of the myelin, the person may now not be able to walk or feel her face. A neurological examination shows numerous abnormal findings, and MRI imaging studies show signs of extensive damage. Now a diagnosis of multiple sclerosis is made.

The problem with the standard health care model is doctors wait for the autoimmunity to destroy a significant amount of tissue before making a diagnosis. This is partly because extensive damage allows for a black-and-white diagnosis. Also, the first line of therapy for autoimmunity is heavy corticosteroids to suppress the immune system, a therapy with significant adverse reactions that cannot be employed without absolute confirmation.

Unfortunately, many people stay in the autoimmune reactivity stage for many years without a diagnosis. Some may never develop enough destruction of their nervous system to be diagnosed, yet they suffer significant signs and symptoms that impair quality of life. Many eventually progress to various neurological diseases, such as multiple sclerosis. Even diseases such as Parkinson's disease and Alzheimer's disease have now been shown to have their roots in long-standing autoimmunity to specific neurological tissues.

If you have a family history of autoimmune disease, a gluten sensitivity or celiac disease, or a significant loss of brain integrity at an early age, you may be suffering from neurological autoimmunity. Additionally, if you have been told nothing is wrong with you because your imaging studies and examination findings do not identify a neurological disease, you may be one of millions of people with an autoimmune reaction against neurological tissue but not a full-blown neurological autoimmune disease.

● ●

Although neurodegenerative disorders usually do not fit the typical model of autoimmunity, researchers are finding many diseases—such as Parkinson's disease, which is not considered an autoimmune disease—may actually be the result of a neurological autoimmune reaction

A recent paper in the Journal of Immunology *found 72 percent of Parkinson's patients had antibodies against neurological tissue.*[6] *Another paper published in the* Journal of Neurochemistry *found 90 percent of Parkinson's patients had autoimmunity.*[7] *Researchers are discovering the immune system may be destroying the dopamine-producing cells of the brain in an autoimmune reaction, just as the immune system attacks insulin-producing cells of the pancreas in Type 1 diabetes.*

● ●

With the worldwide explosion of both autoimmunity and neurological diseases, we know there are thousands of cases of undetected neurological autoimmune conditions today. These are people who have no idea why their brain is failing. Since many of them do not have autoimmunity severe enough to be completely debilitating or diagnosable, the health care system overlooks them despite their complaints. They are on their own and may suffer for years and years. They have seen numerous doctors, some of whom tell them they are strange or weird cases. Many have been told they have a mental disorder and need a psychologist. They begin to doubt themselves and think they are going crazy. In the end, these people—possibly you—suffer endlessly and needlessly because they do not fit current diagnostic models.

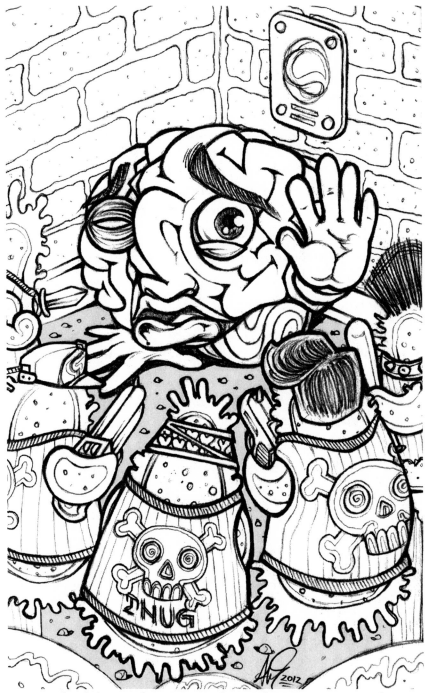

A family history of autoimmune disease, gluten sensitivity, or early loss of brain function can indicate neurological autoimmunity.

TESTING FOR NEUROLOGICAL AUTOIMMUNITY

We identify autoimmunity by measuring antibodies to different body tissues with a standard blood test. In the case of neurological autoimmunity, a test screens for antibodies against the proteins of various nerve cell structures. When antibodies to a specific body tissue are elevated outside the reference range, it indicates the immune system has lost "self-tolerance" and is targeting those tissues for destruction. Many labs offer tests for neurological tissue antibodies, but I have found that Cyrex Labs (Cyrexlabs.com) does the most complete and sensitive evaluation. Their neurological antibody panel tests for multiple sites of autoimmunity, which other labs do not offer as a complete panel. The neurological autoimmunity panel includes:

Myelin basic protein antibodies: autoimmune reactions to the outer covering of nerve cells

Asialoganglioside antibodies: autoimmune reactions to sugar- and protein-chain clusters on the surface of nerve cells

Alpha and beta tubulin antibodies: autoimmune reactions to proteins found in neurons

Synapsin antibodies: autoimmune reactions to proteins found in all nerve cells that regulate synapses

Glutamic acid decarboxylase (GAD) antibodies: autoimmune reactions to the enzyme in the body that produces the inhibitory neurotransmitter GABA

Cerebellum antibodies: autoimmune reactions to the cerebellum, which is involved with balance and muscle movement calibration

All of these neurological tissue antibodies, with the exception of cerebellum and GAD, can cause diverse neurological symptoms anywhere in the body. Symptoms can include cognitive dysfunction, nerve pain such as neuropathy, and non-pain syndromes such as weakness, numbness, or double vision.

Cerebellum autoimmunity may cause all, none, or some of the following symptoms: balance difficulty, vertigo, symptoms of nausea and anxiety, decreased tolerance for alcohol, or an inability to coordinate thoughts. I will discuss GAD antibodies shortly.

If you do not test all of these antibodies you may not properly identify neurological autoimmunity. I have seen many cases in which a patient's doctor tested only one tissue antibody, which was found to be normal, but the complete neurological autoimmunity screen identified an autoimmune reaction to a different tissue.

GAD antibodies

A more commonly recognized autoimmune reaction today is GAD autoimmunity. GAD stands for glutamic acid decarboxylase, an enzyme that triggers the production of the neurotransmitter GABA. GABA is responsible for calming the brain and preventing anxiety-related symptoms. Gluten intolerance, celiac disease, Hashimoto's hypothyroidism, Type I diabetes, and other autoimmune diseases are linked with GAD autoimmunity.

When we eat, our bodies convert glutamic acid from foods to glutamate, an excitatory neurotransmitter. The GAD enzyme then converts glutamate to GABA. When people develop an autoimmune reaction to the GAD enzyme, this conversion to GABA suffers and the result is too much excitatory glutamate and not enough calming GABA. This can lead to symptoms associated with anxiety.

GAD is also found in the pancreas and is involved with the release of insulin, and GAD antibodies are an early marker for autoimmune diabetes. People with a GAD autoimmunity are also more prone to gluten ataxia, a form of gluten intolerance that manifests in the brain causing a variety of neurological symptoms both physical and behavioral. As with Type I diabetes, positive GAD antibodies are an early screening tool for gluten ataxia.

When GAD autoimmunity is present you are at a greater risk for developing autoimmune diabetes, OCD, vertigo, motion sickness, various movement disorders such as facial tics, and a neurological condition called "stiff man syndrome," a severe disease of progressive muscle stiffness.[8][9][10][11][12]

In addition to avoiding gluten, people with positive GAD antibodies should also avoid foods high in artificial glutamates. The most common example of this is a sensitivity to monosodium glutamate (MSG), the additive that gave Chinese food a bad name many years ago and is found in numerous packaged and processed foods. People with positive GAD antibodies can experience a strong reaction to foods high in glutamates with symptoms that include extreme anxiety, nervousness, migraines, and more.

Many labs can test for antibodies to GAD. An autoimmune reaction to GAD is more common among those with a gluten intolerance or celiac disease. In my practice, it is the autoimmune reaction I see most in people with gluten sensitivity. Gluten intolerance and celiac disease should always be considered in the case of persistent symptoms of poor GABA activity. (GABA is discussed more in Chapter Fifteen.)

Autism and GAD antibodies

GAD autoimmunity is a common, well-published mechanism in regards to autism. When some children with autism react neurologically to gluten, this autoimmune response to GAD is the reason why. This also has been considered a theoretical model for severe temper tantrums in some children with autism, as well as for temper tantrums in non-autistic children with gluten sensitivity.

IS YOUR AUTOIMMUNE REACTION SILENT, SYMPTOMATIC, OR AT DISEASE STAGE?

If a blood test identifies elevated levels of antibodies to neurological tissue, you must also evaluate symptoms to determine whether you suffer from early silent autoimmunity, symptomatic autoimmune reactivity, or autoimmune disease.

If you suffer from silent autoimmunity or autoimmune reactivity you must understand there is no known time frame for developing a full-blown autoimmune neurological disease, if at all. You must monitor yourself and work with a practitioner trained in evaluating symptoms or signs of progression.

Remember, the current health care model does not treat silent autoimmunity or autoimmune reactivity until it becomes a disease. Also, many doctors completely dismiss elevated neurological antibodies unless you have developed severe autoimmune destruction. These doctors play the end-stage disease game and early prevention is not part of their model.

But if you have silent autoimmunity or autoimmune reactivity, many diet, lifestyle, and nutritional recommendations may help dampen your autoimmune process, reduce your symptoms, and prevent its progression. It will just take more care and attention on your part to manage what you eat, your lifestyle, stressors in your life, and so forth.

Also, when evaluating a neurological antibody test you may want to consider how high or low the numbers are. Typically, these numbers are not clinically significant because antibodies themselves do not destroy tissue. The antibody is a protein made by immune cells that tags a harmful bacteria or virus for destruction. In the case of an autoimmune reaction, they tag body tissue.

However, researchers have found neurological antibodies differ from antibodies found elsewhere in the body—neurological antibodies themselves are destructive. This is unique in immunology because it means the antibody count indicates the degree of potential destruction that may be occurring.

LIVING WITH NEUROLOGICAL AUTOIMMUNITY

Autoimmunity in general is challenging, but neurological autoimmunity can become serious because brain cells lost to autoimmunity are permanently lost. Neurons are called post-mitotic cells because they do not go through cell division, which means once they are destroyed they are gone forever.

Despite relentless effort by the world's most brilliant researchers, there is no cure for autoimmunity. However, the expression of autoimmunity can be modulated, or "tamed." If you have neurological autoimmunity you must embrace the proper lifestyle, dietary, and nutritional strategies to decrease its expression.

The upside to neurological autoimmunity is that although neuron death is permanent, the brain has great potential for positive plasticity. This means your brain can compensate for neuron loss by developing more efficient communication with other neurons to retain or even improve function. But you must know you may have bad days when something triggers immune activation. These triggers include stress, lack of sleep, a heated argument, a food intolerance, and so on.

In fact, you may need to make significant changes in some areas of your life to preserve your brain health. This could mean changing your job, relationships, where you live, or some other important part of life. It is vital for you to pay attention to what triggers and dampens your autoimmunity—this will empower you to improve the quality of your life and slow down the destruction of your brain. By embracing changes to develop positive plasticity, your neurons can communicate with each other more efficiently and you can maintain or even improve brain function.

● ●

Reyna, a 22-year old college student and former triathlete in the Philippines, was suffering from multiple symptoms that had come on suddenly. They included hypothyroid symptoms, weight gain, extreme fatigue, constant headaches, acne, memory loss, depression, and more. For a year and a half Reyna visited multiple doctors around her country, but her symptoms progressively worsened. She was not responding well to thyroid medications her doctors prescribed despite continual adjustments of the dosage or the type of medication.

Reyna was losing hope and searching for answers when she found Dr. Kharrazian's thyroid book online and ordered a copy. She saw my name in the book and because she had relatives in California, she contacted me and was in my office two weeks later with her mother.

She was only in the United States for a short time so we had to work fast. I ordered blood, stool, and saliva testing and realized her lab tests did not indicate thyroid dysfunction. You can imagine the look on her face when after traveling halfway around the world for thyroid help I told her she did not have a thyroid problem. Instead, the most prominent findings were inflammation, an improper cortisol rhythm, and poor pituitary function, which correlated with her symptoms.

Reyna's symptoms began after a long period of overtraining, undereating, too much stress, and too little rest. The tipping point was a four-day, 370-mile cycling event. In the week following the event she gained 10 pounds and developed the symptoms that continued to plague her until we could address the underlying mechanisms.

"I was inflicting so much abuse on my body without realizing it: training too hard, eating too little, drinking too much coffee, being busy with too many things, and resting too little," said Reyna. "My college schedule was very busy. I had triathlon training in

the morning, classes until the afternoon, and then more training again in the evening. I was in a running or bike race almost every other week and only took one day off every two weeks for rest. I was always too tired to eat more than the bare minimum."

I recommended supplements that dampened inflammation, modulated her immune system, helped regulate her imbalanced circadian rhythm, supported acetylcholine activity and brain health, and supported pituitary function. I also had her adopt a diet free of gluten and sugar.

Most of her symptoms resolved during her two-week visit but we weren't finished, as her labs tests still indicated inflammation. When she returned to California three months later I ordered a 24-tissue antibody test known as the Multiple Autoimmune Reactivity Screen from Cyrex Labs. The test indicated autoimmunity to her gastrointestinal tract, heart, phospholipids, joint tissue, pancreas, and neurologic tissue. We were able to use the nutritional protocols I learned from Dr. Kharrazian to dampen the autoimmune attacks on her body.

Reyna says she now feels better than she did before her symptoms began. She eats a whole-foods diet and strictly avoids sugar, gluten, and fried foods. She takes long, vigorous hikes and does other forms of exercise, although she has not returned to her arduous triathlon schedule. Reyna is also working on a master's degree abroad and is able to enjoy her life like never before.

A large part of her recovery has been learning how to tune into her body. "This journey made me realize the importance of taking care of my body and giving it time to recover and heal itself," says Reyna. "There is definitely no point in abusing it because it is only by taking care of our body that we can take care of our spirit, too."

Mark Flannery, DC, MS, BS, FAAIM, DBCBN, DCCN, CNS
Woodland Hills, California
www.drflannery.com

● ●

LIFESTYLE STRATEGIES FOR NEUROLOGICAL AUTOIMMUNITY: TH-3 AND TH-17

The lifestyle strategies for autoimmunity are based on common sense; however, that doesn't mean people follow them, especially if they do not understand why they should. Knowing what's "under the hood" of your autoimmune condition can help you better understand why that pizza dinner, staying up late too many nights in a row, or getting yourself worked up over politics can tank you. Adopting specific daily strategies can profoundly impact how you feel and theoretically slow down the progression of your autoimmunity.

Immunologists have found two major immune responses that either stimulate or suppress the autoimmune response. These are known respectively as the T-helper 17 (TH-17) and T-helper 3 (TH-3) responses. The TH-3 responses include regulatory T-cells, or suppressor T-cells. As their names imply, these cells can regulate or suppress autoimmunity, so you want to support TH-3.

A TH-17 response stimulates autoimmunity. It's like adding fuel to the fire of autoimmunity, and it's a response you want to avoid activating.

* *

I run my own business and have a great family, but for the past 17 years my health has been a constant struggle and on a downhill spiral. All of my health challenges began after the birth of my second child in 1994. Up to that point I had been the picture of health. I ate the right things and exercised consistently in an effort to avoid the health problems and panic attacks that plagued my mother.

I felt great while I was pregnant with my second child, but within a few months after delivery I started to notice a subtle trembling throughout my whole body and a slight nervousness. That alone was enough to send me into a panic, and over the next few months they blossomed into full-blown panic attacks and very severe brain fog.

I had episodes every day that would leave me exhausted and feeling broken on the inside. But I knew if I could find the right person I could get my health back. Well, that took 17 years.

By the time I met Dr. Noseworthy I had been diagnosed with adrenal failure, low thyroid, and hormone imbalances, and some-

one thought I had celiac disease but wasn't really sure. I was on thyroid medication, bioidentical hormone replacement, and two types of prescription hydrocortisones—and I was still miserable!

The first thing Dr. N did was a very thorough history and exam, and then we looked at my blood work and hormone levels. My hormones were through the roof. He called it "hormone overload," explaining that when hormones are too high you get symptoms of hormone deficiencies when you actually have too much.

I went on a specially designed hormone detox program and went back to see the doctor who originally prescribed them to make some changes. In a few weeks I was significantly better, but still had a long way to go.

By that time the test results came back and Dr. N told me I was battling autoimmune issues. My immune system was attacking my thyroid gland, causing surges of thyroid hormones that would jack up my heart rate and make me shaky on the inside, nervous, and anxious. The other key problem was my adrenals and my brain were also under autoimmune attack. I was making antibodies to my adrenal glands and cerebellum.

After the hormone detox Dr. N recommended special anti-inflammatory nutrients to dampen autoimmunity and improve blood flow to the brain. He explained that once we had the inflammation under control and could balance my immune system, the attack would slow down and my brain would function better. He was right. I noticed small changes in the beginning, but the longer I stuck with it and followed his advice, the better I felt.

I haven't felt this good in a long time. The brain fog is gone and the trembling and anxiety are rare and quite manageable.

a patient of Dr. Noseworthy
Steven A. Noseworthy DC, DACNB, DCCN
Tampa, Florida
www.DrNoseworthy.com

ACTIVATING REGULATORY TH-3 TO DAMPEN AUTOIMMUNITY

Increase opioids

Let's start with the strategies that activate TH-3 cells to dampen autoimmunity. When your body releases natural opioid they activate your TH-3 cells, which are loaded with opioid receptors. Opioids are chemicals that make you feel good.

The best example of an opioid release is the great feeling you get after exercise, known as the "exercise high." To get the best opioid release your exercise has to challenge you and get your heart rate up, even if it's just for a few minutes. The act of pushing yourself, even when you want to quit, creates the opioid release. Just slowly walking on the treadmill while you watch TV will not elicit the best opioid response. On the other hand, you do not want to hurt yourself or overtrain when you exercise. Overtraining activates an inflammatory immune protein called IL-6, which activates TH-17 and promotes autoimmunity.

So the key is balance—push yourself hard enough to get an "exercise high" after your workout, but not so hard that you create an injury or overtrain. You can jump rope, rebound, do jumping jacks, squats, or push ups to fatigue. When you feel you can't go on any longer, do a few more—that's when you release opioids. You will know when you are not overtraining because you will not injure yourself and will be able to recover after your workouts. By accomplishing this you are activating the TH-3 response without activating TH-17, which is critical to dampening the autoimmune response.

Another way to generate opioids is to get "high on life." A positive mental attitude, love, appreciation for life, and positive self-esteem are ways to increase opioids. On the other hand, a negative attitude, violence, poor relationships, and internal mental stress are examples of ways to promote IL-6, which activates TH-17 and promotes autoimmunity. In my own practice I have clearly observed the difference between patients who have a positive mental attitude, love, and family support versus those mired in resentment, blame, and poor relationships.

If you have an autoimmune reaction, it is time to reflect on your life and decide if you are happy and whether you have made peace with any internal demons. As a matter of fact, it may be the most important clinical factor in determining your autoimmunity outcome. No amount of dietary supplements, or medications can change the effects of a negative outlook and internal stress on your autoimmunity. You must do some inner reflection, face your issues, and create a mental environment that makes you "high on life."

Create an immune healthy environment

In addition to personal internal stressors, external stressors such as a bad job, strict deadlines, unrealistic goals, or an environment that places great demands on you activates your TH-17 pathway and promotes autoimmunity. Mental stress, physical stress, or chemical stress all increase IL-6, which activates both the adrenal stress response and TH-17. If you have autoimmunity you must take yourself out of a stressful environment, even if it will lower your finances, change your relationships, or alter your commitments. Your brain health and the quality of your life are worth it.

I remember doing a history recently on a new patient, aged 36. She was a physician who started medical school at age 17. By the time she finished her medical specialty in nephrology she had developed autoimmunity. She had consulted with her medical colleagues, but they had nothing to offer, so she sought alternative strategies in diet and nutritional therapy, which is when she became a patient in my office. She had been diagnosed with Hashimoto's thyroid autoimmunity, and her mother had a history of severe neurochemical and neurological disease.

When I examined her she had already developed signs of significant neurological degeneration, such as ataxia (an inability to walk without swaying and falling), termination tremor (tremor of the hand when reaching for objects), and abnormal signs of neurological attack against her myelin. She knew her brain was not working like it used to, but she was not aware of these findings.

Remember, she was only 36 years old and these findings do not happen normally until your brain becomes significantly compromised. Her history, examination findings, and laboratory tests indicated she was suffering from early neurological autoimmune reactivity but not a frank neurological disease.

In talking to her about her work environment it was clear being on call was a major stressor and potential promoter of autoimmunity in her life.

We sat down together and discussed the importance of slowing down, which was against the very nature of her personality but her lifestyle was a significant risk factor for TH-17 activation.

Stress plays a significant role in autoimmunity, but both alternative and conventional health care providers overlook it. If you have autoimmunity you must figure out ways to decrease your stress load in order to decrease the expression of TH-17. You must create an environment that is protective and supportive for you so you can focus on your passions and increase your opioid activity. You must get out of the vicious unhealthy cycle you are in and really focus on "you."

DIETARY CONSIDERATIONS FOR NEUROLOGICAL AUTOIMMUNITY

Blood glucose levels

In addition to internal and external stressors, if you have autoimmunity you must decrease chemical stressors by optimizing your diet. The most common and significant biochemical stressor today is dysglycemia, or poor blood glucose control due to diet and lifestyle. We have already looked at the importance of blood sugar stability for steady fuel supply for your brain, but now we will discuss blood sugar mechanisms and autoimmunity.

If you have autoimmunity you cannot let your blood glucose spike or drop sharply. When your blood glucose is low from missing meals or eating meals that are low in fiber or protein, your body raises blood glucose by increasing production of inflammatory IL-6. This not only activates adrenal hormones to raise blood glucose, but also stimulates the TH-17 pathways that activate autoimmunity.

If you have autoimmunity you need to prevent your blood glucose levels from going up and down all day like a roller coaster. If you become tired after meals you may be eating too much, eating too many carbs for your body, or not getting enough exercise. If you get shaky, lightheaded, irritable, or crash in the afternoon and feel better after you eat, you are either going too long without eating or you are not getting enough fiber and protein to stabilize your blood sugar.

The biggest clue your blood glucose levels are stable is that you have an appetite at meal times (not just cravings for simple sugars) and when you eat there is no change in your energy levels. Feeling either tired or energized after you eat indicates your blood glucose levels are too high (insulin resistance) or too low (functional hypoglycemia), respectively. You should have no change in energy levels after meals; you should just no longer be hungry.

Avoid gluten and improve gut-brain axis

If you have neurological autoimmunity you must also make sure you do not eat gluten or any foods that cross-react with gluten, as discussed in Chapter Eight. You must improve your the gut-brain axis the best you can and support leaky gut as discussed in Chapter Nine.

If you can make these lifestyle and dietary changes you will probably notice significant changes in your overall health and function as you engage the mechanisms that may slow the progression of autoimmunity. These changes must become part of your life and not just a program you do for a few weeks. Your brain and neurons are counting on it.

NUTRITIONAL SUPPLEMENTS FOR NEUROLOGICAL AUTOIMMUNITY

You cannot simply supplement your way out of autoimmunity. You must also make the necessary lifestyle and dietary changes. We have a "pill culture" today that suggests instead of making diet and lifestyle changes we take a pill to fix the problem. That said, I will recommend various supplements to improve your health and function. At best, taking these various supplements may decrease the expression of your autoimmunity, but they are not a cure. They also work differently for different people, so I cannot predict how they will affect you.

If you have made the appropriate diet and lifestyle changes and want to take it to the next level, various nutritional supplements may help. I will review the current known mechanisms of autoimmunity and the applications of supplementation in the peer-reviewed nutritional literature.

Supplements to avoid

Before we get started on what supplements to consider, let's talk about which supplements to avoid. Based on much research, if you have neurological autoimmunity there is a strong possibility you have a gluten sensitivity. You should avoid any supplements that use gluten as a filler. All nutritional tablets and some capsules use a filler to fill up empty space in the tablet or capsule.

You want to make sure the filler is not gluten or uses a hidden source of gluten such as "modified food starch." Modified food starch may contain gluten. You want to make sure the capsule itself is not made of gluten. Also, some companies that make "whole food" supplements use wheat as a filler based on the model grains are nutritious. Please carefully avoid these exposures because if you have gluten sensitivity and you take supplements with gluten in them, you may make yourself much worse.

You also want avoid supplements that may increase the activity of your autoimmunity, as many supplements stimulate your immune system. The worst thing you can do is take a compound that makes your immune system stronger and have it destroy your brain. After all, autoimmunity is the result of an overzealous immune system.

If you have read my book *Why Do I Still Have Thyroid Symptoms?* you know immunologists have classified autoimmunity into two types of immune dominance, TH-1 and TH-2. The TH-1 system responds immediately to an invader, such as surrounding a splinter with pus. The TH-2 system is the delayed response, which creates antibodies to tag the invader in the future. Either one of these systems can become overly dominant in an autoimmune condition, so we want to restore balance between these systems.

Botanicals that enhance immunity and stimulate TH-1 include echinacea, astragalus, lemon balm (*melissa officinalis*), and maitake mushrooms. Botanicals that stimulate the TH-2 system include pine bark extract, grape seed extract, green tea extract, acai berry extract, and Pycnogenol, a pine bark extract. These are antioxidant compounds with immune activating properties; however, most flavonoids and nutritional antioxidants do not stimulate immunity.

The TH-1 and TH-2 systems work like a seesaw. As one side gets activated the other side may become suppressed. Some individuals with autoimmunity have found some of these compounds may help them or make them worse, depending on the TH-1 or TH-2 dominance they have.

In some cases of autoimmunity we have patients challenge themselves with either TH-1 or TH-2 compounds to see if they have any noticeable adverse responses, but with neurological autoimmunity we typically avoid such challenges because we do not want to risk injuring neurons.

To play it safe with neurological autoimmunity, we stay away from these substances and work on other mechanisms, which I will get to in a moment.

● ●

Jill, 40, was a chiropractor suffering from ataxia. Ataxia is neurological disorder in which a person loses muscle coordination. She had difficulty walking in a straight line and coordinating her muscles for speaking. She had several neurological consults but did not fit a classical disease mode and was dismissed by some of the best neurology departments in the country without any real answers. She was told it may be a neurological genetic disorder but testing would be difficult and unnecessary.

When I evaluated Jill's file it was clear no one investigated autoimmunity of her nervous system. A key finding in her history, however, was that she was gluten sensitive. When she went on a gluten-free diet she noticed significant improvements in her symptoms. This is a typical case history of a commonly overlooked neurological condition called gluten ataxia, a disorder in which an autoimmune attack against the cerebellum and GAD enzymes leads to deterioration of muscle coordination. We later confirmed this with laboratory tests.

Also, when Jill came in for her first visit she brought 30 different supplements she was taking. I immediately identified supplements that stimulated her TH-1 and TH-2 systems and had her stop taking those. I also had her stop drinking her echinacea tea in the morning.

Just removing these immune-stimulating substances caused another immediate leap in her function within the first two weeks. We decided not to challenge her with any other immune supplements because her condition was too fragile. Jill's case is a great example of how identifying and removing immune-stimulating triggers such as herbs or dietary proteins (gluten) can dampen the expression of her autoimmune disorder. Not all autoimmune cases respond this clearly, but many do.

Datis Kharrazian, DHSc, DC, MS

● ●

Supplements to dampen autoimmunity

We have already looked at the effect of diet and lifestyle on TH-3 and TH-17 pathways, but nutritional supplements also impact these pathways. Remember, TH-3 suppresses autoimmunity and TH-17 stimulates it.

Vitamin D

Regulatory T-cells are saturated with vitamin D receptors, and vitamin D has been shown to increase TH-3 activity, thus dampening autoimmunity.[13 14 15] However, with autoimmunity you cannot just take RDA amounts of vitamin D and expect a response. Typical doses of vitamin D for autoimmunity can be anywhere from 5,000 to 10,000 IU per day.

Some may take higher doses, but if you do, you should test your vitamin D levels with a serum 25-hydroxy vitamin D test. Your level should be around 50 ng/mL. Levels above 100 ng/mL may indicate a vitamin D overload. Most people with autoimmunity have low levels of vitamin D when tested. If you have autoimmunity you want to take vitamin D regularly and get some healthy time in the sun every day.

Glutathione

Another strategy to improve your TH-3 response is to take compounds that increase glutathione. Glutathione is an antioxidant made by your body to protect your tissue and it has several key mechanisms to support autoimmunity.[16 17 18] Glutathione preserves and protects neurons against inflammation, supports TH-3 responses, supports regeneration of the blood-brain barrier and the intestinal barrier, and is a natural chelator that can bind to environmental compounds such as heavy metals and pollutants, which may trigger autoimmunity. Although glutathione can be taken as a nutritional supplement, most forms are not absorbed well and do not raise levels within the cells (intracellular). Glutathione can also be taken intravenously, which is effective but can be costly and not easily accessible.

In my practice I use a mixture of botanicals that have been shown to profoundly impact levels of glutathione inside the cells. These natural compounds include Cordyceps, N-acetylcysteine, gotu kola, milk thistle, L-glutamine, and alpha lipoic acid. These are all TH-1 and TH-2 neutral and because they support TH-3, they have the potential to dampen an overactive TH-1 or TH-2 response in autoimmunity. To read more about glutathione go to Chapter Twenty.

Resveratrol and curcumin

Two of the most important plant-based natural compounds for autoimmunity are resveratrol and curcumin, both of which have very powerful anti-inflammatory properties. Resveratrol and curcumin dampen the two major inflammatory pathways in autoimmunity, TH-17 and NF-kappaB, and have been used in foods for thousands of years. [19 20 21 22 23 24 25 26 27]

However, you cannot obtain doses high enough from foods to be therapeutic and dampen autoimmunity. They must be isolated and concentrated in a nutritional product for the best effect. I find the best way to take both resveratrol and curcumin is in an emulsified liquid. Research has shown that as an emulsified liquid they provide up to seven times the impact compared to oral tablets or capsules.

With all of these supplements the dosage is hard to calculate because it is not based on body weight or age. You must use trial and error, starting with a standard initial dose and gradually increasing the amount until you obtain the best results. The biggest mistake autoimmune patients make is they do not take enough of the compounds. It is not uncommon for a patient to take several hundred or several thousand milligrams individually of resveratrol, curcumin, or compounds to support glutathione. In studies researchers used doses as high as 400 mg a day of resveratrol and 800 mg a day of curcumin. However, you may not need these doses; the effective amount varies from person to person.

If you read the thyroid book then you may recall resveratrol is listed as a compound that stimulates TH-2. We have since learned that it's more of TH-17 and NF-kappaB blocker than it is a TH-2 stimulator. Many TH-2 dominant people benefit from resveratrol. However, you may want to dose up slowly on it just to be sure you do not react negatively.

You may also want to take nutritional supplements to support intestinal permeability and flavonoids to dampen the inflammatory microglia in the brain, as discussed in Chapters Nine and Ten. This may seem like a lot of supplements to take, but it may be necessary to dampen neurological autoimmunity.

CHAPTER SUMMARY

• The rates of autoimmunity have exploded worldwide. In autoimmunity the immune system cannot distinguish body tissue from infectious organisms. As a result, it attacks the tissue it was designed to protect as if it were a pathogen.

• A common area of autoimmune attack is the brain and the nervous system. The attack can be against the brain, the spinal cord, or the peripheral nerves that carry information to our hands and feet. When the immune system attacks its own nervous system it is called "neuroautoimmunity" and can create such diverse symptoms as weakness, poor brain function, dizziness, burning sensations in the hands and feet, obsessive compulsive disorder, and more.

• Red flags for possible neuroautoimmunity are symptoms of neurological and brain dysfunction that appear early in life, having another autoimmune disease, or a family history of autoimmune disease.

• In the immunology literature autism is considered an autoimmune disease that develops during pregnancy. This is evidenced by both the presence of antibodies to the fetus' brain in the mother's blood and elevated neurological antibodies in children with autism. Autism and many childhood developmental delays are extreme examples of profound neurological autoimmunity in early life.

• Neuroautoimmunity and autoimmune reactions in general take place in stages.

• The first stage of autoimmunity is called silent autoimmunity. This is the beginning of an autoimmune reaction in which the immune system is attacking body tissue, but does not result in any significant loss of tissue or even symptoms. We can identify silent autoimmunity through elevated tissue antibodies in the blood.

• The second stage of autoimmunity is called autoimmune reactivity. In this stage the autoimmune reactions have progressed to the point that enough tissue has been destroyed so that signs, symptoms, or loss of function are noticeable. However, the condition is not so advanced as to be labeled an autoimmune disease.

• The last stage of autoimmunity is called autoimmune disease. At this point symptoms and loss of tissue are significant. The loss of tissue is also advanced enough to be identified with imaging studies and other tests, such as nerve conduction studies.

• The problem that occurs with autoimmunity in the standard health care model is doctors wait for the autoimmunity to significantly destroy the tissue before making a diagnosis.

• Unfortunately, many people stay in the autoimmune reactivity stage for many years without a diagnosis. Some may never develop enough destruction of their nervous system to be diagnosed, yet suffer significant signs and symptoms that impair quality of life. Many eventually progress to various neurological diseases, such as multiple sclerosis. Even diseases such as Parkinson's disease and Alzheimer's disease have now been shown to be a consequence of long-standing autoimmunity to specific neurological tissues.

• With the worldwide explosion of both autoimmunity and neurological diseases, we know there are thousands of cases of undetected neurological autoimmune conditions today. Since the autoimmunity is not severe enough to be completely debilitating or diagnosable, the health care system overlooks them. They are on their own and may suffer for years.

• We identify autoimmunity by measuring antibodies to different body tissues with a standard blood test. In the case of neurological autoimmunity, a test screens for antibodies against the proteins of various nerve cell structures.

• These neurological tissue antibodies can cause diverse neurological symptoms anywhere in the body. Symptoms can include cognitive dysfunction, nerve pain such as neuropathy, and non-pain syndromes such as weakness, numbness, or double vision.

• Cerebellum autoimmunity may cause balance difficulty, vertigo, symptoms of nausea and anxiety, decreased tolerance for alcohol, or an inability to coordinate thoughts.

• Glutamic acid decarboxylase (GAD) antibody reactions are the most common and create the most specific symptoms. GAD is the enzyme that produces the inhibitory neurotransmitter GABA, which is responsible for calming the nervous system. Elevated GAD antibodies are linked to obsessive compulsive disorder (OCD), motion sickness, vertigo, and a neurological condition called "stiff man syndrome," a severe disease of progressive muscle stiffness. GAD is also found in the pancreas and is involved with the release of insulin, and GAD antibodies are the earliest laboratory marker for autoimmune diabetes. Therefore, when GAD autoimmunity is present you are at a greater risk for developing autoimmune diabetes, OCD, vertigo, motion sickness, and various movement disorders such as facial tics.

• Diet, lifestyle, and nutritional recommendations may help dampen your autoimmune process, reduce your symptoms, and prevent its progression.

• Researchers have found neurological antibodies differ from antibodies found elsewhere in the body—neurological antibodies themselves are destructive. This is unique in immunology because it means the antibody count indicates the degree of potential destruction that may be occurring.

• Autoimmunity in general is challenging, but neurological autoimmunity can become serious because brain cells lost to autoimmunity are permanently lost. The upside to neurological autoimmunity is that although neuron death is permanent, the brain has great potential for positive plasticity. This means your brain can compensate for neuron loss by developing more efficient communication with other neurons to retain or even improve function. But you must know you may have bad days when something triggers immune activation. In fact, you may need to make significant changes in some areas of your life to preserve your brain health. This could mean changing your job, relationship, where you live, or some other important part of life.

• Immunologists have found two major immune responses that either stimulate or suppress the autoimmune response. These are known respectively as the TH-3 and TH-17 responses. The TH-3 responses include regulatory T-cells, or suppressor T-cells. As their names imply, these cells can regulate or suppress autoimmunity, so you want to support TH-3. A TH-17 response stimulates autoimmunity. It's like adding fuel to the fire of autoimmunity, and it's a response you want to avoid activating.

• Releasing opioids is one way to stimulate TH-3 receptors. Opioids are chemicals that make you feel good. The "exercise high" you get after working out is one way to release opioids. Creating a positive attitude and a healthy environment are also important to release opioids and promote TH-3.

• In addition to an angry or negative attitude, external stressors such as a bad job, strict deadlines, unrealistic goals, or an environment that places great demands on you activates your TH-17 pathway and promotes autoimmunity. If you have autoimmunity you must take yourself out of a stressful environment, even if it will lower your finances, change your relationships, or alter your commitments. Your brain health and the quality of your life are worth it.

• Blood glucose levels have a powerful impact on autoimmunity.

• If you have autoimmunity, avoid supplements that contain gluten (which may be some whole-food supplements) and supplements that activate the TH-1 or TH-2 systems.

• Therapeutic doses of vitamin D, glutathione precursors, curcumin, and resveratrol can dampen autoimmunity.

CHAPTER TWELVE
INTRODUCTION TO NEUROTRANSMITTERS

• •

Jack suffered from chronic depression ever since losing his job during the recession. He is very fortunate to have a wife who works full-time and supports him, both emotionally and financially. Cindy's full-time employment was supposed to last only until Jack got back on his feet so they could start a family. However, it has been five years and Jack is still unemployed and depressed. He tried various antidepressants but most didn't help at all, and others only helped for a short while.

Jack could not motivate himself, derive joy from anything, or do anything that required brain function without fatiguing immediately. He had exhausted all pharmaceutical options, and his brain was still not working. Cindy was a champion and began pursuing alternative options for Jack. She would not give up, and eventually they landed in my practice.

After a detailed history and examination, it was clear to me Jack suffered from numerous neurochemical imbalances. Many factors related to his diet and brain chemistry were in need of drastic help. Fortunately for Jack, Cindy was able to help him change his diet and make sure he took his supplements during the day.

Jack began to feel better and became more active and social. As he became more functional he made a major breakthrough and began exercising again. It took many months and many drastic changes to his diet and lifestyle with the support of his wife, but Jack finally came out of his black hole and regained his brain function.

I share Jack's story with you for several reasons. First, Jack is like many people with chronic depression and poor brain function who continue to suffer from chronic depression despite trying all the pharmaceutical options. Second, Jack was fortunate enough to have a family member stick with him and get him the help he needed to improve his brain health. Unfortunately, many people who suffer from chronic depression do not have someone supportive to help them out of their dark hole of depression. Lastly, diet, nutrition, botanicals, exercise, and lifestyle can profoundly impact brain chemistry in a way most medications cannot.

As a matter of fact, exercise alone is one of the most profound ways to increase your brain neurotransmitter levels. It has been consistently found to be as good and even better than medication at relieving depression. Exercise raises brain levels of the neurotransmitters dopamine, norepinephrine, and serotonin, which impact mood. It also increases endorphin levels and increases blood flow to the brain. There are no antidepressants that have been shown to impact the brain in as many positive ways as exercise can.

In the next few chapters I will discuss the basic concepts of neurotransmitters and how diet, nutrition, and natural compounds can influence their function. If your brain is not working, you really need to make sure your neurotransmitter signaling system is functioning well. I will describe each of the main neurotransmitters in detail later, but this chapter will focus on some fundamental concepts of neurotransmitters that may explain why your brain may not be functioning as well as it should.

Datis Kharrazian, DHSc, DC, MS

• •

To understand how best to stimulate the brain, whether it's playing brain games, learning a new language, or taking up a new sport, it's important to understand more about neurotransmitters and how the brain functions and learns. Throughout the next several chapters, I will talk about lifestyle strategies and nutritional compounds that can successfully address breakdowns in these pathways.

NECESSARY STEPS FOR HEALTHY
SYNAPSE FUNCTION [1] [2]

Neurons communicate by discharging a small messenger chemical called a neurotransmitter. The neuron that sends the neurotransmitter is the presynaptic neuron, and the neuron that receives the neurotransmitter is the postsynaptic neuron. To get from the presynaptic to the postsynaptic neuron, the neurotransmitter must travel across a small empty space called the "synaptic cleft." This whole process is called synaptic transmission (or synapse), and brain function can decline when there are breakdowns along this pathway.

Using amino acid supplements to boost neurotransmitter activity has become popular. For instance, people may use tyrosine to boost energy and motivation or 5-HTP to relieve depression. These amino acids serve as precursors to neurotransmitters, providing the raw materials from which neurotransmitters are synthesized.

The ability to boost neurotransmitter production with amino acids has been the subject of several books. It is also a mainstay for some health care practitioners who, using quizzes and looking at symptoms, assess which neurotransmitters are deficient. They then advise which amino acid supplements will boost neurotransmitter levels and activity in the brain. I will talk more about those in coming chapters. However, my clinical experience and research of the literature has shown there's more to it than just boosting neurotransmitter levels...a lot more.

Much can go wrong during a synapse in an unhealthy system. For instance, there can be sufficient neurotransmitters but a problem with the presynaptic or postsynaptic receptor. Or the neurotransmitter doesn't break down or get reabsorbed as it should after the synapse is complete, disrupting future synapses. Neurons may fire too many neurotransmitters at once, or too few.

Inflammation, hormone imbalances, and poor blood sugar handling are some of the factors that can sabotage neurotransmitter function. In the coming chapters I cover not only the use of amino acids and other nutritional compounds that boost neurotransmitter activity, but also the other necessary factors.

A synapse has several requirements for healthy function. Here are three:

- Release of neurotransmitters by the presynaptic neuron. For this to work properly there needs to be a sufficient amount of neurotransmitters.

- Binding of neurotransmitters to a receptor on the postsynaptic neuron.

- Termination of the synapse by the neurotransmitter either breaking down or being reabsorbed into the presynaptic neuron.

Defects in any one of these areas of neurotransmitter activity hinders communication between neurons and brain function. This is most evident when you see a person with obvious neurotransmitter imbalances who does not respond to amino acid supplementation.

For instance, Laura has many of the classic symptoms of serotonin deficiency. She gets depressed and lethargic during winter when the days are short, suffers from PMS, struggles with chronic anxiety, and doesn't find much joy overall in the things she used to like, such as her favorite music or restaurant.

Theoretically, Laura should respond positively to 5-HTP, amino acids that boost serotonin, but she does not. Why? Turns out she is deficient in estrogen, and sufficient estrogen is necessary for the receptor sites on the postsynaptic neurons to take up serotonin. Other factors that can affect postsynaptic neurons are inflammation and autoimmune disease.

EXCITATION OR INHIBITION FROM NEUROTRANSMITTERS

Neurons are either excitatory or inhibitory when they communicate. In a synapse, excitatory neurons excite their target neurons, and inhibitory neurons inhibit their target neurons. These outcomes are determined by whether the neurotransmitter used in communication is excitatory or inhibitory.

The excitatory neurotransmitters are:

- Epinephrine (adrenaline) and norepinephrine (noradrenaline), also commonly known as the "fight or flight" adrenal hormones.

- Dopamine, the "pleasure and reward" neurotransmitter that is produced in large amounts when you fall in love or first engage in addictive behavior, such as smoking, using amphetamines, or gambling.

- Acetylcholine, the "learning and memory" neurotransmitter.
- Serotonin, the "happy" neurotransmitter. Serotonin is commonly associated with feeling calm and relaxed, but technically it is still an excitatory neurotransmitter.

The only inhibitory neurotransmitter is:

- Gamma-aminobutyric acid, or GABA, also known as the "anti-anxiety" neurotransmitter. The most popular anti-anxiety medications act on the GABA pathways.

Although an excitatory neurotransmitter such as dopamine is always excitatory, and GABA is always inhibitory, they still can have opposite effects depending on the neuron pathways with which they synapse. For example, if dopamine excites an inhibitory neuron pathway, the result is inhibition because dopamine is exaggerating the inhibitory response. If GABA, which is always inhibitory, acts on an inhibitory neuron pathway, then you get excitation, since the inhibition is being inhibited. And, of course, if an excitatory neurotransmitter acts on an excitatory neuron pathway, then, as you can imagine, you get more excitation.

Why 5-HTP or GABA supplements aren't relaxing for everyone

Why is this confusing concept important? Because it dispels the commonly held notion that taking GABA supplements will relax everyone, or that tyrosine supplements to boost dopamine will energize everyone. Although they work that way for some people, it's important to realize neurology is not as simple as many would have you believe.

For instance, Julie suffers from fibromyalgia, chronic fatigue, and a slew of other chronic health issues. In an effort to add some relaxation to her stressful life of dealing with chronic pain and health issues, she began taking a supplement that promised to promote GABA activity, a calming, inhibiting neurotransmitter. Yet every time she took it she developed anxiety and insomnia. Although supporting GABA theoretically should have inhibited, or calmed, Julie's brain, the GABA inhibited inhibitory neuron pathways, therefore excited her brain, causing anxiety and insomnia.

● ●

CLASSIFICATION OF NEURON EXCITABILITY

Excitatory neurotransmitter +
excitatory neuron pathway = Excitation

Inhibitory neurotransmitter +
excitatory neuron pathway = Inhibition

Excitatory neurotransmitter +
inhibitory neuron pathway = Inhibition
(because it is amplifying the effect of the inhibitory neuron)

Inhibitory neurotransmitter +
inhibitory neuron pathway = Excitation
(because it is dampening the inhibitory neuron)

● ●

WHEN NEURONS GET TOUCHY AND TRIGGER-HAPPY

Each neuron has a *threshold*, defined as the amount of input needed to cause it respond. When a neuron is at rest (which isn't often), it has a *resting membrane potential* that determines how close it is to threshold, or in other words, how little or how much stimulation is needed to make the neuron fire. If a neuron's resting membrane potential is close to threshold very little input is required for it to fire (by fire, I mean synapse with neighboring neurons in order to communicate). If it is far from threshold a great deal of input is required for it to fire.

Neurons also adhere to the *all-or-none principle*, which states that a neuron either responds completely to communication from another neuron, or not at all. If a neuron is far from threshold it may never get enough input to fire. An example is a dog whistle. We cannot hear it because the frequency of the sound waves does not stimulate our hearing pathways to reach threshold as they do with a dog.

Unfortunately, many people's neurons today do not get enough oxygen, glucose, or stimulation and are either too close to or too far from threshold, both of which are symptoms of a degenerating brain.

A resting membrane potential that is far from threshold and difficult to fire, while less common of the two, can be a problem. An example would be someone who needs to turn the volume on their iPod ever higher because the resting membrane potential of neurons responsible

258

for processing sound are far from threshold. This could perhaps be due to deterioration or an injury to that part of the brain.

In my clinical experience most people struggle with neurons that are too close to threshold. These neurons are "touchy" and fire too easily. One example of this is tinnitus, that annoying, constant ringing in the ears. Many factors can cause tinnitus, but neurons that are close to threshold are one explanation—the auditory neurons are so easily triggered that they process noise that isn't even there.

This could be the scenario for the former roadie of a rock band who was exposed to ear-splitting music night after night for years. Over time the tiny bones in his ear fused from all the noise trauma and stopped sending information from his hearing nerve to his brain. Ten years later, his temporal lobe, the area of the brain that processes sound, has degenerated and is so close to threshold that the neurons fire on their own, and he hears sound that isn't there.

To continue with this example, some people resolve tinnitus by wearing a hearing aid. This sounds counterintuitive. Why would introducing more sounds cause the neurons to fire less readily? Because the hearing aid can actually be a form of therapy, exercising the neurons back to better health. Gently stimulating them while being careful not to overdo it will cause each neuron to generate more energy and hence regain its integrity. As they strengthen, the neurons' resting membrane potential is no longer close to threshold, and they no longer fire in the absence of sound to create tinnitus.

I had a case that illustrated the concept of resting membrane potential in relation to smell. My patient suffered from migraines when she smelled certain things. Simply walking past the perfume counter in a department store would trigger incontinence and a migraine that lasted for days. This is because the neurons responsible for processing smell had degenerated and fatigued to the point that any input overwhelmed their metabolic capacity, causing stress in the rest of her brain and body. In other words, the neurons were too weak to function properly.

I had her buy a kit of essential oils and determine, as safely as possible so as not to trigger a migraine, which oils she could tolerate. Then, with her arms outstretched, she would open one of the oils several times throughout the day. As she continued to practice the exercise each day, she was able to gradually bring the oil closer to her nose. Once she had

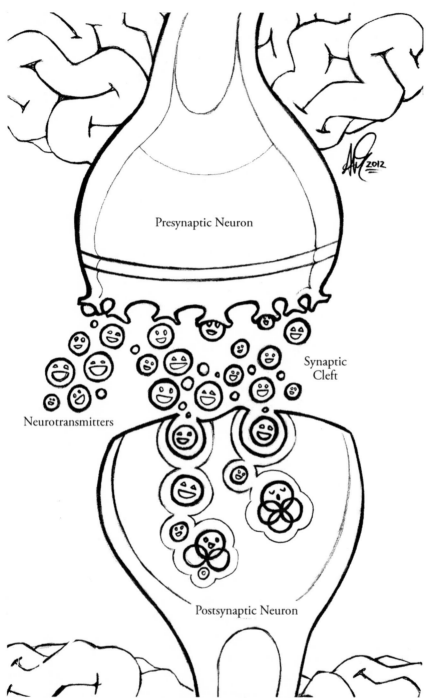

Presynaptic Neuron

Synaptic
Cleft

Neurotransmitters

Postsynaptic Neuron

*Inflammation, hormone imbalances, and poor blood sugar handling
are factors that can sabotage neurotransmitter function.*

"conquered" one oil, she would move on to other oils in the kit—scents she formerly couldn't tolerate. What this exercise did was to gently "exercise" her olfactory neurons so that they increased their production of energy, almost akin to recharging a battery. This increase in energy production allowed the neurons to do their job without fatiguing too quickly.

Resting membrane potential that is close to threshold explains why some chronically brain-degenerated people are so sensitive. These are the people who can't tolerate scents or strong light or sound, and who are intolerant of many foods and supplements. So many of their neurons are so close to threshold that any stimulation in general fatigues them, and symptoms of neurodegeneration develop.

A healthy neuron has sufficient oxygen, glucose, and stimulation, and hence a resting membrane potential that is neither too close to nor too far from threshold. It doesn't spontaneously fire on its own, as with the tinnitus example, nor does it need massive amounts of input to fire.

• •

I find that while I can provide good nutrition advice to my clients, my own family usually doesn't appreciate it. Just recently, my husband, who has had a life-long struggle with mood issues, changed his mind about taking my advice. Here is some background: after many suicide attempts, beginning at age 18, and electro-shock therapy treatments, he was finally diagnosed with manic depression/bipolar spectrum disorder in his late 30s. He was subsequently put on lithium and his mood issues improved significantly.

He continued to cycle in and out of depression and mania, but this happened less often. When he developed lithium toxicity, his psychiatrist switched him to a combination of different medications that he remained on for 15 years. He functioned well as a high school teacher but still suffered prolonged bouts of depression. The mania was less frequent.

As a family, we could always tell before he could when he was heading into a depression. We also knew that when he had his manic episodes he would be severely depressed within a few days' time, after which his mood would improve and he would be emotionally stable for a while.

When I first started my nutrition practice, I was determined to eat a healthy diet and live a healthy lifestyle. That's when I began to notice that my husband's memory was declining, and his craving for sweets was so intense he would eat a loaf of bread and a dozen doughnuts at one sitting. His low blood sugar issues became worse, and he had to eat every two hours or he would get severe symptoms.

While he hadn't been interested in changing his diet thus far, he knew he wasn't doing well. I approached him about allowing me to give him some nutrition advice, and he was amenable. I ran a comprehensive blood panel along with an adrenal profile. As it turned out, he had an autoimmune thyroid condition, which would account for his mood issues and indicate that he was gluten intolerant. He was also prediabetic with clinically high liver enzymes.

Diabetes plays a significant role in my husband's family history; all the men have passed away at young ages from heart disease. He was also experiencing adrenal fatigue with a switched circadian rhythm, which meant that his cortisol levels were low in the morning and remained so throughout the day, returning to normal at night. This accounted for his insomnia and his need for sleeping pills.

Armed with this information, I recommended an anti-inflammatory, low-antigenic diet that included an elimination of all grains, legumes, dairy, caffeine, and chocolate. His supplemental support included gastrointestinal and digestive support, liver detox support, vitamin D, glutathione for immune regulation, vitamin and mineral support, and fish oil.

He was determined to get off medication, which was problematic because, of course, his psychiatrist was adamantly opposed to it. I had read that high doses of inositol were being used successfully in research studies addressing bipolar spectrum disorder, and so I recommended slowly titrated doses of inositol and low doses of 5-HTP to support serotonin activity.

As he tried the diet and the supplemental support, his memory improved and he began to feel better. He even noticed a lift in his mood. Unbeknownst to me, he began to go off his medication, and after six months, he reached his goal of being medication free.

Over the past seven years, we have added dopamine, acetylcholine, DHA, thyroid and immune regulation support, and maintained his vitamin regime. He still has to take his neurotransmitter support every day, but he has had very few depressive or manic episodes in the last seven years.

He has learned how to cook and is committed to his gluten- and food-sensitivity-free diet. Moreover, he has learned how to manage his blood sugar and take better care of himself. As for me, I reap the benefits of having a husband who is happy and vital.

Linda Clark, MA, CN
Fair Oaks, California
www.uwanutrition.com

• •

RELEASING THE RIGHT AMOUNT OF NEUROTRANSMITTER

Other factors that play into a properly functioning synapse are neurotransmitters. For instance, if the presynaptic neuron releases too much of the same neurotransmitter, the receptor site on the postsynaptic neuron will become resistant to it and not allow it in.

Take as an example a person who has high amounts of norepinephrine, an adrenal fight or flight hormone, released during stress. At some point, norepinephrine levels will be so high that receptors on the postsynaptic neuron shut down and refuse it entry. This is a good thing because it prevents stress from going out of control and causing lethally high blood pressure or massive heart damage.

If you're driving on the freeway and someone suddenly cuts in front of you, nearly clipping the nose of your car, this stimulates the presynaptic neurons to release norepinephrine so you can respond to the stressor. In a healthy response, just enough norepinephrine is released so that you can quickly adjust by slowing down. This function not only releases the right neurotransmitter, but it also releases the right amount and replenishes its stores with sufficient amounts should someone cut you off again. This balancing act prevents overstimulation of the postsynaptic neuron so that functions such as breathing and pulse are not at risk.

If this function is not operating well you might have a different response. If you continually release too much norepinephrine you may be startled for hours and hours after the initial stimulation and have difficulty reducing your heart rate and anxiety. You would also have an increased risk for stroke. On the other hand, if you continually release too little of this important stress hormone, you may fail to hit the brakes at all and possibly get yourself into an accident. Of course many other factors play into these two possible scenarios, but poor neuron-to-neuron communication is where it begins.

This mechanism is called *homotropic modulation* and prevents the damaging effects of overstimulation. Unfortunately, it is also what causes us to develop a tolerance to drugs, either prescription or recreational, causing the addict to take more drugs or smoke more cigarettes for the same high.

It's also common to see antidepressants work for about six months to two years, then lose their effectiveness. In fact, new studies show long-term use of antidepressants can permanently desensitize postsynaptic neurons, thus rendering the drugs or even neurotransmitter therapy ineffective.[3]

RELEASING THE RIGHT KIND OF NEUROTRANSMITTER

In the axon of every neuron are terminals that store neurotransmitters for release when needed. It's important that the neuron release the right neurotransmitter for the job. It's also important that the wrong neurotransmitter for the job remain in its terminal. Also, different neurotransmitters will cause different reactions in the postsynaptic neuron. For instance, norepinephrine is excitatory and will excite the neuron. GABA, on the other hand, is inhibitory and will have a calming effect on the postsynaptic neuron. This is called *heterotropic modulation*.

For instance, consider the woman who is not responding to 5-HTP supplements for her obvious serotonin deficiency. We know sufficient estrogen is what keeps receptor sites sensitive to serotonin in females (in men it's testosterone). Likewise, we know both progesterone and thyroid hormones sensitize receptor sites to dopamine. This is another example of heterotropic modulation—multiple signaling compounds have an effect on how a postsynaptic neuron responds.

This again shows why just supplementing with 5-HTP for a serotonin deficiency, or just supplementing with tyrosine for a dopamine deficiency are oversimplified approaches and won't always be effective. What about the role the other signaling compounds play?

Back to the freeway scenario when your neurons just released norepinephrine so you can respond safely to being cut off by a reckless teenage driver (whose frontal lobe is not yet fully developed and who therefore suffers from lack of impulse control). The release of norepinephrine inhibits the release of neurotransmitters that might cause you to feel relaxed or aid in the digestion of food. This is one reason eating while driving is bad for you—when your stress response is engaged, the "rest and digest" neurotransmitters are put on hold, and so is the food in your stomach.

THE RATE OF NEUROTRANSMITTER RELEASE

Our neurons are able to communicate with multiple other neurons at the same time, and the frequency and amount of simultaneous communication influences the action of the neuron.

For instance, the timing and frequency of presynaptic activity affects outcome—an example would be the cumulative effect of smoking a cigarette once an hour, which releases the stress hormone norepinephrine.

Input that happens on a regular, consistent basis is called *temporal summation*. Releasing a small amount of norepinephrine on an hourly basis would begin to affect how the postsynaptic neuron receives that response. As you can imagine, it would overexcite it in the beginning but gradually cause desensitization so that an hourly cigarette is no longer as stimulating (and it depletes you of an important neurotransmitter, dopamine, and robs your brain of oxygen).

Another example would be the effect of smoking a cigarette after your girlfriend texted she is breaking up with you and you just slammed your finger in the car door, all three of which will also release norepinephrine. This is an example of *spatial summation*. Instead of a regular, frequent stimulation this person got blasted by several different emotional and physical stimuli all at once.

A neuron is typically under the influence of both regular input (temporal summation), and input from several different sources at the same time (spatial summation), though not perhaps in such dramatic ways as just mentioned. Nevertheless, the combined effect of these two different styles of input, together with whether the net result of the input is excitatory or inhibitory, all work together to create what is called the *central integrative state*. The central integrative state, or CIS, is a neurological term that simply describes how all these various inputs play out in the neuron's resulting behavior.

For instance, if you look at the hypothalamus, an area of the brain that controls our responses to stress, whether the CIS of this tissue is inhibitory or excitatory will determine whether our stress response is low and tired out, or hyperactive and over responsive (the person who overreacts to every little thing). In affecting neuronal outcome, the CIS also determines not only our hormonal levels and immune function, but our behavior as well.

All of these actions explain the various facets of neuronal communication and explain why there is so much more to improving brain health, mood, or personality than just boosting neurotransmitter levels with amino acid supplements—a popular model today. You can see why a simple model of just giving 5-HTP to boost serotonin levels or tyrosine to boost dopamine levels doesn't address these more complex neurological processes.

Also, although amino acids and other nutritional compounds can affect neurotransmitter activity, it's important to realize brain function is not as simple as take a pill and expect X, Y, or Z to happen. The brain is a highly complex organ we don't yet fully understand. Brain development in utero and during early childhood, life experiences, injuries, toxins, diet and lifestyle, and health imbalances are all factors that can affect the brain in multiple complex ways. Although neurotransmitter support can often promote brain health, it should not be viewed as a one-size-fits-all approach that will work for everyone or every condition.

That said, in the coming chapters I will discuss some of the most influential neurotransmitters, behaviors and symptoms associated with them, and ways to boost their activity.

CHAPTER SUMMARY

• Neurons communicate by discharging a small messenger chemical called a neurotransmitter.

• Boosting neurotransmitter levels with amino acids is a popular approach. However, my clinical experience and research of the literature has shown there's more to it than just boosting neurotransmitter levels.

• Much can go wrong during a synapse in an unhealthy system, including problems with the pre- or postsynaptic receptor, improper break down or reabsorption of the neurotransmitter, or neurons firing too many or too few neurotransmitters.

• Inflammation, hormone imbalances, poor blood sugar handling, and autoimmune disease are some of the factors that can sabotage neurotransmitter function. For instance, sufficient estrogen is necessary for the receptor sites on the postsynaptic neurons to take up serotonin.

• The excitatory neurotransmitters are epinephrine, norepinephrine, serotonin, dopamine, and acetylcholine. The only truly inhibitory neurotransmitter is GABA.

• A neurotransmitter can have an opposite effect depending on the neuron pathways with which it synapses.

• Each neuron has a threshold, defined as the amount of input needed to cause it respond. Many people's neurons today do not get enough oxygen, glucose, or stimulation and are either too close to or too far from threshold, both of which are symptoms of a degenerating brain. In my experience most people struggle with neurons that are too close to threshold. These neurons are "touchy" and fire too easily. One example of this is tinnitus. Many factors can cause tinnitus, but neurons that are close to threshold are one explanation—the auditory neurons are so easily triggered that they process noise that isn't even there.

• Neurons too close to threshold explain why some chronically brain-degenerated people are so sensitive to scents, strong light or sound, and many foods and supplements. So many of their neurons are so close to threshold that any stimulation in general fatigues them, and symptoms of neurodegeneration develop.

• If the presynaptic neuron releases too much of the same neurotransmitter, the receptor site on the postsynaptic neuron will become resistant to it and not allow it in. This prevents the damaging effects of overstimulation, but it also what causes us to develop a tolerance to drugs or other addictive substances.

Chapter Thirteen

ACETYLCHOLINE

SYMPTOMS OF IMPAIRED ACETYLCHOLINE ACTIVITY

- Loss of visual and photographic memory
- Loss of verbal memory
- Memory lapses
- Impaired creativity
- Diminished comprehension
- Difficulty calculating numbers
- Difficulty recognizing objects and faces
- Slowness of mental responsiveness
- Difficulty with directions and spatial orientation

● ●

Carolyn, 36, was a yoga teacher and one of those unfortunate individuals whose life had been changed by a head trauma sustained in a car accident. When she was a junior in college, a drunk driver ran a red light and hit her car as she was driving through an intersection, which sent her head first through the window. She was diagnosed with a mild concussion and given stitches for some lacerations on her head. She was told she was lucky not to have received any life-threatening injuries and given a clean bill of health.

However, she was never the same after the accident. After the accident she suffered episodes of migraines, nausea, and dizzi-

ness. She lost her ability to focus and concentrate and developed such poor brain endurance that she had to drop out of school. She was devastated, as her dream of becoming a marine biologist was crumbling.

She had to move back in with her parents, as she was unable to work. She kept hoping she would recover in few months, but the months turned into years. She consulted with various conventional and alternative doctors, but nobody was able to help her.

One day she tried yoga, and it was the first thing to improve her function. The quiet, restful deep breathing and slow stretching calmed down her overactive brain. After a few weeks of doing yoga she found her headaches began to disappear. She didn't know it at the time, but the slow stretches and deep breathing were activating areas of her brain (cerebellum and parietal lobe) that were injured in the accident and she was rehabilitating her brain with every yoga session. She defined her life with two significant events: the day of the car accident and the day she found yoga. She eventually become a yoga teacher and began to practice meditation, a vegan diet, and regular fasts.

When Carolyn fist came to my office she appeared significantly malnourished. Her skin and hair were dry and her nails unhealthy. She almost looked like an alcoholic, but she did not drink. It was obvious her brain function was impaired because after taking her history for 20 minutes she needed to take a break by closing her eyes and deep breathing for a few minutes.

As I continued the history and exam her eyelids and facial muscles began to droop, and she started to fade due to exhaustion. Despite the great gains she made from yoga, her new vegan diet was void of essential fats and choline. This was critical because choline is essential for the production of acetylcholine, the neurotransmitter necessary for focus, concentration, memory, and brain endurance. She also suffered from daily episodes of low blood glucose as she fasted for part of each day. It was clear that without essential fatty acids for brain food, choline for acetylcholine production, and a steady supply of glucose to fuel brain energy, her brain would not work efficiently again.

Unfortunately, Carolyn was not willing to change her diet but did agree to limit the fasting. I gave her essential fatty acids and compounds to support acetylcholine, which I will discuss in this chapter. Her response to these supplements was immediate and dramatic. Within 30 minutes of taking them her concentration and focus improved significantly.

Carolyn's case involved many factors beyond acetylcholine support, but I share her story because it illustrates how certain dietary restrictions can affect the brain. Although her brain was not working due to her head injury, the potential for yoga to continue to rehabilitate her brain became compromised because her brain chemistry was not ideal. Ideal brain chemistry, which is based on diet and lifestyle, is critical not only for brain recovery but also for ideal brain function. If your brain is not working well and you are having difficulty with memory, focus, and concentration, this chapter on acetylcholine is very important for you.

Datis Kharrazian, DHSc, DC, MS

⦿ ⦿

Whenever I see these cases I know they always start with a person initially losing their photographic and verbal memory. Instead of taking action, they continue to ignore the symptoms until it is too late. Early signs of acetylcholine impairment are the earliest presentations of Alzheimer's disease and dementia, and these symptoms should not be overlooked, especially if they get worse.

Poor acetylcholine activity is a great concern as a significant portion of the U.S. population ages, for symptoms of dementia and Alzheimer's disease are the same as symptoms of acetylcholine impairment. This is because acetylcholine is the most important neurotransmitter for conversion of short-term memory to long-term memory, which happens in the area of the brain called the hippocampus.[1]

Current research shows the hippocampus is the earliest to degenerate in Alzheimer's disease and dementia, meaning acetylcholine impairment should be addressed swiftly.[2] Someone who is in the earliest stages of Alzheimer's disease may vividly recall his wedding 40 years earlier, but draws a total blank when you ask him what he had for lunch an hour ago. She has memory lapses in the middle of conversations and can't remember what you were talking about, or will hem and haw frequently in search of the words perpetually glued to the tip of her tongue. It's also common to see the acetylcholine-impaired person wandering with a confused expression through the parking lot, having completely

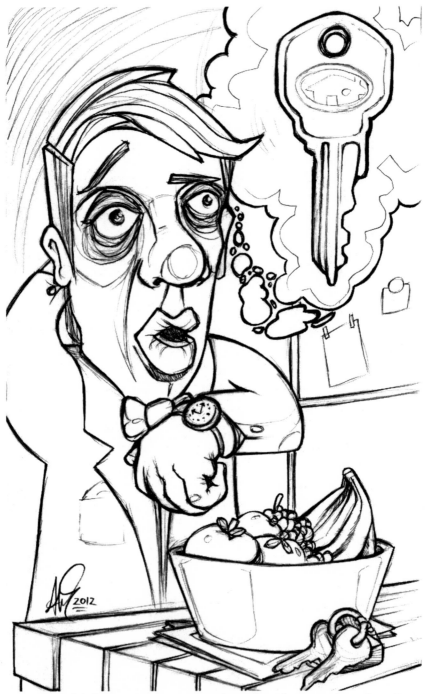

Poor acetylcholine activity can cause memory loss, slow mental speed, getting lost easily, diminished comprehension, and difficulty calculating numbers.

forgotten where he parked. It is only in the end stages of Alzheimer's disease, when it is already too late, that an individual will start to lose established long-term memory.

Basic symptoms of impaired acetylcholine activity include loss of visual memory, or photographic memory. With the loss of visual memory, people have a hard time learning—they can't remember what they read since they can't form images in their minds of the material. They also lose things all the time, as they can't form a picture in their mind of where they left something. Or they see someone and know they know the person, but can't remember who it is since they have lost memory of the person's face.

People with impaired acetylcholine activity also have poor verbal memory and forget words. They have memory lapses, forgetting what they were saying in the middle of conversations and have to start over. Their creativity is impaired, as is their comprehension, and they have difficulty calculating numbers. For instance, they may not be able to count backwards from 100 by sevens (can you?). They also respond slowly to everything that comes at them in life. Have you ever driven behind someone going about 25 or 30 miles per hour on a busy road when everyone else is doing 50 or 60? It doesn't do any good to honk at them as they have no idea they are going so slowly and are incapable of going faster due to slow mental processing.

The hippocampus is also responsible for spatial orientation, or sense of direction. As acetylcholine declines and the hippocampus loses functioning, people lose their spatial orientation and get lost easily. For instance they may pull out of a parking lot they just pulled into and forget whether they had come from the right or left, and which direction they're supposed to be going. Eventually they lose their way around well-traveled routes and forget their way home. So not only do they drive too slowly but they frequently get lost as well, compounding the confusion. This is very scary because it also suggests the earliest presentation of Alzheimer's disease.

Although we expect "senior moments" in older people, they should not be ignored, as they may herald the onset of dementia or Alzheimer's disease. If these symptoms turn up in a younger person, as they frequently do these days, it especially warrants immediate attention, as it indicates potential early brain degeneration. Unfortunately, it seems a person has to get the point where he can no longer remember his children's names to receive diagnosis and treatment in the standard health care model. The decline could have been happening for decades and prevented years earlier.

NUTRITIONAL COMPOUNDS THAT IMPACT ACETYLCHOLINE

If you notice you have symptoms associated with acetylcholine activity or you have a hereditary risk for Alzheimer's disease, taking nutritional compounds to optimize the activity of your acetylcholine pathways may be a good idea. You can also support your acetylcholine function simply because you want to optimize your memory. A brain that is already healthy can support the development of multiple branches of acetylcholine pathways associated with greater memory plasticity and long-term potentiation that may serve one well into the later years.

The nutritional compounds listed below support acetylcholine pathways, slow down acetylcholine breakdown, and have precursors for acetylcholine synthesis. Many of these compounds also have shown promise in protecting against the development of plaques in the brain found in Alzheimer's disease.

One of the benefits of acetylcholine receptors compared to those of the other neurotransmitters is they are not subject to the laws of homotropic modulation. In other words, with repeated exposure the receptor sites will not become resistant to acetylcholine. This is not the case with serotonin, dopamine, or GABA. If the receptor sites of these neurotransmitters receive too much repeated long-term exposure, they begin to become resistant. (This explains why one may need to gradually increase doses of antidepressant or anti-anxiety drugs.)

In fact, the opposite happens with the acetylcholine receptors—it has been found stimulating acetylcholine pathways develops long-term potentiation. In other words, constant stimulation over a period of time actually makes the receptor sites more responsive and sensitive so they need less acetylcholine for the same effect.

L-Huperzine A

L-Huperzine A is a potent compound derived from club moss (Huperzia serreta). It decreases the breakdown of acetylcholine and increases levels of the neurotransmitter in the brain.[3][4][5][6] L-Huperzine A has shown to be an effective aid in memory, cognition, and Alzheimer's.[7][8][9][10] It is one of the most effective compounds and one to first use if you have symptoms of acetylcholine imbalance.

Alpha GPC (L-alpha-glycerylphosphorylcholine)

Alpha GPC is a phospholipid metabolite that is isolated from lecithin. It is probably the best form of choline to raise acetylcholine levels because it is very well absorbed in the gastrointestinal tract and crosses the blood-brain barrier easily, where it is used for the synthesis of acetylcholine. Oral intake of alpha GPC has been shown to increase acetylcholine levels in the brain.[11][12] Alpha GPC compounds significantly improve cognitive capacities in Alzheimer's disease and suggest potential to prevent and delay the progression of the condition.[13][14][15][16][17][18] Alpha GPC has also shown tremendous potential as a nutrient to aid in stroke recovery.[19][20][21]

L-acetyl carnitine

L-acetyl carnitine is an amino acid compound that has a structure similar to acetylcholine. N-acetyl-carnitine binds and activates the acetylcholine receptor. Research has shown that L-acetyl carnitine is effective in improving cognition and has the potential to delay the progression of Alzheimer's.[22][23][24][25]

Pantothenic acid

Pantothenic acid, vitamin B-5, is used in the synthesis of coenzyme A, which is used to transport carbon atoms important for the biosynthesis of acetylcholine. Supplementation of pantothenic acid in an animal study demonstrated the ability to increase acetylcholine levels in the brain.[26][27]

Because my livelihood depends upon my cognitive abilities, I take nutritional compounds to support acetylcholine daily. When I am in an intense period of writing or research, I will up my dose until I feel the desired effects of focus, concentration, and memory that will sustain me through multiple weeks of long days of pushing my brain to its maximum potential.

Because we know homotropic modulation, or a resistance, to acetyl-choline is not a concern, daily use is safe. When my workload is lighter I reduce to a lower daily dose that I maintain for a preventive effect.

Supporting neurotransmitter activity is not dependent upon body size, but instead on the degree to which you have symptoms. As a result, determining your dose requires some trial and error. It typically takes a half hour to an hour after taking acetylcholine support to notice the effects.

Continue to gradually increase your dose until you notice an improvement in your symptoms, such as better mental clarity or improved memory. Then increase the dose again to see whether you experience even more improvement. Once you no longer feel any improvement, go back the previous dose at which you felt improvement. How often you take acetylcholine support also varies with the individual. Some may find they need it three or more times a day, others just once. Some people find if they take too much they develop muscle cramps.

• •

At one of my brain chemistry seminars for health care prac-titioners I mentioned how much acetylcholine support I took each day during an exhausting and intense period of writ-ing new material. Upon hearing this one of the practitioners decided to try the same dose when on deadline with a large and difficult project. She was sleep-deprived, the stress of which was already fatiguing her neurons, and hoped acetylcholine support would help.

The large dose of acetylcholine, while appropriate for me, gave her a bad headache and brain fog and made her jittery and tense. Her brain may have been too fatigued for stimulation of that mag-nitude, and she was forced to finish her project feeling worse than before she started. Remember, dosing is entirely individual. Always start slow and build your dose to avoid any adverse reactions.

• •

What if you crash and burn on acetylcholine support?

Sometimes when people support acetylcholine activity they will "crash," getting hit with intense fatigue or other symptoms. This is due to the neurons being too close to threshold and not able to make enough energy to function properly. Although your brain may need acetylcholine support, it could be so fragile that just a little bit of support sends it over the edge, fatiguing both your neurons and your entire body.

If this crash happens after just the minimum dose, it could actually mean you are in desperate need of support. However, additional support for brain inflammation, brain oxygenation, and neuron support may also be warranted. Compounds for these conditions will dampen inflammation in the brain common with neurodegeneration, give the neurons more support against degeneration, and supply the brain with more oxygen-rich blood (assuming anemia isn't a factor).

So what do you do when you need acetylcholine support but even just a little is too much? You use even less while simultaneously addressing brain inflammation, dysglycemia, and oxygenation.

Additional considerations with acetylcholine support

When some individuals take too much acetylcholine support they experience muscle cramping, nausea, and increased gastrointestinal motility. This is because the neurotransmitter signal for skeletal and gastrointestinal muscle contractions is acetylcholine.

Acetylcholine also activates the vagal motor nuclei, the area of the brain stem that makes you feel nauseous or vomit. People who have failure in communication between their brain and gut may immediately feel nauseous or even vomit when taking low doses of acetylcholine support. In these cases, the strategies to improve neuron health and support the gut-brain axis should be considered seriously.

Another thing that can happen is the additional neurotransmitter support can enforce negative plasticity. For example, if a person has tight calf muscles from training or poor postural tone, the acetylcholine support may stimulate her muscles to cramp before it's able to impact her brain chemistry for memory. Taking acetylcholine support impacts all synapses in the body, not just those in the brain.

● ●

I was in my office before the start of my day when my assistant told me my new patient, Eva, 68, had emailed a letter explaining her symptoms that I was to read before our appointment. In reading Eva's letter I became very concerned about her brain health because the writing was so incoherent. When Eva arrived with her husband she frantically handed me a piece of paper and told me I must read it now. It was the same letter Eva had emailed me, but when I told her I already read it she became confused because she did not remember emailing it.

We sat down to perform a history with her husband's help and within a few minutes she stopped us and frantically told me that she needed me to read a letter. When I told her she had already given me the letter, Eva's husband let out a deep cry of grief realizing how progressed his wife's memory loss had become. After the history and examination I scheduled Eva for an MRI to evaluate her brain. Unfortunately, Eva's MRI indicated that her brain had atrophied and exhibited changes characteristic of Alzheimer's disease. Eva's case is unfortunate because her actual brain volume is now permanently atrophied.

These changes happen very slowly over years, and I'm sure Eva's brain impairment was visible to friends and family in the form of personality changes. Her physicians likely labeled her declining brain function as normal aging. In short, Eva had no chance to save her brain in her medical and family situation. Although we may be able to incorporate some strategies to improve her brain now, it really is too late. She will never live a life without significant impairment from this point forward, no matter what medications or nutrients she takes, and she will continue to decline.

When a case progresses to this level, the people who really suffer are the spouse and family members. I had a long talk about Eva's condition with her husband and encouraged him to seek a support group and plan strategies for her long-term care.

Datis Kharrazian, DHSc, DC, MS

● ●

FOODS RICHEST IN CHOLINE, AN ACETYLCHOLINE PRECURSOR

With serotonin, dopamine, and GABA, deficiencies of dietary precursors typically aren't a factor in this country. Instead, blood sugar imbalances or other issues are more often the issue, as will be discussed in the next few chapters. With acetylcholine, however, precursor deficiency can be a factor in the United States thanks to the popularity of the low-fat diet.

Foods that impact acetylcholine activity are those high in natural fats, particularly animal fats (processed vegetable oils are not beneficial to acetylcholine activity or brain health in general). If the brain needs acetylcholine and is not getting it from adequate dietary fat, then it will break down brain tissue for phosphatidylcholine and phosphatidylserine, two fat-based components of neurons tissue from which acetylcholine can be synthesized. However, breaking down your own neuron tissue to provide acetylcholine does not make your brain very efficient in acetylcholine tasks.

Foods rich in choline

- Liver and organ meats
- Egg yolk
- Beef
- Tofu
- Nuts
- Cream
- Milk with fat (not non-fat or skim milk)
- Fatty cheeses

Like serotonin, dopamine, and GABA, synthesis of acetylcholine can be affected by blood sugar imbalances. Choline, the precursor for acetylcholine derived from dietary fat, is able to cross the blood-brain barrier. Once inside the brain, choline combines with an acetyl group, which is a byproduct of glucose metabolism, and pantothenic acid. For this acetyl group to be available for acetylcholine synthesis, energy production in the brain must be active and healthy.

Factors that affect energy production—blood sugar imbalances or poor oxygenation—can also affect acetylcholine production. Therefore, when I see symptoms of an acetylcholine deficiency, the first thing I'll ask about is whether the person is eating sufficient dietary fats. By sufficient dietary fat I mean that they do not follow a strict non-fat diet or a vegan/vegetarian diet with lack of choline-rich foods. If you eat eggs, beef, nuts, and cheese you are getting enough choline from your diet.

If dietary fat is not an issue, I'll then look to blood sugar and whether hypoglycemia, insulin resistance, or diabetes is disrupting the energy production cycle and, hence, acetylcholine synthesis.

DISTINGUISHING ACETYLCHOLINE DEFICIENCY FROM EARLY ALZHEIMER'S DISEASE

When neither a low-fat diet nor energy production are the issue, then the condition is more serious—the symptoms of acetylcholine deficiency are identical to early Alzheimer's disease from hippocampus destruction. In this case, the person will still benefit from supporting acetylcholine activity as that will help the neurons stay healthy, but it may be too late to undo the damage already done; the neurons involved in acetylcholine pathways are dead or no longer there. If that is the case then you may need to make your existing acetylcholine generating pathways more efficient in order to maintain what neurons you have left.

The neurons richest in acetylcholine activity are those found in the hippocampus, which governs memory and spatial orientation. If this area of the brain is degenerating then you need to develop as much plasticity in this area as possible, support your acetylcholine pathways with nutritional compounds, and adopt the other strategies found in this book for general neuron health.

CHAPTER SUMMARY

• Acetylcholine is the most important neurotransmitter for conversion of short-term memory to long-term memory, which happens in the area of the brain called the hippocampus. Poor acetylcholine activity is a great concern as much of the U.S. population ages—symptoms of dementia and Alzheimer's disease are the same as symptoms of acetylcholine impairment.

• Although we expect "senior moments" in older people, they should not be ignored as they may herald the onset of dementia or Alzheimer's disease. If these symptoms turn up in a younger person it indicates potential early brain degeneration. Unfortunately, it seems a person has to get the point where he can no longer remember his children's names to receive diagnosis and treatment in the standard health care model. The decline could have been happening for decades and prevented years earlier.

• If you have symptoms associated with acetylcholine activity or a hereditary risk for Alzheimer's, taking nutritional compounds to optimize acetylcholine activity may be a good idea. You can also support your acetylcholine function simply because you want to optimize your memory.

• Certain nutritional compounds support acetylcholine pathways, slow down acetylcholine breakdown, and have precursors for acetylcholine synthesis. Many of these compounds have shown promise in protecting against the development of brain plaques associated with Alzheimer's disease.

• One of the benefits of acetylcholine receptors compared to those of the other neurotransmitters is repeated exposure to acetylcholine does not cause the receptor sites to become resistant. This is not the case with serotonin, dopamine, or GABA. In fact, the opposite happens with acetylcholine receptors—constant stimulation of acetylcholine receptors makes them more responsive and sensitive so they need less acetylcholine for the same effect.

• Nutritional compounds that have been shown to support acetylcholine activity include L-Huperzine A, Alpha GPC, acetyl L-carnitine, and pantothenic acid.

• A low-fat diet can rob the brain of acetylcholine as foods that impact acetylcholine activity are those high in natural fats, particularly animal fats (processed vegetable oils are not beneficial to acetylcholine activity or brain health in general). If the brain is not getting acetylcholine from adequate dietary fat, then it will break down brain tissue to synthesize acetylcholine. However, breaking down your own brain tissue to provide acetylcholine does not make your brain very efficient in tasks that require acetylcholine.

• Blood sugar imbalances can affect acetylcholine synthesis.

• The neurons richest in acetylcholine activity are those found in the hippocampus, the area of the brain first affected by dementia you need to develop as much plasticity in this area as possible, support your acetylcholine pathways with nutritional compounds, and adopt the other strategies found in this book for general neuron health.

• The symptoms of acetylcholine deficiency are identical to early Alzheimer's disease from hippocampus destruction. A person will benefit from supporting brain health and acetylcholine activity, but it may be too late to undo the damage already done; the neurons involved in acetylcholine pathways are dead or no longer there. If that is the case then you may need to make your existing acetylcholine generating pathways more efficient in order to maintain what neurons you have left.

• Sometimes when people support acetylcholine activity they will "crash," getting hit with intense fatigue or other symptoms. This is due to the neurons being too close to threshold and not able to make enough energy to function properly. Although your brain may need acetylcholine support, it could be so fragile that just a little bit of support sends it over the edge, fatiguing both your neurons and your entire body.

• Another thing that can happen is that the additional neurotransmitter support can actually support negative plasticity. For example, if a person has tight calf muscles from training or poor postural tone, the acetylcholine support may stimulate her muscles to cramp before it's able to impact her brain chemistry for memory. Taking acetylcholine support impacts all synapses in the body, not just those in the brain.

• Another common adverse reaction in people who have failure in communication between their brain and gut is they immediately feel nauseous or even vomit when taking low doses of acetylcholine support. In these cases, the strategies to improve brain health and support the gut-brain axis should be considered seriously.

• So what do you do when you need acetylcholine support but even just a little is too much for a fragile brain? You use even less, while paying attention to issues of brain inflammation and oxygenation.

CHAPTER FOURTEEN
SEROTONIN

SYMPTOMS OF IMPAIRED SEROTONIN ACTIVITY

- Loss of pleasure in hobbies and interests
- Feelings of inner rage and anger
- Feelings of depression
- Difficulty finding joy from life pleasures
- Depression when it is cloudy or when there is lack of sunlight
- Loss of enthusiasm for favorite activities
- Not enjoying favorite foods
- Not enjoying friendships and relationships
- Unable to fall into deep restful sleep

* *

Melissa, 22, suffered from chronic headaches and gastrointestinal pain, with pain so severe at times she considered suicide. Several different gastroenterologists and internists had evaluated her but could not give her a diagnosis or an explanation for her complaints.

The last specialist Melissa saw accused her of making up her symptoms as a cry for attention. Sadly, this type of response is common in physicians who have big egos and are too incompetent to understand their patient's case. I have heard it many times from my chronic patients and in emails from readers. It is always upsetting that a physician would accuse a patient of such a thing.

When I saw Melissa I was able to properly diagnose her with abdominal migraines. These migraines are associated with imbalances in the serotonin system and its impact on blood flow regulation. In her case the migraines were impacting the vascular system in her gut-brain axis. Her case required a lot of work, but because she was suffering so badly I immediately referred her to a family physician to prescribe her migraine medication. The medication really helped if she took it immediately when symptoms started.

Although she now had a tool to reduce her suffering, the real work had just begun—I had to figure out why she was having the migraines, especially since the medications eventually stop working for many patients, and Melissa was having episodes daily. After a complete evaluation it was obvious many factors contributed to a faulty serotonin system. She had blood sugar issues, magnesium deficiencies, hormonal imbalances, and poor dietary habits.

As we addressed each of these issues over the course of a year, the abdominal migraines became less frequent, to the point Melissa had an attack only once or twice a year instead of almost every day.

I share Melissa's case with you for several reasons. First, although serotonin is associated with depression, imbalances in serotonin can cause many problems, including migraines, chronic constipation, poor cognitive function, flushing episodes, and more. Also, looking at serotonin imbalances from a natural approach requires more than just taking St. John's Wort or 5-HTP.

Proper serotonin physiology is linked to multiple mechanisms. If your brain is not working well and you have symptoms of serotonin imbalances, this chapter is very important for you to understand.

Datis Kharrazian, DHSc, DC, MS

• •

Melissa's case is an example of a lesser-known serotonin mechanism. Many people, however, experience depression as a result of poor serotonin activity. In neurology, depression is simply decreased firing of the frontal lobe, and the frontal lobe is saturated with receptor sites for serotonin—serotonin is a vital ingredient to a well-functioning frontal lobe.

It is overly simplistic to assume all depression stems from a serotonin imbalance. The brain is far more complex than that, and there can be numerous different reasons for depression, including impairment in any of the neurotransmitter pathways or anything that causes the frontal lobe to lose its chemical activity. However, for many people a serotonin impairment is a major contributing factor to poor frontal lobe function, resulting in symptoms of depression.

One of the key symptoms of poor serotonin activity, whether low serotonin or a breakdown in the serotonin transmission pathway, is that the person can't get joy from anything. Symptoms of serotonin imbalance include: Have you lost enthusiasm for your hobbies, interests, favorite foods, or favorite activities? Do you feel overwhelmed with ideas to manage? Do you have feelings of inner rage or paranoia? Do you feel depressed that you are not enjoying your life or that you have lost interest in life? Do you have no appreciation for art? Do you get depressed when it's cloudy or there is a lack of sunlight? Are you not enjoying your friendships and relationships? Are you unable to sleep well? Do you feel dependent on others? Do you feel more susceptible to pain? Do you experience unprovoked anger?

My serotonin-deficient patients have a wonderful-looking life on paper, but they aren't enjoying the benefits. They tell me their life is great, they have a good job, they're financially secure, they have a great family…and yet they're unhappy. In fact, they often feel guilty for being unhappy because they know it doesn't make sense.

Well-meaning but misguided advice from friends and family to think of those who are worse off or to count their blessings do little to replenish depleted serotonin or restore function to misfiring synapses. The person with low serotonin activity can't use intellectual reasoning to find joy in her life. If I ask these patients if they could have any food they wanted, what would they choose, they can't think of anything. They can't think of a favorite song or a favorite type of music. They used to have a hobby, but dropped it because they no longer got anything out of it, or they're not motivated to socialize anymore. If left unmanaged, these symptoms have the potential to worsen into a desperate situation.

Another common aspect of serotonin impairment is that symptoms worsen when the skies turn cloudy or during the short days of winter. I teach in hotel conference rooms around the country, some of which are like dungeons with poor artificial lighting and no windows. As the course wears on, I can see the serotonin-deficient practitioners in the room slowly lose brain function. Without the serotonin synthesis brought on by sunlight, they begin to lose stimulation to the brain and start to fatigue and lose their focus.

Although general brain health, stress, and blood sugar imbalances are first steps in addressing a serotonin deficiency, many people also benefit from direct nutritional support of the serotonin pathway. As was the case with Alena, below, the effects can sometimes be life-changing.

• •

Alena, 40, was in her late 30s when her life fell into a series of back-to-back tragedies. Her dad died after battling cancer for two years, she went through a divorce, she found a good friend dead on his living room floor, and she was in a bad car accident. She remembers this period being dominated by tremendous stress, anxiety, grief, obsessive thoughts, and an inability to sleep.

As a health-conscious vegetarian and a yoga teacher, she assumed she would emerge from the grief and eventually recover. Instead, however, she found herself spiraling ever deeper into depression with thoughts of suicide—anything to stop the never ending pain—creeping into her mental landscape.

"I desperately wanted an off-switch for how I was feeling," Alena says. "I felt like I was going crazy. I was so desperate and felt so horrible."

At an annual physical by her medical doctor, she burst into tears and explained what was going on, and that depression runs in her family. Her doctor told her she exhibited all the symptoms of clinical depression and needed to begin antidepressants and counseling immediately. She also explained to Alena the chemical nature of depression. Alena took her doctor's warnings to heart, but because she prefers a holistic approach, she decided to try natural medicine first and consulted with me.

"Antidepressants were the last resort for me," says Alena. "I wanted to see if what she had would work and if not, I'd just go on antidepressants."

After assessing Alena, I immediately got her started on nutritional compounds to support her serotonin and GABA pathways.

Remarkably, within just a couple of days Alena's depression, anxiety, and obsessive thinking magically lifted. She found that off-switch for which she desperately had been grasping.

"I slept through the night for the first time in three years," Alena says. "It's not that my problems went away, but the obsessive thoughts, dread, despair, and anxiety did so that I could deal with my grief in a more clear-minded manner."

After she stabilized her depression, Alena then noticed that lack of focus and getting easily distracted were affecting her work as a professional photographer, and I gave her some additional support for her acetylcholine pathways (vegetarians, vegans, and low-fat eaters run a risk of acetylcholine deficiency). Overnight she regained her mental clarity and focus while working.

During this time she also switched from a vegetarian diet to a Paleo diet, which is comprised of meats, vegetables, and fruits—no grains or sweets. This helped to significantly diminish her thyroid disease symptoms of a pounding heart, exhaustion, and night sweats, and it further improved her sleep and mood. She also dropped the 10 pounds that had slowly been accumulating on her otherwise slender frame.

After more than a year and a half on the brain chemistry support, Alena wanted to try weaning off the supplements and let her own brain take over. As she lowered her doses of the nutritional compounds to minimal levels, she was buoyed by the results—her good mood stuck around.

"I feel like the brain support saved my life," says Alena. "I was really going down in a destructive way. The experience gave me a perspective of what it's like to be clinically depressed and why people commit suicide. There's never any relief from the pain—it just goes on and on and on. I also have a totally different perspective on my life, the patterns in my life, and the relationships I've had. I realized a huge component of it all was chemical."

Cari Nyland, ND
Portland, Oregon

SEROTONIN 101

Serotonin is manufactured in the raphe nuclei, an area located in the midbrain. Its production is triggered by activation of the tectum, also located in the midbrain. Stimulation of the tectum depends on adequate light, which is why serotonin deficiency is often associated with depression and moodiness during winter, on cloudy days, or with too many days spent inside. If someone spends a lot of time in a dark apartment, all day in a cubicle with poor lighting, or they go to work and come home in the dark, the tectum may not receive enough light stimulation. As a result, the tectum fails to fire into the rest of the midbrain sufficiently, including the raphe nuclei, and serotonin production suffers.

In the scientific literature, low serotonin activity is associated with increased anger and aggressiveness, depression, obsessive compulsive disorder, migraines, irritable bowel syndrome, tinnitus (ringing in the ears), fibromyalgia, bipolar disorder, anxiety disorders, and intense religious experiences.[1][2][3][4][5] This doesn't mean that all migraines or tinnitus issues are serotonin-based; these are just symptoms that have been seen in the research.

On the other hand, excessive levels of serotonin have been associated in the literature with shyness, inferiority complex, nervousness, feeling vulnerable to criticism, fear of being disliked, and a desire for social contact but being too afraid to initiate it.[6] Again, these are common traits that aren't always associated with a serotonin excess.

However, they may be worth considering when one is taking a medication that impacts serotonin levels, such as a selective serotonin re-uptake inhibitor (SSRI) antidepressant. Typically when people take these for long periods of time, their levels of serotonin may get too high and they may begin to exhibit the symptoms of excess amounts. Another risk is that the response to serotonin may become blunted if excess exposure continues for too long. This is due to homotropic modulation, when repeated excess exposure to a single neurotransmitter causes the postsynaptic receptors to lose sensitivity to it.

• •

A 40-year-old woman concerned about losing weight came to see me. She had two young children, traveled often for work, slept poorly, and was in the middle of a nasty divorce. She was taking an over-the-counter nighttime pain medication, allergy medication, antidepressants, and had just finished a round of medication for a sinus infection. She vacillated between high and low blood sugar daily and ate fast food regularly.

Of concern to me was that her symptoms indicated several problems with neurotransmitter production. She assured me that with her SSRI antidepressant she was OK. She wanted to get off it some day but was afraid she would fall apart. Even though she was numb to life, she at least felt like she could cope, which was the most important thing to her at the time, in addition to losing weight. Diabetes ran in her family, and she definitely did not want to follow suit.

I started her on a three-week cleanse with a hypoallergenic detoxification protein powder, blood sugar support, and vitamin D. The cleanse began with a three-to-five-day fast using a drink made from water, lemon or lime juice, maple syrup, and green tea. The fast made her feel so good she didn't want to go back to eating, an indication of severe food intolerances.

Her blood work indicated hypothyroidism secondary to insulin resistance. Insulin resistance causes testosterone to rise in females, which causes an increase in free T3 and T3 uptake. This in turn causes cells to become resistant to T3 hormones, creating symptoms of hypothyroidism. Her blood panel also showed oxidation and extremely low vitamin D levels.

Once she completed the cleanse and lost 10 pounds, she stayed clear of sugar, gluten, and dairy and continued to lose weight and feel good. She felt so good that she opted to discontinue her SSRI. She had already stopped taking her sleeping medication. However, she called because her anxiety began to creep back in and she wanted to try something natural for it, so I gave her nutritional compounds to support serotonin and dopamine. She reported success in both sleeping and mood and stayed with the program for some time until she stopped coming in.

The good news is her renewed health and energy garnered her a newfound social life. The bad news is her new social life sent her nearly back to square one: After a year passed, she called to say she needed help. She wanted to lose the 25 pounds she had gained back as a result of all the eating out she was doing as part *of her new social life. She didn't date or see friends while on the SSRI because of how numb it made her feel, so she didn't want to go back to taking it. However, her anxiety was now "through the roof." She knew the food issue was conquerable and necessary on her own and she was prepared to take that on. Back on serotonin and dopamine support, her life was cheerful, serene, and active once again.*

Kari Vernon, DC
Scottsdale, Arizona
www.karismaforlife.com

● ●

ESTROGEN AND SEROTONIN

Excess serotonin can also be associated with excess estrogen, which is sometimes seen with the use of oral contraceptives or estrogen creams. Estrogen increases the activity of the serotonin receptor and increases overall serotonin activity in the brain. Therefore, when someone presents with symptoms of high serotonin, excess estrogen should be considered. This goes the other way as well—low estrogen levels, also common, can likewise cause low serotonin activity and symptoms of deficiency.

Estrogens (there are three forms of estrogen) increase the sensitivity of the serotonin receptor sites.[7] A very common example of this is the woman who is postmenopausal and unable to produce the amounts of estrogen her body needs. As a result she may become depressed or lose some of her mental cognition, such as the ability to do math, learn new things, or remember well.

At this point she may see her primary care doctor, who prescribes an antidepressant. If it's a medication that impacts serotonin activity, it may help for a while. Or she may go on estrogen replacement therapy and find this helps for a while. However, with both these approaches she runs the risk of long-term complications: a tolerance to antidepressants may develop, or levels of estrogen in the body become too high, causing cellular resistance to the hormone and hence symptoms of estrogen deficiency.

Because of the role estrogen plays in healthy serotonin activity, taking nutritional compounds that support serotonin may help only somewhat or not at all if estrogen is deficient. In this case a hormone panel that charts estrogen levels can be very useful. As I mentioned in my thyroid book, I am very reluctant to use bioidentical hormones for hormonal deficiencies without first investigating mechanisms. I prefer to discover the cause of the estrogen deficiency, such as poor adrenal function, and address that.

However, due to the importance of estrogen for brain function, if a perimenopausal or postmenopausal woman is unable to resolve her estrogen deficiencies through functional medicine, I feel bioidentical hormone replacement is warranted. In this case it's important to use natural, bioidentical hormones instead of synthetic ones because the bioidentical hormones show up on lab tests (synthetic do not), so that levels can be monitored. Also, because taking estrogen can deplete the methyl donors necessary for serotonin synthesis, it's also important to supplement with these if you use estrogen. These include methyl B-12, SAMe, or MSM (methylsulfonylmethane).

• •

I recently started working with a 35-year-old woman who came to me complaining of extreme depression and a complete lack of libido. It was obvious from the very second that she walked into my clinic that she was not well. Her eyes lacked the sparkle of a happy and thriving person. She looked exhausted. And she appeared to have been crying on the way to the appointment. Needless to say, her marriage was under considerable strain.

I learned that eight months earlier she underwent a complete hysterectomy due to a 10-pound tumor growing on her ovaries. She has since declined any hormone replacement therapy from her medical doctor and only takes some basic herbal support.

In reviewing her intake questionnaire it was obvious that she suffered from symptoms of insulin resistance. She also complained about being overweight, which was further impacting her blood sugar imbalance. The hormonal declines due to the removal of the ovaries was also taking its toll in many different ways—low estrogen impacts serotonin, which can be tightly connected to her main complaint of depression.

As a clinician I feel treating the root of the problem is extremely important, but in some cases treating the symptoms first can be even more important. After reviewing her symptoms I found that the vast majority of her complaints came from the serotonin section, though GABA was impacted as well. As a first step, even before ordering more blood tests, I sent her home with some nutritional compounds to boost serotonin activity. I felt that this patient needed some immediate help.

I saw her the next week to go over her blood chemistry report and was met with a completely different patient. She walked in with much more energy, and the sparkle in here eyes was apparent. There were even smiles. She admitted to still struggling, but overall felt much better. She even started to eat breakfast again. She was more present than before and willing to take on the dietary changes to manage her insulin resistance, which was confirmed by a high fasting blood sugar level. I believe that working with her further on insulin resistance will impact neurotransmitter function in general. I was eager to see what her next blood chemistry report would reveal about her progress.

In my last consultation with her I asked her how she felt about the serotonin support. She replied, "The day after starting I felt like someone gave me a big hug and I have felt that way ever since." You can't ask for a better testimonial that.

Jim Chialtas, LAc, MTCM
San Diego, California
www.laurelacupuncturesd.blogspot.com

● ●

5-HTP VERSUS TRYPTOPHAN

In the natural medicine world practitioners debate as to whether it is better to supplement with 5-HTP or tryptophan—both amino acids that are precursors to serotonin—when wanting to boost serotonin production. Some people prefer tryptophan because it has been shown to more easily cross the blood-brain barrier than 5-HTP. Others prefer 5-HTP because it is only one step away from being converted to serotonin, whereas tryptophan is two steps away, so 5-HTP has more potential to boost serotonin levels, but both work.

I sometimes give a combination of both 5-HTP and tryptophan to cover the bases of blood-brain barrier transport and conversion. I also use the following botanicals to increase receptor site sensitivity, ensure the breakdown of used serotonin, and provide necessary cofactors for serotonin production: St. John's wort, SAMe, P-5-P (a form of B-6), niacinamide, magnesium citrate, methyl B-12, and folic acid.

Studies show both 5-HTP and tryptophan increase levels of serotonin and can be helpful in addressing depression, persistent nightmares, fibromyalgia, chronic headaches, migraines, and mood disorders.[8][9][10][11][12]

OTHER NUTRITIONAL COMPOUNDS THAT IMPACT SEROTONIN

St. John's wort has been shown to act as a natural serotonin reuptake inhibitor. This means it allows serotonin to hang out in the synaptic cleft longer, therefore increasing its activity on postsynaptic receptor sites and boosting serotonin transmission.[13][14][15][16][17][18][19]

SAMe is used to transfer a methyl group to boost serotonin production and increase serotonin levels. Several studies have shown it to be effective at easing depression. In fact, it's a very popular treatment for depression in Europe and other parts of the world.[20][21][22][23][24][25]

The other nutrients—magnesium, P-5-P, niacin, methyl B-12, and folic acid—are necessary for the synthesis of serotonin. All of these nutritional compounds together can help encourage healthy serotonin production.

* *

There is a myth that the tryptophan from Thanksgiving turkey dinner is what makes you sleepy. What makes you sleepy is the insulin surge from overeating, not the tryptophan. You can take several capsules of tryptophan at doses that far exceed the tryptophan load you would ever get from eating turkey and it will not cause you to get sleepy.

When your body cannot utilize the excess glucose you eat, it converts the glucose into fat. This conversion uses significant energy, which makes you tired. You are more likely to get sleepy from the pie, stuffing, and other high carbohydrate foods than from anything else. You can bet the people at the Thanksgiving dinner who only eat turkey and vegetables do not fall asleep. But those who had stuffing and pie and overate carbohydrates are the ones passing out.

● ●

SEROTONIN AND FOODS

Many nutritionists have proposed we become deficient in serotonin because we do not eat enough foods rich in tryptophan, such as shrimp, mushrooms, snapper, halibut, chicken, scallops, spinach, turkey, lamb, beef, liver, and salmon. They have also gone as far as to make menus for people with low serotonin activity.

I can tell you from clinical experience and a review of the literature that just raising these foods in your diet won't do much to boost serotonin levels. For one thing, with the exception perhaps of poorly practicing vegans or junk-food vegetarians who are completely protein deprived, most Americans eat enough protein-rich foods to supply precursors for all their amino acids. The Standard American Diet (SAD) is not deficient in protein or amino acids. As a matter of fact, the SAD is overly abundant in meats, milk, cheese, and other sources of proteins that contain amino acids necessary to make neurotransmitters. The main issue with amino acids in the United States is how you utilize them.

The bigger issue is whether the precursors make it into the brain and are able to be synthesized into serotonin. Again, this is where general brain health, stress, and blood sugar imbalances determine how well the brain is able to uptake and use serotonin precursors.

● ●

I worked with a 38-year-old man for depression for a year. He had been on a selective serotonin reuptake inhibitor (SSRI) antidepressant for five years. Despite taking his medication he complained of feeling unmotivated and irritable, both of which were relieved to some extent with exercise. He was sad 40 percent of the time and felt much worse without his medication. He felt his depression was always in the background and impeding his rela-tionships. He wanted to get off the antidepressant but felt he could not. He had been a vegetarian for 18 years and does not eat dairy. An intake form indicated he suffered from both hypoglycemia and insulin resistance.

His memory has significantly declined in the past five years, and he complained of weight gain around the hips. A salivary adrenal panel showed an abnormal sleep-wake cycle, and his blood work indicated hypothyroidism and hypochlorhydria, a condition of insufficient stomach acid. A testosterone test came back with results at the low end of normal.

We worked on balancing blood sugar and his adrenal function for three to four months with diet and nutritional compounds. He included more fat and protein in his diet while lowering his carbohydrates and started to include fish but still no red meat. His follow-up adrenal test came back much more normal, and he said his memory improved quite a bit.

At this point he felt confident enough to wean himself off his medication. His symptoms still showed weakness in the serotonin area, and I gave him nutritional compounds to support serotonin activity as we backed off on some of the blood sugar and adrenal support (however, he maintained his blood-sugar stabilizing diet). He has now been off his medication for three months and is doing great.

Dagmar Ehling, MAc, LAc, DOM(NM), Dipl OM, FABORM
Durham, North Carolina
www.orientalhealthsolutions.com

● ●

A SWEET LOOK INTO SEROTONIN PRODUCTION

While supplementing with nutritional compounds to support serotonin activity may be necessary at times, the real question to consider is why serotonin activity is impaired. A major cause is poor utilization of tryptophan for serotonin production. Tryptophan is an essential amino acid that cannot be synthesized in the body and must be supplied by the diet. The SAD supplies plenty of tryptophan so serotonin issues are rarely from consumption, but rather from the inability to transport tryptophan across the blood-brain barrier.

The transport protein used to carry tryptophan across the blood-brain barrier is called "large neutral amino acid transporter" (LNAA). Abnormal insulin surges from constant blood sugar fluctuations will alter the transport of LANA and the ability to maintain ideal serotonin function.

Although the SAD of eating excess sugar, animal products, and carbohydrates is not deficient in tryptophan, it does promote abnormal glucose and insulin surges that compromise tryptophan transport across the blood-brain barrier and hence serotonin production.

• •

I have been in the natural health care field for more than 10 years. I recently had surgery to replace my right knee, the result of an injury sustained 35 years ago. After surgery and all the medications it entailed, I grew progressively irritable and depressed. This is highly unusual for me, as I am an energetic, happy person by nature. I thought about some of the mechanisms involved in my mood shift and what I had learned from Dr. Kharrazian and started taking nutritional compounds to improve the activity and synthesis of serotonin. Within five days my dark cloud of irritability and depression had lifted and I was feeling back to my normal optimistic self.

Terence A. Trinka, OD CN BCNP
Conifer, Colorado
www.rockymountainthyroidcenter.com

• •

IRON AND SEROTONIN

Once tryptophan or 5-HTP cross the blood-brain barrier they must be made into serotonin. As mentioned earlier, tryptophan, found in protein-rich foods, is two steps away from serotonin. First tryptophan converts to 5-HTP and then to serotonin. These conversions are entirely dependent on sufficient levels of iron, which makes an iron deficiency another factor to consider with poor serotonin activity.

Iron anemia, of course, is a dead giveaway. Some symptoms of iron-deficiency anemia (as there are several types of anemia), include the whites of the eyes turning a bluish color, a pale face, nail beds that are pale instead of pink, a compulsion to chew ice or dirt, or chronic fingernail biting. Women with heavy menstrual periods are at risk, as are endurance athletes who may experience excessive red blood cell breakdown. Women with uterine fibroids often become iron deficient as the fibroids take up most of the body's iron. People with parasites such as pinworms develop iron deficiencies, as do those with malabsorption issues.

Iron deficiency anemia is very common in those with a gluten intolerance or celiac disease as gluten destroys the lining of the small intestine, causing malabsorption. Hypothyroidism can also impair the body's ability to absorb iron, as can low stomach hydrochloric acid, which is often associated with an H. pylori bacterial infection.

If you have chronic serotonin symptoms or are dependent on natural serotonin support compounds to function, you must rule out iron deficiency. Please make sure you have a complete blood count and an iron panel completed by your practitioner to rule out any issues with iron metabolism interfering with serotonin production.

OTHER NUTRITIONAL COFACTORS FOR SEROTONIN PRODUCTION

Besides iron, other nutrients are important for serotonin synthesis. These are P-5-P (pyridoxal-5-phosphate), an active form of B-6, niacin, methyl B-12, folic acid, and magnesium. With the prevalence of fast-food diets and processed foods today, deficiencies in these important cofactors are widespread.

A severe magnesium deficiency may hamper conversion of 5-HTP into serotonin; you see magnesium deficiencies in those taking diuretics, a first-line therapy for high blood pressure. Athletes who overtrain can also become deficient in magnesium.

Methyl donors such as methyl B-12 are important for the conversion of 5-HTP to serotonin. Studies show people who take SSRIs for long periods of time become deficient in methyl donors and P-5-P. Those considering weaning off their antidepressant medication may need to supplement with these cofactors to cover deficiencies acquired during use of the medication.

Lack of methyl donors are found in those who take estrogen replacement therapy, such as birth control pills or estrogen creams. They can also be low in those with insufficient stomach hydrochloric acid or those with H. pylori infections—a bacterial infection in the stomach that causes low stomach acid. Additionally, chronic alcohol use can reduce the levels of P-5-P. (And it doesn't matter what kind of alcohol. Expensive fine wines are still considered alcohol).

• •

Since the age of 12, I suffered from depression. Several times in my adult life I trialed medications to help combat severe depression. My first trials, at age 32, were very poorly tolerated—I would vomit almost immediately after taking them. Finally, at age 34, I was able to tolerate one antidepressant that I remained on for about nine months, although it caused very intense symptoms: significant weight loss, significant insomnia, sadness, suicidal ideation, depersonalization, a sense of unreality, and these weird "brain zaps," which have been well described by many other individuals treated with SSRIs. I sought therapy but I was never consistent with treatment.

I continued without medications most of my adult life. I was a parent, a student, and then a professional, a volunteer, and an active athlete. I did all this with the constant burden of incredible sadness. Interestingly, from ages 35 to 37, I had made good progress in therapy, putting behind me many of my younger struggles, but the sadness persisted.

My depression is not the only story here, though. Starting at age 18, I had what neurologists call an "idiopathic benign tremor" or "familial tremor." Fear, anger, or adrenaline caused me to shake very visibly in both my hands and sometimes my neck. I had been prescribed a beta blocker and while it was certainly helpful for acute symptoms, sometimes it would give me a headache and it did not address the cause of the problem. It just provided symptomatic treatment.

In December 2008, at the urging of Dr. Glen Zielinski, I tried nutritional compounds to support serotonin activity. In one week of taking them the sadness lifted. One who has not lived through it cannot understand the relief of overcoming depression. Gone were the suicidal thoughts I would have just driving to work or walking through the supermarket. After spending all of my adult life in a cognitive fog, I finally felt like I could think, remember, and concentrate.

Dr. Zielinski identified several metabolic issues that were negatively impacting my well-being. Prior to the success of the sero-

tonin support I had rejected them because they seemed too difficult to address. He told me hypoglycemia was exacerbating my tremor and my capacity to manufacture neurotransmitters. I would frequently fast throughout the day and eat only at night.

He performed tests to assess for antigliadin antibodies and discovered that I had a gluten sensitivity. He told me how this affected both my mood and the neurology of the tremor. After some coaxing I stopped eating gluten. Two years later I eliminated most dairy from my diet. Dr. Zielinski also asked me to perform many neurorehabilitative exercises to help me reduce my tremors.

The tremors are still present, but only rarely and quite minimally. I take the beta blocker maybe once or twice a month, if that, compared to my almost-daily use a few years ago. The depression has stayed away. It's been almost four years of a solid non-depressed mood.

Melanie, age 41, patient of Dr. Zielinski
Glen Zielinski, DC, DACNB, FACFN
Lake Oswego, Oregon
www.northwestfunctionalneurology.com

● ●

When considering the cause of a serotonin deficiency, you must first address the three deal breakers: general brain health, stress, and blood sugar imbalances. If you are eating ample protein, then you must additionally consider whether you are sufficient in estrogen, iron, and the other nutritional cofactors.

Are you postmenopausal and suffering from an estrogen deficiency? Do you have an undiagnosed gluten intolerance or uterine fibroid that may be making you anemic? Do you take birth control pills or use estrogen creams that may be creating excess levels of estrogen and depleting you of methyl donors? Has your overall diet been poor and possibly lacking in the necessary nutrients for serotonin conversion? Do you drink alcohol daily or take medications that may be interfering with serotonin activity?

SUPPORTING YOUR SEROTONIN PATHWAYS

Once these factors have been addressed, serotonin support may still be necessary to jump-start its production in the brain. Or, as in the case of Alena and some of the other people featured in this chapter, immediate relief is sometimes necessary before delving into the deal breakers and cofactors. In summary, here are the nutrients I use to support serotonin: 5-HTP and/or tryptophan, SAMe, St. John's wort, niacinamide, P-5-P, folic acid, methyl B-12, and magnesium.

Dosing

The big question is always, "How much do I take?" My answer is as much as you need to experience a benefit. Supporting neurotransmitter activity is not dependent upon body size, but instead on the degree to which you have symptoms. As a result, determining your dose requires some trial and error.

I suggest starting with 75 mg of 5-HTP or tryptophan. (You may also choose to experiment with either one as some people get different reactions to each). It typically takes a half hour to an hour to notice the effects, although for more severe symptoms such as Alena's depression and suicidal thoughts, the full effects can take two to three days.

Continue to gradually increase your dose until you notice an improvement in your symptoms. Then increase the dose again to see whether you experience even more improvement. Once you no longer feel any improvement, go back to the previous dose at which you last felt improvement.

How often you take serotonin support also varies with the individual. Some may find they need it three or more times a day, others just once.

● ●

Ever since a head injury that temporarily blinded her when she was 8 years old, Cassandra, 26, suffered from headaches, stomach aches, and chronic digestive issues. She vacillated between constipation that would last for two weeks and cause extreme discomfort, and chronic diarrhea that kept her constantly on alert for the nearest bathroom. Bloating, an inability to digest what she ate, and headaches were also a part of her daily life.

I tried various nutritional remedies on Cassandra. The remedies would work for a couple of weeks before the same old problems cropped up. Then I went to Dr. Kharrazian's class on brain chemistry and came back with a new idea: boost Cassandra's serotonin activity. Serotonin is necessary in the gut, and Cassandra's childhood head injury had caused lasting neurological damage affecting gut function.

"She put me on serotonin support along with some other things to support digestion and estrogen, and it worked perfectly within a few days," says Cassandra. "For the first time since I was a child I feel like a normal person, and I know what it's like to have a normal day now."

Cassandra has been taking the serotonin support for three months now and says she wakes up feeling great and has more energy in general. She doesn't have to worry about where a bathroom is all the time and says she can also think more clearly and feels less frazzled—important for a woman who runs two businesses.

"I've even noticed my nails grow faster and my eyelashes are longer and thicker, probably because I'm getting more nutrients from better gut function," she says. "I am truly thankful."

Lisa Merritt, DC, ND
Charlotte, North Carolina
www.weddingtonwellness.com

● ●

What if you crash and burn on serotonin support? Sometimes when people support serotonin or one of the other neurotransmitters they will "crash." In other words, they will suddenly feel slammed with intense fatigue. This is due to the neurons being too close to threshold and not able to make enough energy to function properly. Although the person's brain may need serotonin support, it is so fragile that just a little bit of support sends it over the edge, fatiguing the neurons and hence the individual.

If this crash happens after just the minimum dose, it could actually mean you are in desperate need of support. However, additional support for brain inflammation, brain oxygenation, and general neuronal function may also be warranted. Compounds for these conditions will

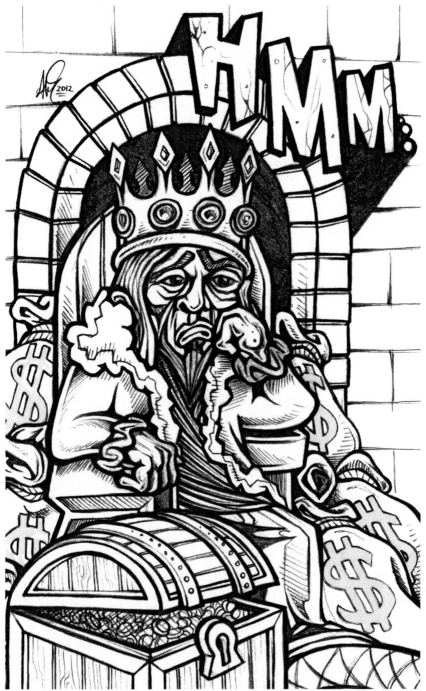

Many serotonin-deficient people have good jobs, secure finances, and great families, yet they're unhappy and feel guilty about it.

dampen the inflammation in the brain that is commonly seen with neurodegeneration, give the neurons more protection against degeneration, and supply the brain with more oxygen-rich blood (assuming anemia isn't a factor).

Another thing that can happen to the fragile brain is that additional neurotransmitter support can actually encourage negative plasticity. For example, a person with obsessive compulsive disorder (OCD) driven by poor serotonin activity may actually find supporting serotonin makes her OCD worse. The same factors are at work as in the individual who crashes.

So what do you do when you need serotonin support but even just a little is too much? You use even less, while simultaneously addressing brain inflammation, dysglycemia, and oxygenation.

Earlier I gave an example of how tinnitus, that annoying ringing in the ears, can sometimes be caused by the auditory neurons being too close to threshold. In other words, they are so weak and unstable due to poor health that they fire too easily and perceive noise that isn't even there, hence the ringing. The way some people restore function to those neurons is not to completely isolate them from sound, but rather to use a hearing aid that gently stimulates them with small amounts of more sound so that they rebuild strength and begin to function properly again.

It's the same concept with very low doses of serotonin precursors for those who "fry out" rather quickly with support. The lower doses gently stimulate and strengthen the neurons so they can function better on their own and slowly handle increasing amounts of input, whether it is from serotonin-boosting compounds or life in general.

PROPER BREAKDOWN OF SEROTONIN IS IMPORTANT

The breakdown and clearance of serotonin is another vital part of neurotransmitter activity in the brain. As I mentioned earlier, three things are necessary for healthy neurotransmitter activity: the brain's ability to make the neurotransmitter, the ability of the neurotransmitter to bind to the receptor site, and the ability of the neurotransmitter to be broken down and cleared. If the serotonin can't be degraded and broken down for clearance from the synaptic cleft, then new serotonin can't bind to the postsynaptic receptors. The result is faulty transmission.

Two specific enzymes are involved in the breakdown of serotonin: 5-hydroxyindoleacetic acid (5-HIAA) and monoamine oxidase (MAO). One thing to consider is whether these enzymes are getting what they need to function properly, namely magnesium, methyl donors, and B vitamins.

Certain medications can inhibit these enzymes as well, especially a class of antidepressants called MAO-inhibiting drugs (Marplan, Nardil, Parnate, Manerix, and Emsam). MAO-inhibiting drugs work for depression because they slow the breakdown of serotonin and epinephrine and norepinephrine, our fight-or-flight adrenal stress hormones. This class of drugs increases levels of both serotonin and these adrenal hormones to address severe depression.

The danger is when SSRIs, drugs that increase the amount of serotonin in the synaptic cleft, are used in conjunction with MAO-inhibiting drugs, which slow the breakdown of serotonin. Used together they can lead to "serotonin syndrome," a rare condition caused by excess serotonin.

Serotonin syndrome, which occurs when there is too much serotonin in the synaptic cleft, usually comes on suddenly and causes a broad, diverse range of neurological symptoms. Symptom onset is usually rapid, often in association with a new medication, and can include confusion, hallucinations, agitation, headaches, coma, shivering, sweating, fever, hypertension, tachycardia, nausea, diarrhea, muscle twitching, and tremors.

Eating foods high in tyramine, such as smoked, pickled, spoiled, cured, or fermented meats, can contribute to the risk of serotonin syndrome in people taking MAO-inhibitors. Though rare, the same is true for those taking certain natural compounds in conjunction with MAO-inhibiting drugs. These include St. John's wort, 5-HTP, tryptophan, yohimbe (a male-enhancing herb), and boswellia.

● ●

Since the birth of my last child five years ago I had seizures, depression, constant migraines, and my memory was so poor I had to take a notepad everywhere I went just so I could remember my tasks for the day.

I went to many internists and neurologists, and all they had to offer were medications with side effects that made me feel worse. I was at the end of my rope. I literally no longer wanted to live.

A friend told me Dr. Redd was a student of Dr. Kharrazian and he could help. At my first appointment Dr. Redd spent a lot of time with me doing neurological testing. He also did a blood test, a food intolerance test, an intestinal permeability test, and had me fill out an assessment form. Almost all my answers to questions were outside the normal range.

Dr. Redd had me take home pills to do a GABA challenge and after the first dose my symptoms intensified. Dr. Redd said I had a blood-brain barrier problem and a significant amount of brain inflammation. He said we needed to work on the barriers of my brain and my intestinal tract, and that we also needed to decrease the inflammation in my body.

I started taking compounds to support oxygenation of my brain, quench brain inflammation, repair the gut lining, and address general inflammation. He also had me avoid gluten, dairy, and eggs.

Within two weeks my symptoms improved drastically, and two months later when I did the GABA challenge again I had no problems. It was amazing to see the difference in only two months. I redid the assessment form, and it was a lot better as well.

The only problem remaining was my serotonin activity, as I was still having some depression. To help support this, Dr. Redd gave me nutrients for serotonin activity, adrenal function, and inflammation for another two months. After that, I filled out the assessment form for the third time, and it was almost perfect.

I no longer get seizures or migraines. I can remember things without a notepad. My future looks bright again, and I am happy to be alive! My neurologist and internist were shocked by both the results and the fact that they were achieved in such a short period of time.

I am so grateful to Dr. Redd. I'm also grateful to Dr. Kharrazian for all his efforts in doing research and teaching doctors how to help their patients more effectively. I owe my life to these doctors!

Julie, a patient of Dr. Redd

Joshua Redd, DC

Salt Lake City, Utah

www.drjoshuaredd.com

● ●

SEROTONIN, MELATONIN, AND SLEEP DISTURBANCES

One of the more common symptoms of poor serotonin activity is poor sleep. This can mean an inability to sleep deeply or stay asleep, insomnia, persistent nightmares, and restless sleep. While many different things can cause sleep problems, poor serotonin activity should be considered.

Healthy sleep is dependent upon healthy melatonin activity. Melatonin is a sleep hormone that relies on serotonin for proper function. Other clues that point to a melatonin issue are depression, moodiness, lethargy, or migraines brought on by too much darkness or poor light.

Serotonin is converted into melatonin in the brain's pineal gland, the most serotonin-rich tissue in the body. In addition to helping us sleep, melatonin regulates the sleep-wake cycle and metabolic and behavioral changes in response to the seasons. Melatonin is also one of the hormones that regulates female reproductive hormones, helping determine when menstruation begins, the frequency and duration of menstrual cycles, and when menopause begins.

Secretion of melatonin is stimulated by the dark and inhibited by light. The conversion of serotonin to melatonin involves two enzymes: N-acetyl transferase (NAT) and 5-hydroxyindole-O-methyltransferase (5-HIOMT). These enzymes depend upon methyl donors and the adrenal hormone norepinephrine.

Normally we relate adrenal hormones, our stress hormones, with an inability to sleep. Although this can be true when adrenal hormones are too high in response to chronic stress, levels that are too low, such as in the case of adrenal fatigue, can hinder the conversion of serotonin to melatonin as norepinephrine triggers one of the enzymes responsible for this conversion.

Melatonin and norepinephrine

Factors that can eventually depress norepinephrine levels are the same ones that initially raise stress hormones too high. Chronic caffeine and nicotine consumption, blood sugar imbalances, food intolerances, chronic inflammation, gut infections or parasites, chronic viruses, overtraining, and chronic lack of sleep are examples of factors that can eventually fatigue the adrenal glands and the production of stress hormones. The result is a double-edged sword: a chronically tired person who cannot sleep well and grapples with depression. Over time, the chronic stress and repeated release of these hormones can exhaust adrenal hormone production and the brain's regulation of these systems.

Another factor that affects levels of norepinephrine is darkness. Each day as the sun gets lower in the sky, the pupils enlarge to allow in more light. The release of norepinephrine is a is a sympathetic response that dilates the pupils in response to a darkening day, which begins the conversion of serotonin to melatonin. This explains why when you look at the sleep-wake cycle, also called the circadian rhythm, melatonin levels are lower in the day and higher at night. However, people with adrenal fatigue may be low in norepinephrine and have trouble converting serotonin to melatonin. As a result, sleep is a struggle.

In my practice it's not uncommon to see patients who overtrain, drink too much caffeine, smoke regularly, suffer from undiagnosed food intolerances (which release histamine, impacting norepinephrine levels), take recreational drugs, or eat too many sugars and starches.

Nutrient deficiencies, such as in vitamin C or the amino acid tyrosine, can also affect norepinephrine levels. Frequently these people also have trouble sleeping. It could be because all these habits impact the body's ability to maintain appropriate levels of norepinephrine. In these cases, it's important to address overall adrenal function.

Melatonin and methyl donors

Also important for melatonin production are folic acid, methyl B-12, betaine, and other methyl donors. Methyl donor deficiencies are linked with H. pylori infections (a bacterial overgrowth in the stomach), low stomach hydrochloric acid, hypothyroidism, the use of antacid medications, oral contraceptives, or estrogen replacement therapy. If this is an issue, supplemental methyl donors may be helpful. This can be especially true in the elderly whose levels of stomach acid are lower.

Melatonin and cortisol

Another adrenal hormone that impacts melatonin levels is cortisol. Clinically we see an inverse relationship between cortisol and melatonin—as cortisol levels climb too high, as is common in those with insulin resistance, melatonin levels drop. People with insulin resistance typically struggle with insomnia.

Like melatonin, cortisol has a daily cycle that governs our sleeping and waking habits. In a healthy person, cortisol is highest in the morning so one wakes alert and refreshed. How many people do you know who actually wake up feeling that way? Throughout the day, levels gradually lower until they are lowest at night so one retires feeling drowsy and ready to sleep. Again, how many people do you know who are wide awake come bedtime?

During the night, cortisol slowly rises again. One of its functions is to break down glycogen, a form of energy stored in the muscles and liver, into glucose to supply the brain and body with energy during the night while you sleep. This process begins during the night when the body enters a fasting state and continues until morning, keeping your body fueled with a steady supply of glucose.

As it's doing this, the level of cortisol eventually rises high enough to wake you up, also sensitizing receptors in the brain for the other adrenal hormones. Then, as the day wears on and the sky darkens, epinephrine dilates the pupils and facilitates the conversion of serotonin to melatonin while cortisol steadily lowers (assuming methyl donors are sufficient).

This whole scenario explains why you can't look at sleep disturbances, and hence melatonin issues, without also considering cortisol levels and function. Many people, especially those with insulin resistance, have cortisol levels that are chronically high. Some people have cortisol that is low in the morning and high at night or their levels dip and surge throughout the day or are chronically low, in which cases norepinephrine levels may also be too low to aid in the conversion of serotonin to melatonin. In all these cases, melatonin production will be disrupted and sleep disturbed.

The pitfalls of taking melatonin supplements to sleep

One thing that will clue you in to whether you have melatonin issues is how well melatonin works for you as a sleep aid. If it works great that's a big clue you have melatonin issues.

As a conservative functional medicine practitioner I do not recommend melatonin supplements but instead prefer to address the root cause of the problem. Once you start supplementing with melatonin you risk throwing off the delicately balanced circadian rhythm even more.

Clinically, I have seen very skewed melatonin salivary profiles in my patients who take melatonin that can take months to normalize. Instead, I look at whether cortisol levels are too high, which would drive down melatonin production. It's also important to consider whether serotonin is sufficient enough for conversion to melatonin.

Is adrenal function healthy enough so that appropriate levels of norepinephrine are available for the conversion process? Could a methyl donor deficiency be hampering the conversion process? Although sleep disorders are a deep and complex topic, these factors should always be considered. As a side note, however, I can't tell you how many people have restored healthy sleep patterns simply by reducing the amount of sugars and carbs they eat. Blood sugar imbalances not only eventually hinder serotonin activity, but also create chronic stress that impacts norepinephrine levels.

CHAPTER SUMMARY

• In neurology, depression is simply decreased firing of the frontal lobe, and the frontal lobe is saturated with receptor sites for serotonin. Serotonin is a vital ingredient to a well-functioning frontal lobe. However, it is overly simplistic to assume all depression stems from a serotonin imbalance.

• Symptoms of poor serotonin activity include feelings of depression, loss of pleasure in life, inner rage and anger, depression from lack of sunlight, and being unable to fall into a deep restful sleep.

• The production of serotonin is triggered by activation of the tectum, which depends on adequate light. This is why serotonin deficiency is often associated with depression and moodiness from lack of light.

• Risks of long-term use of SSRIs include excess serotonin or building a tolerance to the drug.

• Estrogens increase the sensitivity of serotonin receptor sites. High estrogen levels can cause symptoms of serotonin excess and estrogen deficiency can cause symptoms of low serotonin activity. Because of the role estrogen plays in healthy serotonin activity, taking nutritional compounds that support serotonin may help only somewhat or not at all if estrogen is deficient. In this case a hormone panel can be very useful.

• Studies show both 5-HTP and tryptophan increase levels of serotonin and can be helpful in addressing depression, persistent nightmares, fibromyalgia, chronic headaches, migraines, and mood disorders.

• The following botanicals can increase receptor site sensitivity, ensure the breakdown of used serotonin, and provide necessary cofactors for serotonin production: St. John's wort, SAMe, P-5-P (a form of B6), niacinamide, magnesium citrate, methyl B12, and folic acid.

• The production of serotonin depends on sufficient levels of iron, which makes an iron deficiency another factor to consider with poor serotonin activity. Other nutrients important for serotonin synthesis are P-5-P, niacin, methyl B12, folic acid, and magnesium. With the prevalence of fast-food diets and processed foods today, deficiencies in these important cofactors are widespread.

• When considering the cause of a serotonin deficiency, you must first address the three deal breakers: general brain health, stress, and blood sugar imbalances. If you are eating ample protein, then you must additionally consider whether you are sufficient in estrogen, iron, and the other nutritional cofactors.

• MAO-inhibiting drugs slow the breakdown of serotonin and epinephrine and norepinephrine. This class of drugs increases levels of both serotonin and these adrenal hormones to address severe depression. Using SSRIs with MAO-inhibiting drugs can lead to "serotonin syndrome," a rare condition caused by excess serotonin.

• Serotonin is converted into melatonin in the brain's pineal gland, the most serotonin-rich tissue in the body. Low cortisol can hinder the conversion of serotonin to melatonin and cause difficulty sleeping. If cortisol is too high melatonin levels drop. Once you start supplementing with melatonin you risk throwing off the delicately balanced circadian rhythm.

CHAPTER FIFTEEN
GABA

SYMPTOMS ASSOCIATED WITH GABA IMBALANCES

- Feelings of anxiousness or panic for no reason
- Feelings of dread
- Feelings of inner tension and inner excitability
- Feelings of being overwhelmed for no reason
- Restless mind
- Hard to turn your mind off when you want to relax
- Disorganized attention
- Worry about things you never had thought of before

• •

Carol was diagnosed with a rare condition called burning mouth syndrome. She experienced a continuous burning pain on the tip of her tongue and the roof of her mouth. She had seen various specialists but they always concluded her symptoms were a mystery.

In addition to the constant burning, Carol suffered from constant nervousness and episodes of anxiety. Over the years she coped with her symptoms by consuming alcohol beginning each afternoon. Carol was suffering greatly, and alcohol was the only thing that helped. Although many people mistook her for an alcoholic I knew she wasn't. It was very clear Carol was simply doing whatever it took to alleviate the daily suffering.

When I evaluated Carol I saw that the tip of her tongue and the roof of her mouth were scraped away. An examination made it clear Carol's burning mouth syndrome was secondary to a movement disorder called motor tics. Tics are a neurological disease in which a person has a buildup sensation to perform a certain movement, which brings relief. With a tic this happens over and over again. It is caused by disease in part of the brain called the basal ganglia. Carol could not stop the urge to scrape the roof of her mouth with her tongue all day. She would try to stop, but then the urge to do it would build up so much the tic became worse.

Carol's examination findings indicated she had loss of function of her basal ganglia and cerebellum. These are areas of the brain with very powerful GABA activity. GABA is an inhibitory neurotransmitter that calms neurological pathways. I then tested Carol for gluten sensitivity and neurological autoimmunity. The results showed very high antibodies to gluten and to GAD, an enzyme in the brain that makes GABA. In other words, her inability to suppress the scraping of the roof of her mouth were related to an autoimmune condition that prevented the production of GABA and a gluten intolerance.

I put Carol on an autoimmune diet and gut-repair program, gave her exercises to rehabilitate her basal ganglia, and gave her natural compounds to support GABA pathways. Everything seemed to help her overall brain function, anxiety, and nervousness, but it only reduced her tic disorder somewhat. Her suffering was so significant she could not stop her alcohol abuse. Alcohol suppressed her brain, calmed her symptoms, and alleviated the pain.

I had a long discussion with Carol and her husband about seeking a neurologist specializing in movement disorders to try various medications to either support GABA activity or suppress dopamine activity, but she decided to stay with her current regimen, which unfortunately included excessive alcohol abuse.

I share Carol's case with you because it is an extreme case of GABA pathway dysfunction. When neurological pathways fail it can cause various expressions of the dysfunction that are not a part of the standard diagnosis list. As a clinician, I wished I could have seen her 10 years earlier, before she progressed to where she is now.

Not all people with GABA dysfunction develop the degree of suffering Carol had. The most common GABA issues are anxiety, nervousness, and insomnia. Uncontrollable movement disorders, such as restless leg syndrome, tics, sound sensitivity, light sensitivity, constant worry, and emotional attacks for no apparent reason are common with GABA impairments.

If your brain is not working and you feel you cannot calm down or shut down your brain, this chapter is very important for you.

Datis Kharrazian, DHSc, DC, MS

● ●

People with poor GABA activity tend toward anxiousness and panic, and can have an ongoing sense of dread. They may have a knot in their stomach and become easily overwhelmed, even if they don't necessarily have that much going on (although the restless GABA-deficient person tends to take on too many things).

GABA-deficient people tend to worry about many things needlessly. It's because their minds are restless and hard to turn off, and their attention is disorganized, darting from one thing to the next. Feelings of inner tension and overexcitability are other symptoms of poor GABA activity.

GABA-deficient people like to fall asleep with the TV on. In fact, it's not uncommon to find this person reading a magazine while watching TV, talking on the phone, and texting, because she can't focus on one thing at a time. GABA people are frequently late for appointments because they are too disorganized as they are trying to get out the door, constantly distracted by different things to get done before leaving.

GABA issues are quite common. The anti-anxiety drug Xanax® works on GABA pathways by increasing receptor site sensitivity, and it is one of the most commonly prescribed drugs today. When anti-anxiety medications were first introduced there was an overwhelming demand for them from Americans. As with serotonin and dopamine deficiencies, a GABA deficiency can easily be brought on by stress, blood sugar imbalances, or other lifestyle and diet-related issues. However, GABA warrants special attention compared to the other neurotransmitters.

Some people have a lifelong, genetic inability to synthesize GABA, whereas others can have a GABA deficiency induced by a gluten intolerance or an autoimmune disease. Also, it's worth noting here that those GABA supplements you see on the health food store shelves are theoretically worthless for most people. Due to its large molecular size GABA cannot cross the blood-brain barrier unless the blood-brain barrier is damaged.[1]

Instead, one must use precursors for GABA synthesis in the brain and other compounds to support GABA receptor activity. If straight GABA works on calming and relaxing your mind, that is an indication that your blood-brain barrier may be compromised, or "leaky." A healthy blood-brain barrier only allows compounds that are nanoparticles, or very small, to cross.[2]

Compounds such as neurotransmitters are too large to cross a healthy blood-brain barrier. A leaky brain is capable of allowing dangerous foreign materials into the brain that could trigger inflammation, such as environmental toxins or undigested food particles. This is why we use GABA supplements to assess whether an individual has a leaky brain—if straight GABA works at calming and relaxing you, that's a sign you have a leaky blood-brain barrier. Last time I checked the shelves at my local health food store the GABA had sold out, a sad testament to the permeable state of the average American brain.

● ●

A 35-year-old woman came in one year after delivering a baby. She had always been anxious but it had gotten worse during the last six months. She complained of insomnia and panic attacks coupled with tachycardia or a racing heart. Her heart palpitations could last all day and were worse when she was under stress.

She experienced anxiety when she had arguments with her partner, saw a scary movie, or read a scary story in a magazine. Even though she was eating regularly with snacks in between meals, her symptoms worsened when she would not eat enough or was late with a meal.

We balanced her hypoglycemia by changing her diet and by adding in nutritional compounds to support her blood sugar, and adrenal adaptogens and phosphatidylserine to support her adrenal health. She felt much better within a month, but the insomnia and palpitations persisted. At that point she started on nutritional compounds to support GABA activity, DHA and EPA, and methyl B-12.

Not only did she now sleep through the night, but also her palpitations, anxiety, and panic attacks completely disappeared. She reported that her memory was vastly improved (even though she hadn't complained about it prior) and her moods were very stable, even when she was faced with situations that previously would have caused her to become anxious.

Dagmar Ehling, Mac, LAc, DOM
Durham, North Carolina
www.orientalhealthsolutions.com

● ●

NUTRITIONAL COMPOUNDS THAT SUPPORT GABA ACTIVITY

Although several factors often underlie poor GABA activity, which I will discuss later, various nutritional and herbal compounds have proven very effective in boosting and balancing overall GABA activity. These key ingredients are valerian root extract, lithium orotate, passion flower extract, L-theanine, P-5-P, magnesium citrate, zinc, and manganese.

Valerian root

Valerian root has been well known as an effective sedative in managing insomnia, restlessness, and anxiety for at least several centuries. Studies have confirmed these properties. Research shows it increases the sensitivity of the GABA receptor site, and has been shown to bind to GABA receptor sites, increasing the sensitivity of GABA in the brain. Valerian root extract, or valeric acid, has also been shown to slow down the breakdown of GABA.[3][4][5][6][7][8][9][10][11][12]

Lithium orotate

Not to be confused with lithium carbonate, the drug that is used to treat bipolar disorder, lithium orotate is a naturally occurring mineral that is essential to the body. Studies have found that people drinking water with low levels of lithium show higher incidences of mental hospitalizations, violent crimes, and drug addiction. Lithium appears to work by increasing GABA receptor site sensitivity.[13][14][15][16][17][18]

315

Passion flower extract

Passion flower works like lithium orotate and valerian in that it increases the sensitivity of the GABA receptor sites. Passion flower extract has historically been used for anxiety, insomnia, seizures, and hysteria.[19 20 21 22 23 24 25]

L-theanine

L-theanine is an amino acid that has a very similar structure to GABA. It is found in many teas, especially relaxing teas such as chamomile. L-theanine crosses the blood-brain barrier and has been found to raise GABA levels in the brain.[26 27 28 29 30]

Taurine

Like L-theanine, taurine is an amino acid with a molecular structure similar to GABA and has been shown to impact GABA activity.[31 32 33 34 35 36]

P-5-P, magnesium, zinc, manganese

P-5-P, magnesium, zinc, manganese are cofactors necessary for the synthesis and breakdown of GABA.[37]

Dosing

Together these compounds have a swift and powerful impact on GABA activity. Most people typically don't need to take GABA long term if they address the three deal breakers: general brain health, blood sugar imbalances, and brain oxygenation.

Dosing for GABA support is the same as it is for serotonin—you take as much as you need to experience a benefit. Supporting neurotransmitter activity is not dependent upon body size, but instead on the degree to which you have symptoms.

As a result, determining your dose requires some trial and error. It typically takes a half hour to an hour after taking GABA support to notice the effects. Continue to gradually increase your dose until you notice an improvement in your symptoms. Then increase the dose again to see whether you experience even more improvement. Once you no longer feel any improvement, go back the previous dose at which you felt improvement.

How often you take GABA support also varies with the individual. Some may find they need it three or more times a day, others just once.

● ●

Holly always had trouble finding the right words to relay her thoughts and feelings. She had been a low-fat vegetarian for many years, including through the birth of four children, and now wonders if she didn't get enough of the nutrients necessary for good brain function, or if she was eating too many carbohydrates. Trying to connect her thoughts to language became even more difficult under stressful, emotional, or chaotic situations.

After filling out the Dr. Kharrazian's neurotransmitter questionnaire and scoring high for poor GABA activity, she began taking nutritional compounds to support GABA. She noticed almost immediately how much more eloquently she could communicate in comparison to before. She says she felt like a hand was reaching into her brain, picking out words, and setting them on her tongue. The relief of this new ability to connect her thoughts to words quicker and more easily has truly changed her life for the better.

She wonders too if GABA has increased her ability to focus, or if perhaps she just has more brain energy to focus now that her brain is not working so hard to find the right words. She also noticed her short-term memory has improved. Regardless, she says she feels more stable and grounded than she has in a long time.

Datis Kharrazian, DHSc, DC, MS

● ●

What if you crash and burn on GABA support?

As is the case with serotonin support, sometimes when people support GABA activity they will "crash," getting hit with intense fatigue. This is due to the neurons being too close to threshold and not able to make enough energy to function properly. Although the brain may need GABA support, it is so fragile that just a little bit of support sends it over the edge, fatiguing the neurons and hence the individual.

If this crash happens after just the minimum dose, it could actually mean this person is in desperate need of support. However, additional support for brain inflammation, brain oxygenation, and neuron support may also be warranted. Compounds for these conditions will dampen inflammation in the brain common with neurodegeneration, give the neurons more support against degeneration, and supply the brain with more oxygen-rich blood (assuming anemia isn't a factor).

Another possibility is that the additional neurotransmitter support can actually support negative plasticity. For example, a person with extreme anxiety or panic attacks driven by poor GABA activity may actually find supplementing with GABA precursors and cofactors makes them worse.

So what do you do when you need GABA support but even just a little is too much for a fragile brain? You use even less, while paying attention to issues of brain inflammation and oxygenation.

● ●

I have a patient who arrived at my office suffering from depression, anxiety and panic attacks. She had been experiencing these mood issues since 1965, a period of more than 45 years. During this time, her symptoms were managed with benzo-diazepines and a variety of antidepressants.

We did the appropriate tests and set up a treatment plan to address her diet, gut health, and general brain health. Three months later, she told me how very different she felt. I'll let her say it in her own words:

"My thinking is so different now. Things that used to bother me, I look at and laugh and say, 'Wow, that used to really bother me!' And my husband and I are getting along. Before I came in to see Dr. Elliott, I was about to walk out and get a divorce. I used to itch every night on my arms and my legs, and that's gone. All my aches and pains are gone, too. And here I thought it was all just part of getting old."

Travis J. Elliott, N.D.
Portland, Oregon
www.drtraviselliott.com

● ●

GABA PRODUCTION

Whereas serotonin is made in specific areas of the brain, GABA is so critical to brain health it is made in all the neurons. GABA production is a byproduct of energy production in the brain, produced in what is called the GABA shunt—when glucose is metabolized for energy, one of its byproducts, glutamate (a salt form of the GABA precursor glutamic acid), is converted into GABA as needed. Once the GABA is used for its calming influence, it then converts back into a substance that is sent back into the energy-production cycle.

The GABA shunt can go two ways. It can convert glutamate into GABA, which is calming, or it can continue to manufacture glutamate, the brain's major excitatory neurotransmitter. Every cell in the brain has the ability to fire the shunt toward either an inhibitory or excitatory direction, in other words towards GABA production or more glutamate.

As you can imagine, many anxiety-ridden Americans prefer that shunt produce more GABA for its calming effects. Anxiety disorders are at an all time high, as are prescriptions for medications to alleviate them. The last thing many Americans need is a highly excitable, anxiety-prone brain. So how can we assure we produce enough GABA and avoid producing too much glutamate?

* *

Paul arrived at my office having an intense anxiety episode during which he shook with tremors from head to toe. He was taking quite a bit of anti-anxiety medication but couldn't seem to improve. After taking his health history and listing his physical complaints, we concluded he had poor neurotransmitter function and his brain was overexcited and could not slow down. He was sleeping 16 to 18 hours a day and still felt exhausted.

We began support for his neurotransmitters, primarily dopamine and GABA to help him during his depressed states, and with nutrients necessary for proper brain chemistry activity. His anxiety began to calm within a few days.

After a month, Paul needed anti-anxiety medication only on rare occasions. His mood became stable and he began putting his life back together. We also tested him for an autoimmune reaction to his neurochemistry. It is my opinion that the level of inflammation from his immune system reaction was the driving force behind his problems.

As we have worked to address the underlying mechanism behind the inflammation, there have been great improvements. Paul maintains a positive attitude, refuses to give up, and fully

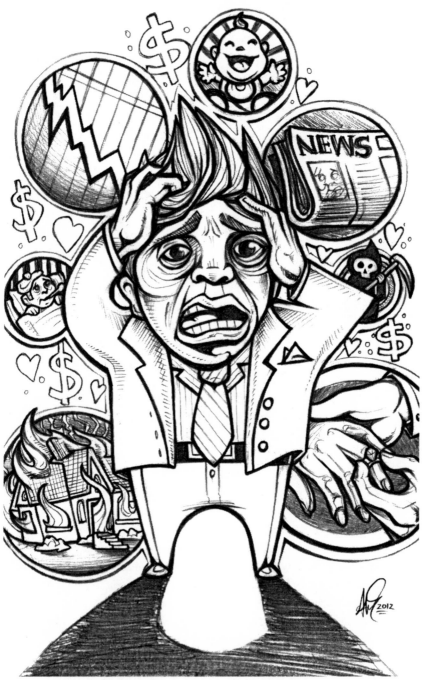

People with poor GABA activity suffer from anxiety, panic, and dread, become easily overwhelmed, and have restless minds.

intends to bring himself out of disability. It is patients like this that
make me excited to be a doctor and do what I do.
   David Arthur, DC, FACFN, DACNB, BCIM, DCCN
   Denver, Colorado
   www.DrDavidArthur.com

● ●

AUTOIMMUNE GABA DISORDER

Many people with GABA-related issues are also gluten-intolerant.[38] More relevant is the fact that gluten intolerance, celiac disease, and autoimmune diseases can trigger an autoimmune reaction against the enzyme responsible for making GABA, called glutamic acid decarboxylase (GAD), which I also discussed in Chapter Eleven.

Our bodies convert glutamic acid in foods to glutamate, which is excitatory. The GAD enzyme then converts glutamate to GABA, which is calming. GAD autoimmunity prevents this conversion and the result is excess excitatory glutamate and not enough calming GABA.

Celiac disease, Hashimoto's hypothyroidism, and Type I diabetes raise the risk of GAD autoimmunity.[39] If GAD antibodies turn up positive on a lab test, it may be an early screening tool for Type I diabetes.

People with a GAD autoimmunity are also more prone to gluten ataxia, a form of gluten intolerance that manifests in the brain. As with Type I diabetes, positive GAD antibodies are an early screening tool for gluten ataxia.[40]

People with positive GAD antibodies should avoid eating gluten and foods high in artificial glutamates, such as MSG. Many people with positive GAD antibodies can react to foods high in glutamates with symptoms that include extreme anxiety, nervousness, migraines, and more.

This mechanism should be considered when people have an autoimmune disease and symptoms of poor GABA activity, especially if those symptoms have been happening for a long time.

AUTISM, GLUTEN, AND GAD ANTIBODIES

GAD autoimmunity is also a well-understood mechanism in autism that explains why some children with autism react neurologically to gluten. It is also a theoretical model for severe temper tantrums in some children with autism, as well as for temper tantrums in non-autistic children with gluten sensitivity.[41]

BLOOD SUGAR AND GABA

When it comes to GABA impairment our old friend blood sugar regulation once again takes center stage. Since GABA production starts with the role of glucose in energy production, conditions such as hypoglycemia, insulin resistance, and diabetes can lower glucose levels in the brain and decrease GABA production. When glucose levels in the brain fall, overall energy production lowers, and so does GABA production.

ANEMIA, LACK OF OXYGEN, AND GABA

The other important factor for GABA production is whether energy production works in each cell. If energy production is hampered in any way, the GABA shunt may send glucose into glutamine production instead of GABA. Lack of oxygen is one factor that can disrupt this energy cycle. Energy production is like a fire that needs fuel (glucose) and air to burn. Anemia can rob the brain of sufficient oxygen to fan the fire of energy production, and it's common to see GABA deficiency symptoms in individuals with anemia.

Poor blood flow to the brain is another cause of insufficient oxygen. As I mentioned earlier in the book, people with poor blood flow to the brain also have poor blood flow to the hands and feet, which are chronically cold and show signs of nail fungus and pale nail beds. They may also have high blood pressure or be consuming too much nicotine or caffeine. In these cases, increasing blood flow and oxygenation of the brain is one way to support healthy GABA activity.

• •

Michelle, 54, is a menopausal woman who was found passed out on the kitchen floor by her husband. Michelle had previously presented to her medical doctor complaining of anxiety and difficulty sleeping. He prescribed her two anxiety medications and an antidepressant. She said the medications turned her in to a zombie, and after passing out in the kitchen, she had had enough and chose to quit taking them. Her symptoms of anxiety and insomnia soon returned, so a friend referred her to our clinic.

Michelle's history revealed inadequate protein intake and excess consumption of simple carbohydrates. Her symptoms indicated compromised GABA activity. Additionally, a physical examination revealed tenderness in her lower abdomen. Blood work showed markers for anemia, the possibility of inflammation, and a vitamin B-1 deficiency.

I advised her to increase her protein intake and consume only low-glycemic carbohydrates, such as from leafy green vegetables, and recommended a gluten-free diet to address her abdominal tenderness and inflammation. I also had her take nutritional compounds to support her B deficiency, anemia, and low GABA activity.

At her return visit one week later her symptoms were nearly gone. She had little anxiety and was sleeping through the night. The following week she said her symptoms were gone and she was completely well. She has not returned to her medications and her tolerance to stress has greatly improved.

Richard Belli, DC, DACNB
Sacramento, California
www.spectrumak.com

TOXICITY AND GABA

Overexposure to toxic chemicals or metals is another factor that can impede the energy production cycle of each cell and hence GABA production. Sometimes when people suffer such exposures or react badly to environmental pollutants, it can permanently damage brain and nervous tissue and hence this energy production cycle. It is not uncommon to see people who have had serious exposure to an environmental neurotoxin end up with severe GABA deficiency symptoms.

In fact, the most common neurotransmitter imbalance that accompanies neurotoxicity is GABA-related. These people may need lifelong supplemental GABA support. I had a patient recently who needed permanent GABA support after being exposed to large amounts of pesticides that produced lifelong GABA impairment and fostered anxiety and panic.

GENETIC GABA CONVERSION DISORDER

Some people have a genetic disorder that impacts the production of GABA, thus causing increased anxiety. This disorder affects the enzyme glutamic acid transaminase, which is responsible for converting glutamic acid to GABA. This is a consideration for someone who has had lifelong GABA deficiency symptoms or a history of anxiety in the family.

How do you know if a persistent GABA deficiency is genetic? You can do a simple challenge with a supplement bought from a health food store, alpha-ketoglutaric acid, a glutamate precursor. If I suspect this disorder I'll have my patient take 3,000 to 4,000 mg of alpha-ketoglutaric acid. For someone with no genetic GABA abnormality, taking this supplement will not produce much in the way of symptoms. If anything, it will just energize them slightly, as if they had just eaten something sugary, but it will not cause anxiety or irritability. For the person with the genetic disorder, however, this surge of glutamates combined with the genetic inability to convert them to GABA will cause symptoms of excitability, nervousness, anxiety, and other GABA-deficiency symptoms. For this person, taking GABA support on a regular, lifelong basis may be helpful.

● ●

Julie could be heard frequently gasping in alarm throughout the day, and twisting about in a panic searching for something she had just misplaced. "Where are my keys?" she would suddenly exclaim, or "Where are my sunglasses? What did I do with my wallet?" or "Oh my gosh I'm running late!"

She seemed to be a human blur, constantly racing from one thing to the next, rarely able to focus on one task very long before the thought popped into her head that she needed to work on something else.

Unfortunately, her racing never allowed her to relax, and bouts of anxiety—when it seemed as if total doom was imminent— popped up regularly. If something really rattled her, she fell into a full-blown panic attack. It seemed the only time she got any rest was when her system collapsed into the flu or pneumonia, or even a temporary bout of exhaustion-induced depression. Julie suffered from a gamma-aminobutyric acid (GABA) impairment, the main neurotransmitter responsible for keeping the brain calm.

Datis Kharrazian, DHSc, DC, MS

AUTOIMMUNE THYROID CAN MIMIC GABA DEFICIENCY

Autoimmune thyroid disease is very common in this country, affecting millions of Americans, and was the subject of my first book, *Why Do I Still Have Thyroid Symptoms?* It's important to point out that sometimes a flare up of an autoimmune thyroid condition can produce symptoms similar to a GABA deficiency. When the immune system attacks the thyroid gland it spills excess thyroid hormone into the bloodstream, ramping up metabolism. Symptoms include nervousness, anxiety, insomnia, and a pounding heart—all of which look like a GABA deficiency. Even though this might not be a true GABA deficiency, taking GABA support may still help quell the symptoms of a flare up. If you have a history of thyroid problems or want to screen for thyroid autoimmunity, ask your doctor to order thyroid antibodies with a routine blood test.

Less than a week after she began taking a multivitamin that included alpha-ketoglutaric acid, Patricia began sleeping only about four hours a night. Despite so little sleep she was wired all day. Worse, however, was a constant feeling she wasn't getting enough air and a feeling of pressure and tightness in her chest. She had to yawn and take deep breaths frequently to fight this feeling of "air hunger."

She searched online and found air hunger can be a symptom of anxiety. Luckily she knew about the alpha-ketoglutaric challenge and the possibility that her GABA pathways may be compromised due to genetics. Her father struggled his whole life with anxiety issues, had been hospitalized once, and took anti-anxiety medications for 30 years.

Patricia stopped taking her multivitamin. Within a day the air hunger had ceased and she went back to sleeping seven or eight hours. To test her theory she waited a week and tried the multivitamin again. Her symptoms returned within a couple of hours and lasted the day.

Although she has symptoms of GABA impairment, she thought she could manage her symptoms through supporting her brain health and managing her blood sugar. However, given her father's history and the possibility that she may suffer from a genetic inability to make sufficient GABA, she began supplementing with nutritional compounds to support GABA.

She was pleasantly surprised to find the support boosted her focus and concentration and allowed her to handle a busy workload and family life in a calmer and more relaxed manner.

Datis Kharrazian, DHSc, DC, MS

● ●

THE LEAKY BRAIN CHALLENGE

As I mentioned earlier, supplements that contain straight GABA technically shouldn't work. The blood-brain barrier only allows nano-sized particles to cross into the brain and GABA is too big.[42][43] GABA precursors and cofactors, however, can cross into the brain where they can be synthesized by the neurons into GABA or can enhance GABA pathways.

If taking straight GABA does have the desired effect of making you calmer and more relaxed, then you know you have a leaky blood-brain barrier and dangerous particles can enter your brain from food, water, or the environment. Another possible symptom is for the GABA to increase feelings of anxiety, irritability, or panic, which could indicate neurons are too close too threshold.

This mechanism allows us to test for leaky brain. When I suspect a compromised blood-brain barrier in my patients I give them the leaky brain challenge: Take 1,000 mg of straight GABA (no other added precursors) during the day—not at night near bedtime—and monitor your reaction over the next several hours. Take the GABA on an empty stomach. If you feel calmer, sleepy, or more relaxed, this indicates a leaky blood-brain barrier and a susceptibility to damaging brain inflammation from undesirable substances that can leak into the brain.

I address what to do about a leaky blood-brain barrier in Chapter Ten. If taking the GABA makes you more anxious or irritable, this also indicates a leaky blood-brain barrier. In this case eating something with protein can help relieve these symptoms.

Feeling no change after taking GABA is a good sign that your blood-brain barrier is intact and functioning well. Taking GABA should produce no symptoms at all as the GABA "bounces off" a healthy blood-brain barrier.

● ●

When Sarah was 51 she had surgery to remove a brain tumor. The surgery was long and complicated due to a hemorrhage, and it took her months to recover. After her surgery she was not able to have a bowel movement without using suppositories, colonics, or enemas.

Her doctors didn't take the problem seriously—they told her to drink more water, walk more, or that it was due to the hypothyroid condition she developed after her operation. However, Sarah knew it was important to figure out why her bowels stopped working.

She eventually came to see me. She failed the GABA challenge, an indication her blood-brain barrier was compromised. From this and other symptoms, I knew her general brain health could use support. I started her on vitamin D, methyl B-12, and high levels of DHA. Her bowel movements returned to normal and she was able to lower the dose of her thyroid medication.

Mark Flannery, DC, FAAIM, DCBCN, DCCN, CNS
Woodland Hills, California
www.DrFlannery.com

● ●

CHAPTER SUMMARY

• People with poor GABA activity tend toward anxiousness and panic, and can have an ongoing sense of dread. They may have a knot in their stomach and become easily overwhelmed, even if they don't necessarily have that much going on (although the restless GABA-deficient person tends to take on too many things).

• GABA issues are quite common. The anti-anxiety drug Xanax® works on GABA pathways by increasing receptor site sensitivity, and it is one of the most commonly prescribed drugs today.

• When anti-anxiety medications were first introduced there was an overwhelming demand for them from Americans.

• Whereas serotonin is made in specific areas of the brain, GABA is so critical to brain health it is made throughout the brain. Some people have a lifelong, genetic inability to synthesize GABA, whereas others can have a GABA deficiency induced by a gluten intolerance or an autoimmune disease. As with serotonin and dopamine deficiencies, a GABA deficiency can easily be brought on by stress, blood sugar imbalances, or other lifestyle and diet-related issues.

• Gluten intolerance, celiac disease, and autoimmune diseases can trigger an autoimmune reaction against the enzyme responsible for making GABA, called glutamic acid decarboxylase (GAD). Other diseases that commonly predispose one to a GAD autoimmune reaction are Hashimoto's autoimmune thyroid disease and Type I diabetes. Since GABA production starts with the role of glucose in energy production, hypoglycemia, insulin resistance, and diabetes can lower glucose levels in the brain and decrease GABA production. Overexposure to toxic chemicals or metals is another factor that can impede the energy production cycle of each cell and hence GABA production.

• People with a GAD autoimmunity are more prone to gluten ataxia, a form of gluten intolerance that manifests in the brain causing a variety of neurological symptoms both physical and behavioral. Positive GAD antibodies are an early screening tool for gluten ataxia.

• Due to its large molecular size GABA cannot cross the blood-brain barrier unless the blood-brain barrier is damaged. If taking straight GABA makes you calmer and more relaxed, then you know you have a leaky blood-brain barrier and dangerous particles can enter your brain from food, water, or the environment. Another possible symptom is for the GABA to increase feelings of anxiety, irritability, or panic, which could indicate neurons are too close too threshold. Feeling no change after taking GABA is a good sign that your blood-brain barrier is intact and functioning well. Taking GABA should produce no symptoms at all as the GABA "bounces off" a healthy blood-brain barrier.

• People with positive GAD antibodies should avoid eating foods high in artificial glutamates. The most common example of this is a sensitivity to MSG. People with positive GAD antibodies can experience a strong reaction to foods high in glutamates with symptoms that include extreme anxiety, nervousness, migraines, and more.

• Various nutritional and herbal compounds have proven very effective in boosting and balancing overall GABA activity: valerian root extract, lithium orotate, passion flower extract, L-theanine, P-5-P, magnesium citrate, zinc, and manganese.

CHAPTER SIXTEEN

DOPAMINE

SYMPTOMS OF POOR DOPAMINE ACTIVITY

- Inability to self-motivate
- Inability to start or finish tasks
- Feelings of worthlessness
- Feelings of hopelessness
- Lose temper for minor reasons
- Inability to handle stress
- Anger and aggression while under stress
- Desire to isolate oneself from others
- Unexplained lack of concern for family and friends

• •

Henry and his wife, Katrina, had been seeing a marriage counselor and were on the brink of divorce. Katrina described her husband as moody and no fun to be around and said he had turned into a different person since they married seven years ago. The Henry Katrina married liked trying new things, going out to dinner, and traveling. But in the past couple of years Henry had gained about 40 pounds, developed sleep apnea, and begun taking an antidepressant, hypertension medication, cholesterol-lowering medication, and antacids.

During his downward spiral Henry also had stopped exercising and started to eat poorly. His stress levels at work become much worse because he could never set healthy deadlines with his boss.

Henry's health took a drastic turn for the worse when he accidentally overdosed on his hypertension medication and passed out. He fell on his head and lost consciousness for a few seconds, basically suffering a brain injury that exacerbated his mood and health problems.

When I examined Henry he demonstrated slow mental speed and poor memory. He also showed an absence of deep tendon reflexes, loss of smell and taste, and hypokinesia, or slow movements. Although Henry did not have a neurological disease it was obvious his brain was not working well, especially considering he suffered a recent head trauma. Henry also presented with all the symptoms of impaired dopamine. He had no motivation, could not handle stress anymore, and felt worthless.

Dopamine-impaired patients are red flags for me because they lack the brain chemistry to follow a program. Their faulty dopamine system makes them non-compliant patients. This concerned me because Henry needed to address many health issues to improve his brain health and dopamine system. His circulation was poor, he was not producing adequate digestive enzymes, he was pre-diabetic, and he did not exercise.

I sat down with both Henry and Katrina and told them how poor dopamine activity makes self-motivation difficult. I asked Katrina if she could please hang in there for a few more months and help Henry stay on track with his supplements and dietary changes. I also told Henry not to complain when Katrina pushed him to follow the regimen, and that he needed to listen to her.

I immediately placed Henry on natural compounds to impact his dopamine system, and had him start a basic exercise program and a diet to reduce his blood sugar levels. The first month was extremely difficult for Henry, but as time went on he began to lose weight and increasingly relied less on Katrina to follow his diet. Henry noticed that if he forgot to take his dopamine support he could not get through the day.

As time went on he was able to improve his blood glucose, lower his blood pressure, improve his circulation, and quit taking his antacid medications. These are all key mechanisms directly involved with how the body makes dopamine, which I will discuss in this chapter.

I share Henry's case because many people who have an impaired dopamine system may need compounds that impact dopamine function to kick start motivation, but they are still a band-aid approach. The mechanisms that lead to dopamine impairment must be addressed in order to make a significant clinical difference.

If you have difficulty motivating yourself, doubt yourself, have poor self-worth, and have other symptoms of impaired dopamine, this chapter is very important for you to understand.

Datis Kharrazian, DHSc, DC, MS

● ●

It pains me to think of all the people who believe their feelings of hopelessness and worthlessness are a true reflection of who they are, or who think the things that trigger their temper tantrums are valid—something their children, spouse, or coworker did—when instead they may be merely suffering from a dopamine deficiency. Once you learn how to support your brain you become much more efficient in life, not to mention more pleasant to be around.

Dopamine is associated with the "pleasure system" of the brain and allows us to feel enjoyment and a sense of reward in order to motivate performance. It also helps us with focus and attention, and the ability to feel pleasure. People with low dopamine experience hopelessness, worthlessness, and an inability to handle stress. They may have self-destructive thoughts. They snap for minor reasons and become angry and aggressive under stress, then feel bad about themselves for losing control so easily. They have a desire to isolate themselves from others and an unexplainable lack of concern for friends and family. They are distracted easily and have a hard time finishing tasks. They may feel the need to stay alert by consuming caffeine or indulging in foods and behavior that give them immediate pleasure so they can get a dopamine fix.

One of the defining characteristics of low dopamine is lack of motivation. Unlike serotonin-deficient people who can't seem to enjoy anything, dopamine-deficient people find enjoyment in things but can't get motivated to do them. For instance, they can't be bothered to go see their favorite band or go to their favorite restaurant, although they would enjoy themselves if they did.

Dopamine is most commonly known for its association with Parkinson's disease, a disease brought on by destruction of the brain's substantia nigra, where dopamine is made, and long-term dopamine deficiency. However, dopamine has numerous functions in the brain related to motor coordination, motivation, and reward.

It helps regulate prolactin, a hormone involved with lactation, reproduction, and libido. It is involved with modulating mood, attention, and learning, and drives the pleasure center of the brain. This is evident in animal studies on dopamine. In these studies animals can push a lever that delivers dopamine or one that delivers food and water. These animals will choose dopamine over food and water until their death, thanks to dopamine's pleasure-producing effects, known as reward delivery.

This helps explain why their human counterparts, those addicted to drugs, gambling, alcohol, sex, the internet, extreme sports, and so on, behave in pretty much the same way. Although recreational drugs and other addictive habits act on multiple neurotransmitters, dopamine is most heavily involved. It's that surge of dopamine we get from a drag on a cigarette, a turn at the table in Las Vegas, and even from checking our Facebook page that hooks us and keeps us coming back for more.

Some of the drugs used to treat Parkinson's disease are dopamine agonists, meaning they enhance dopamine activity. Unfortunately, the surge of dopamine activity created by these drugs also creates very addictive, pleasure-seeking personalities, particularly for gambling. In fact, I've heard talk among neurologists about requiring patients who go on the drug to freeze their bank accounts so they don't gamble away their assets. It should be noted that natural compounds suggested in this book do not create the same reactions as the medications used to open up the dopamine receptors for Parkinson's disease.

• •

A 33-year-old man came to my office suffering from fatigue, poor sleep, an inability to stay focused, and emotional mood swings. He had just given up coffee, drugs, and alcohol but was still struggling to quit smoking and had strong cravings for starchy foods and sugars. His symptoms showed a serious need for a complete brain overhaul.

I started him on a three-week cleanse with an anti-inflammatory diet and a hypoallergenic detoxification protein powder while

I ordered blood work. I also gave him several supplements to regulate blood sugar symptoms and nutritional compounds to support his dopamine pathways. After three weeks he felt tremendous and had lost the first 20 pounds of what would become 80 pounds over the next nine months. As he reintroduced foods he had eliminated on the cleanse, he noticed that the dopamine support was key in eliminating his addictive behavior. He was aware that gluten made him "crazy," but he would eat it anyway, especially if he felt like drinking. If he stayed with the dopamine support, the urge to choose such a harmful food disappeared and, consequently, so did the urge to drink.

He is now working consistently and has put his life back in order. He is back to being the happy-go-lucky guy he once was.

Kari Vernon, DC

Scottsdale, Arizona

www.karismaforlife.com

● ●

Dopamine is also a key player in emotional health, and it's not uncommon to see people with poor dopamine activity suffer from depression, social anxiety, and anhedonia, an inability to experience pleasure.[1][2][3][4][5] In fact, sometimes people confuse low libido with anhedonia. Sexually they may function fine but they experience no pleasure in sex or intimacy and hence lose interest.

Dopamine and depression

Neurologically speaking, depression is simply decreased firing of the frontal lobe.[6] Dopamine is an important and necessary neurotransmitter for frontal lobe function, and some of the more popular antidepressants work on the dopamine pathways. The depression caused by poor dopamine activity is much different than that caused by low serotonin.

People with low dopamine still have the ability to enjoy things, such as their friendships, hobbies, or favorite foods. Their mood is just low in general and they have a hard time getting motivated to do anything. They feel worthless and hopeless about their lives, which isn't necessarily the case with low serotonin, but if they can actually get spurred on to do something, they enjoy themselves. Of course, people can suffer from both low dopamine and low serotonin, and many do.

Dopamine and mental function

Dopamine is also involved with learning. It can either excite the brain into a more active state to engage in new information, or it can dampen the brain to achieve the attention span necessary for more fine-tuned focus and concentration. Learning disorders and attention deficit disorders are commonly associated with (though not limited to) poor dopamine activity.[7][8][9] Conversely, high levels of dopamine are associated with psychosis, schizophrenia, hyper-social activity, and high libido.[10][11] Anti-psychotic medications are typically dopamine blockers.

Dopamine and hormones

Another common presentation of low dopamine is heavy menstrual cycles in women or low testosterone in men, as well as low libido, erectile dysfunction, and an inability to gain muscle mass. In these scenarios depression may also be part of the symptomology. This is partly because in men and women dopamine stimulates luteinizing hormone (LH), a hormone that triggers the release of progesterone in women and testosterone in men.[12]

When I see low progesterone and low LH in women I always look for dopamine symptoms. If I see low testosterone in a man and see that LH is low, again I will consider dopamine. (Just giving him testosterone in this scenario can further depress LH levels, creating a vicious feedback loop.)

Dopamine can affect progesterone and testosterone levels, and these hormones can likewise affect dopamine activity. Just as estrogen is necessary for appropriate uptake of serotonin, dopamine uptake requires healthy levels of progesterone in women and testosterone in men to function well. When a female patient presents with low progesterone and also tells me she snaps at her children and loses her temper easily, feels hopeless or worthless, and has other low dopamine symptoms, then I know poor neurotransmitter function may be a factor in her low progesterone.

Dopamine and motivation

Another issue with the dopamine-deficient person is that he or she tends to be non-compliant. For a practitioner wanting to transition patients into a new diet, dopamine-deficient patients are especially problematic. When I get a patient with low dopamine, it's a red flag to me that they may not do a single thing I ask. If I ask this patient why he came to see me, the answer is typically, "Because my wife made me." It's not that such a person doesn't want to comply, or that things don't make sense to him, it's just that his motivation and drive are so low that he can't muster the energy to do what's required.

This can also be the patient who bounces from practitioner to practitioner, looking for the magic cure. Yet, upon investigation, it turns out she didn't follow through with any of those other practitioners' protocols. Although underlying issues most likely drive a dopamine deficiency, I may start with dopamine support right away with these patients to boost their motivation so they can follow through with the rest of the protocol. I also involve the spouse or another family member in their care and create a strict schedule of when they need to take their dopamine nutritional compounds, leaving as little as possible to their own direction.

* *

Using Dr. Kharrazian's mode of assessment has been a real blessing to many of our patients who are graduate students at Duke University. These students can be decades older than the undergraduates, which means poor neurotransmitter activity is more likely to present itself.

One such student, Janet, was a 50-year-old graduate student in a three-year program. Although her overall health was excellent, she found her mental function declined significantly toward the end of each semester. Her symptoms included feeling isolated, having a hard time finishing tasks, feeling frustrated when stressed, and not being rested after adequate sleep, which only added to the stress of an already challenging program.

In filling out Dr. Kharrazian's brain questionnaire, her symptoms suggested her dopamine pathways were malfunctioning. I gave her nutritional compounds to support dopamine function and she now finds her mind as sharp at the end of the semester as she does

at its outset. This has worked consistently for both semesters so far. It's a delight to see how pleased she is about her improvement.
   Kenneth Morehead, MSOM, LAc, DAONB
   Durham, North Carolina
   www.orientalhealthsolutions.com

• •

NUTRITIONAL COMPOUNDS THAT SUPPORT DOPAMINE ACTIVITY

When general brain health, stress, and blood sugar imbalances, all of which will deplete dopamine, are addressed and dopamine levels still remain low, some additional support may be called for. A variety of natural compounds have been shown to be very effective in raising dopamine levels and supporting dopamine activity.

The herbs that directly stimulate dopamine synthesis are *mucuna pruriens*, also known as cowhage, and the amino acids D, L-phenylalanine, beta-phenylethylamine, and N-acetyl L-tyrosine. Vitamin B-6 (P-5-P), selenium, blueberry extract, and alpha lipoic acid provide cofactors and additional support.

Mucuna pruriens

Studies strongly suggest that the components in *mucuna pruriens*, particularly L-dopa, convert to dopamine in the brain; L-dopa has been shown to cross the blood-brain barrier. In fact, *mucuna pruriens* has been used as a botanical for neurological disorders, and current research shows it has anti-Parkinsonian effects. Flavonoids in *mucuna pruriens* have been shown to protect the substantia nigra, where dopamine is made in the brain, and the nigrastriatal pathways, major routes of dopamine delivery to other areas of the brain. *Mucuna pruriens* has been used for decades for neurological diseases and tremors in other parts of the world, particularly in Eastern Europe.[13][14][15][16][17][18]

Beta-phenylethylamine (PEA)

Another effective precursor to dopamine is beta-phenylethylamine (PEA), a natural compound that easily crosses the blood-brain barrier and has been shown to stimulate and modulate the release of dopamine in the brain. PEA has been shown to improve attention and learning and relieve depression. PEA also influences endorphins, which help with feelings of pleasure.

Not surprisingly, a common natural source of PEA is chocolate. Many times people with low dopamine will rely on chocolate to boost their mood, especially when their brain is fatigued. They may be reading or studying too much, or at a long, information-packed seminar, and their brains will start to fatigue as the activity and stimulation exceeds what their neurons are capable of sustaining. That's when the severe chocolate cravings kick in—all they want to do is eat chocolate and they just won't feel right until they do. Some people are addicted to the chocolate for the sugar of course, but for others it's PEA's influence on the dopamine pathways that hooks them.[19 20 21 22 23]

Falling in love also stimulates dopamine. It's why you often hear that eating chocolate triggers the same chemicals as falling in love. When people fall in love their dopamine levels go up and it seems nothing in the world bothers them. A person deeply in love with her newfound soulmate may walk out and find her car was totaled during the night. She'll shrug her shoulders and respond, "Oh well, it's just a car."

Meanwhile her dopamine-deficient peer across town, who has been married for 10 years and raised three kids while working full time, may walk out and find a bird pooped on her newly washed car. She flies into an explosive rage, ruining her new heels while kicking the nearest tree in a fit. These are examples of how varying levels of dopamine can affect two otherwise reasonable people. Ample dopamine allows people to tolerate things that go wrong, while low dopamine has them snapping over minor provocations.

Blueberry extract, selenium, alpha lipoic acid, N-acetylcysteine

When considering dopamine support, one of the key things to consider is the integrity of the substantia nigra, the area in the midbrain where dopamine is made. Antioxidants have been shown to protect the substantia nigra. Plenty of research has been done on the role of antioxidants in fighting Parkinson's disease, and blueberry extract tends to shine above the rest as an antioxidant particularly protective of the substantia nigra. Glutathione is another powerful antioxidant, and alpha lipoic acid, selenium, and N-acetylcysteine all have been shown to raise glutathione levels.[24 25 26 27]

D, L-Phenylalanine (DLPA)

D, L-Phenylalanine (DLPA) is an essential amino acid that is a precursor to dopamine. By essential, I mean humans must have it in their diets. It is found primarily in meats, fish, eggs, and dairy products. Vegans or vegetarians may be more prone to a dopamine deficiency.

Phenylalanine has a D form and an L form. The L form is converted to dopamine, while the D form is used to produce the dopamine modulator PEA, which I discussed earlier. The combination of both is referred to as DLPA and has been found effective in managing depression, mood, and pain. DLPA also prevents the breakdown and degradation of endorphins, the brain's pleasure chemicals.[28][29][30][31][32]

N-acetyl L-tyrosine

Studies have shown that supplementation of the amino acid N-acetyl L-tyrosine results in increased blood plasma and brain levels of dopamine. Studies also show that depletion of dietary tyrosine decreases dopamine levels in both human and animal study subjects.

Tyrosine is a precursor to not only dopamine but also the adrenal catecholamine hormones epinephrine and norepinephrine. These are our stress fight-or-flight hormones, and supplementing with just L-tyrosine can overly energize a person and cause anxiety, sleeplessness, and irritability. However, if N-acetyl L-tyrosine is used, which includes the two-carbon acetyl group, it tends to activate the dopamine pathways more than the catecholamine pathways.[33][34][35][36][37]

Vitamin B-6—P-5-P

Vitamin B-6 is an important cofactor in the synthesis of dopamine and other major neurotransmitters, and a vitamin commonly depleted by the stress and poor diets of many modern Americans. P-5-P is a more available form of B-6.[38][39][40][41]

Dosing

The rule of thumb for dosing with dopamine support is the same as it is for the other neurotransmitters—you take as much as you need to experience a benefit. Supporting neurotransmitter activity is not dependent upon body size, but instead on the degree to which you have symptoms. As a result, determining your dose requires some trial and error.

It typically takes a half hour to an hour after taking dopamine support to notice the effects. Continue to gradually increase your dose until you notice an improvement in your symptoms. Then increase the dose again to see whether you experience even more improvement. Once you no longer feel any improvement, go back the previous dose at which you felt improvement.

How often you take dopamine support also varies with the individual. Some may find they need it three or more times a day, others just once.

What if you crash and burn on dopamine support?

As is the case with serotonin and GABA, sometimes when people support dopamine they will "crash," succumbing to intense fatigue. This is because their neurons are too close to threshold, aren't able to make enough energy, and therefore do not function properly. Although the brain may need dopamine support, it is so fragile that just a little bit of support sends it over the edge, fatiguing the neurons and hence the individual.

If this crash happens after just the minimum dose, it could actually mean this person is in desperate need of support. However, additional support for brain inflammation, brain oxygenation, and neuron support may also be warranted. Compounds for these conditions will dampen inflammation in the brain common with neurodegeneration, give the neurons more support against degeneration, and supply the brain with more oxygen-rich blood (assuming anemia isn't a factor).

Another possible outcome is that the additional neurotransmitter support can actually support negative plasticity. For example, a person with hair-trigger rage driven by poor dopamine activity may actually find supporting dopamine actually makes her temper worse.

So what do you do when you need dopamine support but even just a little is too much for a fragile brain? You use even less, while paying attention to issues of brain inflammation and oxygenation, as I mentioned above.

DIETARY PRECURSORS AND DOPAMINE

Foods that theoretically impact dopamine typically contain high amounts of phenylalanine, and these are primarily animal products (meats, eggs, and cheeses), as well as oats and chocolate. Phenylalanine is an essential amino acid that must be supplied by our diet because our body cannot synthesize it. Dopamine deficiencies due to diet may be an issue for vegans and vegetarians, as relying on non-animal products such as oats and chocolate for their dopamine needs is not sufficient.

For the average American a dietary lack of dopamine is not an issue. In fact many people are over consuming foods rich in dopamine and serotonin precursors. However, because so many other issues are at play in a dopamine deficiency, dietary consumption of foods high in the amino acid phenylalanine are not typically effective with the exception of vegan and vegetarian diets.

· ·

When I'm under more stress than usual I tend toward a dopamine pattern. When I was writing the course material for my brain chemistry classes I had to squeeze long hours of research and writing in between my lecture schedule and office hours.

As the days wore on and the number of pages increased I could feel my neurochemistry slipping out of balance. I started to feel like everything I was working on was worthless, that everyone would hate it, and that I was a failure as a practitioner and educator. My wife pointed out I was snappy and more irritable than usual, getting angry about the dumbest things. Because of my schedule, time with my family is precious and brief, and yet I was holing up in my office more than usual, preferring to be alone.

Luckily by then I had a substantial enough understanding of the brain to realize what was going on. The extreme stress of the demands I had placed on myself were creating a dopamine deficiency. Because I had a deadline to meet I wasn't able to mend my brain with a vacation in Hawaii. Instead, I supported my dopamine pathways with some key herbal and nutritional compounds and watched all those symptoms fade away, resulting in more energy and focus to complete the task at hand.

Datis Kharrazian, DHSc, DC, MS

· ·

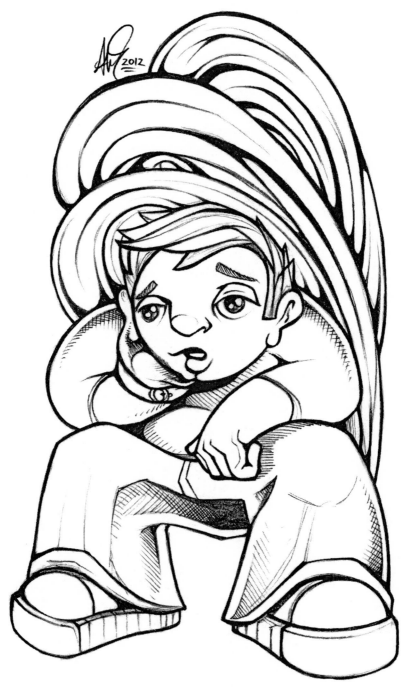

*People with poor dopamine activity feel hopeless and worthless,
handle stress poorly, and suffer from lack of motivation.*

FACTORS THAT AFFECT DOPAMINE TRANSPORT AND SYNTHESIS

The factors that can hamper dopamine activity include medications, insufficient cofactors due to nutritional deficiencies, blood sugar imbalances, and hormonal imbalances.

Two popular antidepressants affect dopamine pathways and are categorized as dopamine selective reuptake inhibitors (DRIs). A positive response to these drugs is a strong indication that dopamine activity is compromised. As with the use of SSRIs for serotonin-related depression, DRIs can eventually deplete the body of important cofactors necessary for dopamine synthesis and activity, as well as create a resistance to dopamine.

BLOOD SUGAR AND DOPAMINE

Phenylalanine is a precursor to dopamine. It's transport across the blood-brain barrier depends on proper liver function and blood sugar balance for transport by the "large neutral amino acid transporter" (LNAA) proteins.

The liver converts phenylalanine into tyrosine for transport into the brain. This conversion requires a healthy liver. People with hepatitis, liver sclerosis, fatty liver as a result of insulin resistance or diabetes, or any other liver disease may have problems with this conversion process and may exhibit symptoms of a dopamine deficiency.

The dopamine used by the brain must be made in the brain. As with serotonin, this function depends on the LNAA transport proteins delivering the precursors for dopamine into the brain.

The effectiveness of this transport, however, depends upon *appropriate* insulin secretion—not too much or not too little. For the person with insulin resistance or hypoglycemia, which is arguably the majority of Americans, appropriate insulin responses are uncommon and dopamine synthesis in the brain can suffer.

Many people secrete high amounts of insulin to help the body cope with carbohydrate-rich diets and sweets. It is not uncommon to see both dopamine and serotonin imbalances with uncontrolled blood sugar spikes. This is why we always address blood sugar imbalances before we jump into direct neurotransmitter support.

IRON AND DOPAMINE

In the brain, tyrosine is converted to dihydroxyphenylalanine (DOPA). This process also requires B-6 (P-5-P), folic acid, iron, and sufficient oxygen. Anemia, which starves the brain of sufficient iron and oxygen, can hamper the production of dopamine. This could help explain why people with anemia experience such symptoms as loss of motivation and depression.

Other symptoms of iron-deficiency anemia (as there are several types of anemia) include the whites of the eyes turning a bluish color, a pale face, and nail beds that are pale instead of pink. The person may chew ice or dirt, or bite his or her fingernails chronically. Women with heavy menstrual periods are at risk, as are athletes who do a lot of endurance running and training—the prolonged and intense physical activity causes excessive red blood cell breakdown so that the individual may have higher demands for iron than the average person.

Women with uterine fibroids often become iron deficient as the fibroids take up most of the body's iron. People with parasites such as pinworms develop iron deficiencies, as do those with malabsorption issues. Iron deficiency anemia is very common in those with a gluten intolerance or celiac disease as gluten destroys the lining of the small intestine, causing malabsorption. Hypothyroidism can also impair the body's ability to absorb iron, as can low levels of hydrochloric acid in the stomach, which can also be associated with an H. pylori infection.

OXYGEN

Oxygen is also critical for the synthesis of dopamine in the brain. Any type of anemia, such as B-12 anemia, folic anemia, pernicious anemia, and iron anemia can affect levels of oxygen in the brain. Anemia should always be considered when symptoms of a dopamine deficiency are evident. Other factors that can affect the delivery of oxygen to the brain include smoking, severe stress, severe metabolic issues, or brain degeneration. Cold hands and feet and chronic fungal nail growth are symptoms that could point to lack of oxygen to the brain.

FOLIC ACID AND P-5-P

Another key factor for the synthesis of dopamine is tetrahydrobiopterin (THB). THB is the byproduct of folic acid that is produced by healthy gut bacteria, an example of how healthy digestive function benefits the brain. Gut infections and insufficient healthy gut flora can actually hamper the brain's production of dopamine.

B-6 is another cofactor necessary for dopamine synthesis and B-6 deficiencies are also very common today—for instance regular alcohol consumption can deplete P-5-P levels, as can blood sugar imbalances. P-5-P, the active form of B-6, is necessary for the synthesis and breakdown of dopamine in the brain.

BREAKDOWN AND CLEARANCE OF DOPAMINE

Just as important as the production of dopamine is its breakdown and clearance from the synaptic cleft so that new, more effective dopamine can take its place. This process requires magnesium and methyl donors, such as betaine, folic acid, and methyl B-12. A severe magnesium deficiency may hamper this breakdown and clearance; you see magnesium deficiencies in those taking diuretics, a first-line therapy for high blood pressure. Athletes who overtrain can become deficient in magnesium also. Methyl donor deficiencies are also common today.

Studies show people who take SSRIs or DRIs for long periods of time become deficient in methyl donors and P-5-P. Those considering weaning off their antidepressant medication may need to supplement with these cofactors to cover for deficiencies acquired during use of the medication.

Lack of methyl donors are also found in those who take estrogen replacement therapy, such as birth control pills or estrogen creams. People with low levels of stomach hydrochloric acid or who have H. pylori infections may also be low in the cofactors.

• •

Anneka consulted me after six years of suffering with severe anxiety, insomnia, fatigue, brain fog, depression, and difficulties staying focused. In addition, she felt a constant pressure in her head. Not only was it hard for her to function, no one could figure out what was wrong with her, and her symptoms were affecting her marriage and family life. Anneka said she didn't remember a day when she felt normal.

Anneka was a classic neurological patient on medications for anxiety, sleep, and depression. After assessing the results of her neurological and endocrine tests, I found she was deficient in acetylcholine and dopamine. She also had high cortisol levels throughout the day.

I immediately put her on therapeutic doses of nutrients to support acetylcholine and dopamine activity. We gave her DHA for the brain inflammation and pressure, and nutrients to support the hypothalamus-adrenal-pituitary axis. Within one month, her symptoms improved. Anneka now says almost every day is a good day, and she feels better than she has in six years.

Joshua Redd, DC
Salt Lake City, Utah
www.drjoshuaredd.com

CHAPTER SUMMARY

• Symptoms of poor dopamine activity include poor motivation or drive, feelings of worthlessness and hopelessness, loss of temper for minor reasons, inability to handle stress, and a desire to isolate from others.

• Dopamine is most commonly known for its association with Parkinson's disease, a disease brought on by destruction of the brain's substantia nigra, where dopamine is made, and long-term dopamine deficiency. However, dopamine has numerous functions in the brain related to motor coordination, motivation, and reward. It helps regulate prolactin, a hormone involved with lactation, reproduction, and libido. It is involved with modulating mood, attention, and learning, and drives the pleasure center of the brain.

• The dopamine-deficient person tends to be non-compliant due to lack of motivation. Dopamine-deficient patients can be problematic for practitioners.

• Dopamine is heavily involved in addiction.

• For the average American a dietary lack of dopamine is not an issue. In fact many people are overconsuming foods rich in dopamine and serotonin precursors. However, because so many other issues are at play in a dopamine deficiency, dietary consumption of foods high in the amino acid phenylalanine are not typically effective with the exception of vegan and vegetarian diets.

• The factors that can hamper dopamine activity include medications, insufficient cofactors due to nutritional deficiencies, blood sugar imbalances, and hormonal imbalances.

• Two popular antidepressants affect dopamine pathways and are categorized as dopamine selective reuptake inhibitors (DRIs). A positive response to these drugs is a strong indication that dopamine activity is compromised. As with the use of SSRIs for serotonin-related depression, DRIs can eventually deplete the body of important cofactors necessary for dopamine synthesis and activity, as well as create a resistance to dopamine.

• Phenylalanine is a precursor to dopamine. It's transport across the blood-brain barrier depends on proper liver function and blood sugar balance for transport by the "large neutral amino acid transporter" (LNAA) proteins.

• THB, the byproduct of folic acid that is produced by healthy gut bacteria, is necessary for the production of dopamine. Gut infections and insufficient healthy gut flora can hamper the brain's production of dopamine. B6 is another cofactor necessary for dopamine synthesis and B6 deficiencies are very common today.

• The breakdown and clearance of dopamine requires magnesium and methyl donors. A severe magnesium deficiency may hamper this breakdown and clearance; you see magnesium deficiencies in those taking diuretics, a first-line therapy for high blood pressure. Athletes who over train can become deficient in magnesium also. Methyl donor deficiencies are also common today.

• Anemia, which starves the brain of sufficient iron and oxygen, can hamper the production of dopamine. This could help explain why people with anemia experience such symptoms as loss of motivation and depression.

• The herbs that directly stimulate dopamine synthesis are mucuna pruriens, also known as cowhage, and the amino acids D, L-phenylalanine, beta-phenylethylamine, and N-acetyl L-tyrosine. Vitamin B6 (P-5-P), selenium, blueberry extract, and alpha lipoic acid provide cofactors and additional support.

Chapter Seventeen
THE HORMONE-BRAIN CONNECTION

SYMPTOMS OF HORMONE IMBALANCE IN MEN (ANY AGE)

- Low libido
- Fluctuations in mood, brain function, and focus
- Loss of muscle mass
- Sweating attacks (hot flashes in men)

SYMPTOMS OF HORMONE IMBALANCE IN WOMEN IN PERIMENOPAUSE

- Fluctuating menstrual cycle lengths
- Hot flushes and spontaneous sweating
- Fluctuations in mood, brain function, and focus

SYMPTOMS OF HORMONE IMBALANCE IN WOMEN IN MENOPAUSE

- Vaginal dryness, itching, or pain
- Deterioration in mood, brain function, and focus
- Loss of bone density
- Mental fogginess after perimenopause

Lucy, 44, suffered from poor memory, poor mental endurance, and episodes of vertigo. She could no longer remember basic phone numbers and was having difficulty remembering people's names. She began changing her daily routine to compensate for her lack of brain function and carried a notepad every place she went so she could write down the things she could no longer remember.

She also had episodes of vertigo that would last several minutes and made it feel like the world was twirling around her. She saw many different physicians and was prescribed seasickness medication for her vertigo and told her memory loss was due to getting older.

Lucy was 45 minutes late for her first visit with me because she had trouble following the directions we gave her. She also brought in a tape recorder so she would not forget anything we discussed. It was obvious before I even did a history and exam that Lucy's brain was not healthy. During the exam she couldn't recall numbers I had given her to remember and she was unable to count backwards from 100. She had significant balance problems and she had difficulty perceiving vibration with a tuning fork and temperature in both of her feet. Although she did not have any signs of peripheral nerve disease, her brain clearly was not functioning well.

I ordered an MRI, and it showed small blood vessel disease throughout her brain. In other words, her brain was degenerating because her blood vessels were unhealthy and could not carry blood to the brain efficiently. These findings were worrisome for a woman only 44 years old.

So what happened to Lucy? Lucy had been a strict and poorly practicing vegan since her late 20s. She had stopped menstruating in her 30s, and she was not even sure if she was menopausal at this point. Lucy's cholesterol was also 98 (normal total cholesterol is around 200). This was important because cholesterol is necessary to make all the major steroid hormones crucial for brain health. Her brain had literally been void of hormones for almost two decades.

Her hormone lab results showed very low levels of reproductive hormones and high FSH levels. This meant she was postmenopau-

sal at this point and did not even know it. Her chronic hormone deficiency was probably a key factor of her accelerated brain aging.

Lucy's management plan included a drastic change in her diet, bioidentical hormone replacement, and various supplements to help support her brain health. I also gave her brain and balance exercises to activate her brain pathways.

Unfortunately for Lucy, some of her loss of brain function is permanent. The brain needs hormones to function and when deprived of them it ages quickly. The changes we made for Lucy helped improved her brain function and potentially slowed degeneration. If you have hormone symptoms and your brain is not working well, understanding the impact hormones have on brain health is very important.

Datis Kharrazian, DHSc, DC, MS

● ●

Hormones significantly impact brain health. This is bad news for many Americans, whose hormones seem to be in a permanent state of disarray. Contrary to popular belief, premenstrual syndrome (PMS) is not normal or healthy; it's a symptom of a hormonal imbalance. This helps explain the cramps, breast tenderness, irritability and moodiness, sometimes to an extreme degree, that many women experience before their periods.

The same can be said for perimenopause, the transition into menopause that can be so dramatic it's a source of cultural amusement yet often intense private suffering. My perimenopausal patients can be the most difficult to work with but I also have the most compassion for them. It's as if an otherwise nice and normal woman sits handcuffed at the back of her brain while a demon entity takes over, causing her to lash out at loved ones, break down into hysterics, or develop anxiety, depression, and insomnia. These women feel remorse and shock for uncontrollable behavior that seems to pop up out of nowhere, or extreme distress over a sudden onslaught of physical and mental symptoms.

At the reproductive end of the hormonal spectrum, female infertility is at an all-time high, largely due to high testosterone levels and polycystic ovarian syndrome (PCOS) that affects an estimated 15 percent of women.[1] Women struggle with menstrual cycles that last too long, don't come at all, or catch them off guard by varying in length and duration.

Men are increasingly under attack from their own imbalanced hormones as well. Erectile dysfunction affects 15 to 30 million men, with the rate having tripled in the last 20 years.[2] Male "breasts" and "hips" are becoming increasingly common as men's estrogen levels soar too high, even in teenage boys. Meanwhile testosterone is plummeting, robbing men of their virility, but perhaps even more importantly, their motivation and general well-being. Low testosterone is behind the unfortunate descent many men make into being a "grumpy old man."

Aging, too, produces a decline in overall hormone levels, which in turn can affect brain function. Unhealthy aging is really just rapid brain degeneration. What does it mean to age poorly? This is the person who can't remember well, can't concentrate, can't focus, can't learn, and who also loses autonomic function, such as bladder control or good digestion. This is also the person whose posture noticeably worsens. (Interestingly, posture is neurologically based. As people lose various aspects of their nervous system integration, this changes the tone of their spine, their heads move forward like a turtle's, and their walking gate becomes impaired.)

Recognizing the impact of hormones on brain function, anti-aging clinics and doctors pump hormones into aging people (unfortunately not taking into account the effects of excess hormones on the brain). Meanwhile, the vital roles of brain degeneration and brain inflammation, both of which have a powerful effect on aging, go overlooked.

So what do hormonal imbalances have to do with the brain? Everything! When hormones become imbalanced you lose neurotransmitter activity, which affects how you feel, function, and view your life. In other words, the more balanced your hormones are, the more half-full your glass looks. Hormonal imbalances also significantly impact brain inflammation and degeneration and considerably speed aging of the brain.

In this chapter I'll go over concepts of how hormones affect brain health and how you can achieve better brain health through better hormone health.

* *

Denise, 46, complained of severe brain fog, moderate depression, word-finding difficulties, and poor memory, especially short-term memory. She was moody and yelled at her kids and her husband a lot. She said she had no libido. She also had insomnia, sleeping at night about two hours, then waking up and being unable to go back to sleep for about two hours. She would then sleep two hours and do it all over again.

She hadn't had a menstrual period for over two years, which meant she was in menopause. Her serum estradiol was less than 19, her progesterone was less than 0.5, and her testosterone was 23. She said she fatigued easily and had a hard time concentrating at work.

She was given transdermal estradiol and progesterone in a rhythmic dosing schedule. Within days she called to tell me she was feeling much better. At a follow-up visit a month later she told me she was continuing to improve. She can concentrate at work and is getting her work done. She is finding work easier because she is much more stress-tolerant (due to the effects of estradiol on serotonin).

She has a much easier time remembering names of people. Her home life has improved. She is more patient with the children (teens). Her husband called to thank me for giving him his wife back. She says her libido is coming back. She tells me her skin is smooth again and it glows. Her coworkers are commenting about how good she looks. Her hair is growing again and is full and looks good. She now sleeps all night without waking up for the first time in more than three years. She feels rested in the morning. She is very happy.

Robert Mathis, MD
Santa Barbara, California
www.baselinehealth.net

• •

HORMONES AND NEUROTRANSMITTERS

In Chapter Twelve I talked about heterotropic modulation, the idea that in order for a neurotransmitter to synapse with a neuron, several compounds are necessary for that transmission to take place. One of those compounds is a hormone—estrogen, progesterone, or testosterone. For example, the following hormones have powerful effects on specific receptor sites:

- Estrogen impacts serotonin receptors in men and women
- Progesterone impacts GABA receptors in men and women
- Estrogen impacts dopamine receptors in women
- Testosterone impacts dopamine receptors in men
- Estrogen impacts acetylcholine receptors in women
- Testosterone impacts acetylcholine receptors in men
- Thyroid hormones impact all neurotransmitter receptors in men and women

It's important to know this when looking at symptoms of neurotransmitter impairment as poor neurotransmitter activity may stem from a hormonal imbalance. Thus addressing that imbalance is paramount to better brain health. For instance, simply upping nutritional compounds to boost serotonin activity may help but won't go the distance in an estrogen-deficient woman.

HORMONES AND INFLAMMATION

Neurons and microglia cells, the brain's immune cells, also have receptor sites for hormones. Healthy hormone levels have been shown to facilitate neuron branching and plasticity, dampen brain inflammation, slow degeneration, and play a role in neuronal migration, the movement of neurons from one place to another to participate in activity and repair.[3][4][5][6][7]

● ●

I initially sought treatment with Dr. Flannery because I was diagnosed with osteopenia. I also was not sleeping well and would wake up with a pounding heart at 3 a.m. every morning.

My medical doctor prescribed hormone replacement therapy. I became aware of the long-term negative effects of taking hormones through my own research and decided I wanted to take a different approach. I wanted to get off the medication but worried about further bone loss.

Dr. Flannery was concerned with my forgetfulness and memory loss. I had always struggled with schoolwork and learning since

I was a little girl (I am now 67) and thought that was normal. Dr. Flannery insisted that these symptoms were not normal.

He ordered several tests to find the cause of my symptoms. Along with the blood test he ordered a stool test and a saliva test. I did not want to spend the money on the stool test as I did not have any digestive problems. I was shocked when the stool test revealed I had four different infections! The saliva test confirmed I had a problem with my cortisol levels. Dr. Flannery explained my insomnia was due to the imbalance in my cortisol.

Within two weeks of starting my protocol I was sleeping again and noticed I had more energy during the day. My children noticed my memory was better. I realized I could dial phone numbers without looking them up in my address book. I had never done that before.

I am so grateful that Dr. Flannery addressed the memory problem I had always accepted as normal. By the way, my last bone density test was normal.

Dr. Flannery's note: This patient was supported with a combination of prescription medication and botanicals for her gastrointestinal infections. Once the infections resolved, natural compounds were used to repair her intestinal lining. Blood sugar and cortisol balance were supported using natural herbal compounds with a high dose phosphatidylserine cream. Memory function improved using compounds that support healthy levels of acetylcholine in the brain, high dose DHA, and phosphatidylserine.

a patient of Dr. Flannery
Mark Flannery, DC, FAAIM, DCBCN, DCCN, CNS
Woodland Hills, California
www.DrFlannery.com

HORMONES AND BRAIN SHAPE

Research on individuals undergoing sex changes has provided us with some interesting observations on how hormones affect the shape and structure of the brain. The male brain is anatomically different than the female brain. Men have a larger hypothalamus than women, and the female brain has more grey matter, which governs sensory perceptions (seeing, hearing, emotions, memory, speech) and muscle control, while men have more white matter, which is essential for relaying information and for cognitive function.

The frontal lobe, our emotional control center and the neurological seat of our personality, also differs between the sexes. The male frontal lobe has more receptor sites for testosterone whereas the female frontal lobe has more receptor sites for estrogen. Right away you can see how deficiencies in these hormones might affect one's personality. The frontal lobe also generates motivation and drive, and it's common to see a woman who is low in estrogen also suffer from depression and poor motivation. The same holds true for men who are low in testosterone.

When people undergo a sex change they take large amounts of hormones to develop the characteristics of the opposite sex. Researchers have looked at brain MRIs of these people before, during, and after hormone treatment. In one study of eight subjects undergoing a male-to-female transition and six subjects undergoing a female-to-male transition, researchers found their brain shape changed.

The men receiving high amounts of female hormones began developing more female-like brains. The women receiving high amounts of male hormones developed a larger hypothalamus, and both the volume of grey and white matter shifted. Granted, these are heavy hormone doses, but in just four months the subjects' brains actually changed to take on the shape and structure of the opposite sex, a powerful testament to the influence of hormones on the brain.[8]

Clinically, it's very common for a health care practitioner to see both women and men with skewed hormone levels. Many men have either too much estrogen or too little testosterone, or both. Many women are deficient in progesterone and either have too much or too little estrogen, and quite often too much testosterone. It's interesting to think that these hormonal shifts may actually be changing the shape of their brains. If men are developing breasts and women are going bald and growing beards, it's not at all far-fetched to consider their brain shape may be changing, too.

BLOOD SUGAR AND HORMONES

Given how drastically hormonal imbalances affect the brain, it is paramount to work to bring these levels back into balance. The answer, contrary to popular belief, does not necessarily lie in hormone replacement therapy. Hormone replacement therapy can create dangerously high levels of hormones that can cause a host of other problems, such as receptor site resistance and poor communication between the brain and the hormone glands. Instead, it's better to address the root cause of the hormonal imbalances, which the majority of the time is our favorite culprit, blood sugar imbalances from a high carbohydrate diet.

HIGH ESTROGEN IN MEN

When a man eats too many carbohydrates too frequently (again, symptoms are feeling tired after eating and/or craving sugar) insulin surges increase an enzyme called aromatase. Found in body fat, aromatase converts testosterone to estradiol, a form of estrogen. As aromatase is chronically activated thanks to a high-carb diet and estradiol levels climb, insulin resistance grows—the excess estradiol causes insulin receptor sites to become resistant so blood sugar levels stay high. This is in turn spikes aromatase in a vicious cycle.

One of the most common scenarios I have seen across the country is men with aromatase overactivity taking testosterone gel, which ends up converting into estrogens. Their lab tests show very little change in testosterone but significant elevations in estrogens. Many of these men suspect their testosterone gel was actually an estrogen gel because they are not aware of the aromatase conversion mechanism. They may develop more female characteristics, such as breasts, hips, or crying more easily.

This is commonly seen in prediabetic and hypoglycemic men, or in men who take insulin shots. It's not uncommon in these scenarios for estrogen levels to be five to 10 times higher than normal, which affects neurotransmitter activity, inflammation, and degeneration in the brain. It's quite possible that over time their brain shape changes and these men experience changes in their motivation, drive, and personality.

● ●

A 34-year-old male came into my office. He said he was losing his mind and couldn't think or function anymore, to the point where he had to quit college. He said his life was falling apart socially and physically.

In the past he saw his doctor for symptoms of low testosterone, and his doctor gave him testosterone injections. As it turns out, he received way too much testosterone and had developed testosterone resistance. This creates all the same symptoms of a testosterone deficiency. I ordered a hormone panel, an adrenal panel, and a salivary hormone panel.

While we waited for his lab tests to come back, I got him started on nutritional compounds to address insulin resistance, which was an issue for him, adrenal adpatogens for poor adrenal function, vitamin D, and methyl B-12. When I got his testosterone panel back it showed his testosterone levels were off the charts, so we weaned him off testosterone and did nutritional therapy work to clear the excess testosterone from his system.

Because testosterone is so important for brain health and dopamine activity, and because his resistance to testosterone was depriving his brain of this vital hormone, I knew his brain needed help. I gave him nutritional compounds to quench brain inflammation and boost dopamine activity. I also gave him compounds to boost acetylcholine activity as he demonstrated so many acetylcholine deficiency symptoms. He felt a huge improvement right away.

When he had gone to see his doctor I have no doubt his testosterone was low. However, it was most likely low due to a blood sugar imbalance, which was an issue for him. By getting his blood sugar under control through diet and proper nutritional compounds, his hormones were able to normalize.

Now he is a totally different person and is back in school and feeling well. His mother even called me to thank me for giving her her son back.

Joleene Anderson, DC, DCBCN
Winter Haven, Florida

• •

HIGH TESTOSTERONE IN WOMEN

Conversely, the most common thing practitioners see in women is elevated testosterone. As with men, insulin surges from high-carb diets increase a hormone-converting enzyme called 17,20 lyase, which increases testosterone production. Women who have high testosterone also tend to be insulin resistant because the excess testosterone blunts the receptor sites for insulin, thus creating a vicious cycle just as in men. Common symptoms include PCOS, excess facial hair, and thinning hair on the scalp. The high testosterone also knocks estrogen and progesterone levels out of balance, affecting neurotransmitter activity in the brain. As a result drive, motivation, and personality are affected.

HORMONE SYNTHESIS IN THE BRAIN

Microglia cells, the brain's immune cells, contain enzymes that can trigger the synthesis of hormones.[9][10][11] Sufficient hormone levels are so important to healthy brain function that these microglia cells make hormones on an ongoing basis. Therefore, the brain receives hormones from two areas: the body's endocrine (hormone) system, which includes the various hormone-producing glands, and the brain's microglia cells. The endocrine system produces the majority of the hormones the brain uses, which enter the brain through the blood-brain barrier.

These hormones are like the paint on a large paint brush going back and forth across a wall. The brush misses patches here and there. It's the hormones made by the microglia cells that fill in the small gaps. The endocrine system has the largest hormonal influence on the brain, whereas the microglia hormones exert small and subtle influences.

CHOLESTEROL AND HORMONES

To make hormones, however, these microglia cells need certain precursors. One of the first things they need is cholesterol (in fact, all hormone production depends on adequate cholesterol). This is a concern today as the trend in cardiology is to push cholesterol levels below 100. To a functional medicine practitioner, this is very disturbing. We believe cholesterol under 150 is too low for healthy hormone, brain, and immune function. For me personally, below 100 is way too low.

We practitioners have seen patients who successfully maintain such low cholesterol and suffer from poor cognition and memory. In my practice, these patients' chief complaint is depression. They may not realize it correlates because it comes on so gradually. Cholesterol provides the precursors to make phospholipids, a fatty compound that makes up much of the brain.

A look at these basics of human physiology shows that low cholesterol can have disastrous consequences on the brain. I believe the harmful effects of excessively low cholesterol levels will be evidenced in the scientific literature in the years to come.

ADRENAL STRESS AND BRAIN HORMONES

Another substance microglia cells use to synthesize hormones is dehydroepiandrosterone (DHEA), a steroid hormone. The microglia cells use DHEA to make testosterone and estrogen, so, like cholesterol, an adequate level of DHEA in the brain is important for good brain function. DHEA is made throughout the body, including by the adrenal glands, the liver, in the testes to make testosterone in men, and in the ovaries to make estrogen in women. However, the majority of DHEA released into the body comes from the adrenal glands.

Unfortunately, due to the various stressors people cope with today—including hectic lifestyles, blood sugar imbalances, and chronic health issues—many people suffer from poor adrenal function and hence low DHEA output. Although DHEA is necessary, supplementing with DHEA is only recommended for a short period of time and when lab testing shows chronic adrenal fatigue. Unnecessarily supplementing with DHEA can exacerbate the conversion of testosterone to estrogen in men and the production of testosterone in women.

Pregnenolone steal

Pregnenolone is another substance the endocrine system and the brain use to make hormones. As the adrenal glands start to fail due to chronic stress, a mechanism called "pregnenolone steal" goes into action. In pregnenolone steal, the body "steals" pregnenolone from cholesterol to make more cortisol as the adrenals fatigue. Normally, pregnenolone is a precursor to sex hormones, such as progesterone and testosterone. As a result of pregnenolone steal, however, pregnenolone consistently is shunted toward cortisol production instead of sex hormone production, causing hormonal imbalances. This mechanism is a common underlying cause of PMS, infertility, male menopause, and PCOS.

What's the most common cause of pregnenolone steal? You guessed it again, blood sugar imbalances. High-carbohydrate diets and the ensuing insulin surges are extremely taxing to the body, keeping it in a constant state of stress. Throughout the book I have talked about the various other ways blood sugar imbalances stress the body, adding to the problem. The end results are hormone deficiencies, hormone imbalances, and the deleterious effects of such imbalances on the brain.

So between the standard health care model driving people's cholesterol dangerously low and chronic stress causing low DHEA and pregnenolone steal, the brain's microglia cells are unable to make enough hormones to meet the brain's needs. Functions that suffer as a consequence include neuronal transmission, myelination (the protective coating glia cells offer to neurons), synaptic activity, neuronal repair, and neuronal migration (the movement of neurons to areas where they're needed for activity or repair).

Therefore, when a patient comes to me with some obvious neurological issues, I'm not going to just look at how to support his or her neurons or neurotransmitters. Given how significant hormone health is to brain health, common sense requires me to address hormonal health as well (and immune health, too, as you have learned). I'm going to look at whether diet and blood sugar imbalances, such as hypoglycemia or insulin resistance, are an issue. I also look at cholesterol levels and adrenal function.

* *

Marilyn, 45, was a divorced mother of three who had suffered from severe depression for the last seven years. She lived with and depended on her mother because she was unable to work. She could only stay awake for about two hours a day, and then only after drinking six cups of coffee.

Marilyn had had a total hysterectomy 10 years earlier for uncontrolled uterine bleeding and was given no hormones after the surgery, throwing her into abrupt surgical menopause. Within two years of the surgery she had become very depressed and ended up divorced from her husband of 20 years. Her doctor prescribed the following: an antidepressant, thyroid medication, 1 mg of estradiol, and 200 mg of progesterone daily. Her depression worsened and her antidepressant dosage was increased substantially, although her symptoms of depression did not improve. Three years ago another MD increased her estradiol to 2 mg and her progesterone to 400 mg daily. Her depression, emotional mood swings, and fatigue became even worse and she attempted suicide on a couple of occasions. She was given two electric shock therapies but refused the other 11 her doctor recommended.

Marilyn had spent about $30,000 seeking advice from a number of different doctors but continued to suffer tremendously. She came to see me a few months after her last suicide attempt.

Based on lab testing, I increased her estradiol and decreased her progesterone dosages and began slowly tapering her off her antidepressant. I placed her on a strong nutritional program that included a detoxification protein shake several times a day and nutrients to support glutathione, inflammation, and adrenal function. I also switched her from a synthetic T4-only medication to a natural thyroid hormone that also supported T3.

By day 23 of the protocol she was able to stay awake all day. Her mood progressed from depression to "I feel much better," and her fatigue lifted. She felt well enough that she was able to celebrate Christmas with her three daughters for the first time in seven years.

She later called to tell me she had moved to Florida, has a full-time job, is doing well, and even wanted to write a book about her experience.

Had she not come into the office and had a chance to work on the underlying mechanisms and adjust her hormone therapy, she likely would have been institutionalized for the rest of her life.

Robert Mathis, MD
Santa Barbara, California
www.baselinehealth.net

● ●

THE MENSTRUATING WOMAN AND THE BRAIN

I don't think we need a scientific study to establish that fluctuating hormones in a menstruating woman can impact the brain. Many women struggle with moodiness, irritability, and personality changes related to their cycles, and many men have partners or daughters who also struggle. It's not the way Mother Nature designed women but rather another unfortunate consequence of modern life's effects on the human body.

Although most of us have real-world examples of PMS in our everyday lives, studies have also verified the PMS-brain connection. One study looked at MRI measurements of brain activity in women throughout their menstrual cycle. They found different activity in their brain correlated to surges of different hormones. For instance, many women experience personality changes when they go on estrogen hormone medications, such as oral contraceptives. When mood and personality change, this indicates an influence on the brain.[12]

There is very little research on PMS, the brain, and neurotransmitters. Additionally, we avoid hormone therapy for menstruating women who are not perimenopausal. Most hormone imbalances for PMS are due to stress physiology, adrenal imbalances, dysglycemia, compromised liver biotransformation of hormones, or essential fatty acid responses.

Studies have shown estrogen to be very protective of the brain. This does not give one license to run out and get a prescription for hormone replacement therapy, as that has been shown to raise the risk of embolisms, strokes, and other complications. Also, estrogen replacement therapy has not been shown to be protective of the brain in menstruating women. However, for postmenopausal women or women going through menopause who have steep dips in estrogen or chronically low estrogen, estrogen replacement therapy can be very protective of the brain. The need should first be determined with a clinical workup and appropriate testing, and the patient should be monitored regularly to ensure levels don't climb too high.

As women go into perimenopause and menopause, communication between the ovaries and the brain's pituitary gland (the command center for hormones) often begins to lose coordination and become disorganized. The result is abnormal spikes and drops of estrogen. This affects brain function, which in turn affects personality and behavior, typically for the worse as the areas of the brain related to mood and personality are rich in serotonin receptors.[13] Estrogen is also linked to verbal and spatial memory, fine motor skills, and depressive illnesses.[14] If estrogen declines too steeply or rapidly, one of the first things to pop up is depression and loss of some cognitive function, such as spatial memory, and fine motor skills.

Suddenly a woman can't remember where she parked or left her keys, she forgets her way home, or she loses things all the time. Or the painter, quilter or athlete suddenly finds it more difficult to manage finger dexterity or hand-eye coordination. Handwriting may worsen, too. If the estrogen deficiency goes on long enough it could result in permanent degeneration to these areas of the brain and their related functions.[15][16]

In addition to its role in sensitizing receptors to serotonin, estrogen (estradiol specifically) also helps neurons grow new dendritic spines so each neuron has a higher density of activity.[17] As I explained in Chapter Two, dendritic spines receive input from other neurons through the post-synaptic receptors. This is important because as we age we lose neurons; however, one way we can maintain good brain function is to grow new dendritic spines so connections with other neurons can increase. Sufficient estrogen in women keeps this function healthy and active.

Estrogens also have a powerful dampening effect on microglia cells, the brain's immune cells.[18][19] These immune cells are difficult to turn off once they're activated and destroy surrounding neural tissue in an inflammatory response. It doesn't help that there are 10 microglia cells for every neuron. Estrogen and other hormones help keep this immune response under control, preventing brain inflammation and degeneration.[20][21]

More dastardly is the fact that low estrogen levels in women actually cause inflammation in the body and brain. Studies show a drop in estrogen (estradiol specifically) levels during perimenopause and menopause increases inflammatory cytokines—the immune system's messengers that create inflammation. These cytokines cross the blood-brain barrier and get into the brain where they activate the brain's microglia cells. Low estrogen increases the number of cytokine receptors in the brain and their sensitivity, enhancing the inflammatory response even more so. So not only does a drop in estrogen make it hard for the brain to dampen inflammation, it also instigates inflammation in the first place.

Women in this situation may find themselves fatiguing more easily, even from routine activities such as driving or reading. They may experience brain fog or a feeling their brain is "on fire." Their circadian rhythm gets thrown off and they have trouble falling asleep, staying asleep, or waking up.

As if all this wasn't bad enough, the research also shows that estrogen-deficient women lose the ability to make glutathione, the body's most potent, stress-fighting antioxidant; bone marrow activity is inhibited, increasing their risk of osteoporosis; and estrogen deficiency skews their fatty acid balance so that they have the profile of someone who is eating a lot of deep-fried foods even if they eat really well. This means they have a greater demand for anti-inflammatory essential fatty acids (omega 3, DHA, and EPA, which are found in fish oil and krill oil, and gamma-linoleic acid, which is found in evening primrose, black currant, and borage oil).

Low estrogen also sensitizes a woman to stress so that it doesn't take much to trigger a stress response. This is the mother who goes ballistic because one of her children left a shoe in the middle of the living room floor, or breaks down into hysterical sobs when she gets pulled over by a cop for failing to use her turn signal.

An estrogen deficiency has also been shown to degrade the gut barrier and the blood-brain barrier. Permeability of both of these tissues allows pathogens, undigested proteins, and other invaders to escape into the bloodstream and the brain, further promoting inflammation. The GABA challenge, mentioned in Chapter Ten, can be used to determine whether a leaky brain is an issue.

In summary, low estrogen has been found to increase brain inflammation and degeneration through the following actions:

- Fails to dampen activated microglia cells in the brain

- Increases cytokine activity, cytokine receptor numbers, and cytokine receptor sensitivity

- Lowers ability to make glutathione, a potent stress-fighting antioxidant

- Skews fatty acid balance toward pro-inflammatory status, regardless of diet, and increases need for anti-inflammatory fats

- Increases bone marrow activity, raising the risk of osteoporosis

- Enhances the self-perpetuating stress response. In Chapter Ten I talked about how chronic stress makes the brain more sensitive to stress and more efficient at responding to it, so that a very small stimulus can trigger a huge stress response (PTSD is a great example of this, when an unexpected loud noise triggers a panic attack in a war veteran).

- Degrades the intestinal lining and blood-brain barrier (leaky gut and leaky brain)

These factors are at the heart of so many distressing symptoms women experience when going through menopause, including the extreme irritability, brain fog, forgetfulness, depression, fatigue, anxiety, stress, insomnia, and a worsening of existing conditions.

This scenario also explains why menopause raises the risk of such inflammatory conditions as heart disease, stroke, osteoporosis (yes, technically osteoporosis is the product of inflammation), dementia and Alzheimer's disease, arthritis, and autoimmune disease. What's even more distressing is that studies show once estrogen levels are restored, the inflammatory cytokine system continues to stay upregulated.[22][23]

As you can imagine, if a woman enters perimenopause with an existing inflammatory condition and experiences these common dips in estrogen, her condition will get worse. Chronic joint pain will worsen; an autoimmune thyroid condition that was relatively stable prior to perimenopause may suddenly take a turn for the worse and trigger other autoimmune diseases, such as pernicious anemia.

A woman may have unknowingly been eating foods every day to which she was intolerant. Suddenly perimenopause has her reacting to practically every food she eats so that every meal leaves her feeling sick. Minor issues with brain fog turn nearly debilitating, or a woman feels her brain is on fire.

In Chapter One I talked about the ways brain degeneration can sabotage autonomic function. This is a common scenario in the estrogen-deficient woman in perimenopause and menopause. The midbrain, which controls autonomic function, is saturated with receptors for IL-6, one of the more dastardly cytokines.

IL-6 goes up significantly with estrogen deficiency, which means rampant activation of the midbrain. As a result, issues that pop up include digestive problems, high blood pressure, bladder control problems, dry eyes or dry mouth—signs that an inflamed, degenerating brain is now affecting autonomic function. Some people simply call this aging, but it's really a cascade of inflammation attacking the body and brain.

This scenario is especially distressing for the woman who is doing everything right. She's done the elimination/provocation diet and knows which foods to eat. She has balanced her blood sugar by getting on a lower-carb diet, and she's disciplined about getting enough exercise and getting to bed on time. And yet she's still plagued by digestive issues, symptoms of hypoglycemia or insulin resistance, sleep disturbances, or chronic pain and inflammation. It's because these estrogen-deficiency cytokine surges are disrupting stress pathways in the brain, not allowing the body to calm down.

It's scenarios like this that make functional medicine so much more difficult today—the health of modern people is mired in so many complications these days, making them harder than ever to manage.

● ●

In one study researchers injected lipopolysaccharides (LPS), a pro-inflammatory compound from bacteria, into the brains of rats to induce neuroinflammation. In one group of rats, they followed the LPS injection 24 hours later with an injection of estradiol. In another group they preceded the LPS injection by 48 hours with an injection of estradiol. The rats who received the estradiol injection prior to the LPS injection showed the highest reduction in inflammation.

This study shows how having sufficient levels of estrogen in the brain can protect it against inflammatory assaults (humans deal with LPS too, though not through cerebral injections). If a person's hormone levels are healthy and normal, her potential for brain degeneration is diminished. If she had a head injury or a stroke, it could mean the consequences are not as bad for her as they are for someone whose estrogen levels are too low.[24]

● ●

TAMING THE INFLAMMATION

For the menopausal woman whose estrogen is too low, estrogen replacement therapy could be lifesaving. Again, this is not a wanton license to run out and get on replacement therapy without a genuine, demonstrated need. However, when the need is there, as it frequently is these days due to the damage of long-term stress on women's hormonal systems, it can give a woman her life back. Studies show an inverse relationship between estrogen replacement therapy and the incidence of Alzheimer's disease.[25] For a menopausal woman showing obvious signs of brain decline, it is a critical area to consider.

That said, estrogen replacement therapy is often not enough when this inflammatory cascade rushes through the body like a river of lava. A woman must also address the inflammation. Diet is, of course, critical. Regulating carbohydrate intake so you don't feel sleepy or crave sugar after a meal is important, as is doing an elimination/provocation diet to remove foods from your diet that create an inflammatory response.

Gluten is pro-inflammatory for most people, and many others have problems with dairy, corn, eggs, soy, or even grains in general. I've had good success clinically with a monosaccharide diet, akin to dairy-free versions of the Gut and Psychology Syndrome (GAPS) diet, the Specific Carbohydrate Diet (SCD), or the Cedars-Sinai diet. These diets are essentially free of all grains, starchy vegetables (such as potatoes, turnips, and jicama), all sweeteners except honey, and most forms of dairy.

I urge you to research these diets, as there is much more to it. Not only are they great low-carb diets, they also eliminate most of the common allergens and are very anti-inflammatory and restorative to the gut.

Other dietary strategies include avoiding processed fats, such as vegetable oils and hydrogenated oils, and focusing on ample amounts of clean, healthy fats from organic, pastured animal foods, wild seafood, and nuts and seeds. This book is not really a diet book, as I feel there are already plenty of great resources out there to help you as long as you follow certain guidelines. I leave it to the reader to find the diet that suits him or her best.

Nutritional strategies to modulate inflammation include nutrients to dampen microglia activation, nutrients to oxygenate the brain, and nutrients to mitigate brain degeneration, as we have discussed in previous chapters.

THE ADRENAL GLANDS AND PERIMENOPAUSE

Theoretically, the adrenal glands take over hormone production in menopause once the ovaries begin to fail, but because they are often in poor shape these days by the time a woman hits menopause, they are not up to the task. Supporting the stress response system is an integral component of managing perimenopausal and menopausal inflammation.

As I mentioned in Chapter Five, it's not necessarily the adrenal glands that need support, but instead the stress pathways in the brain. The

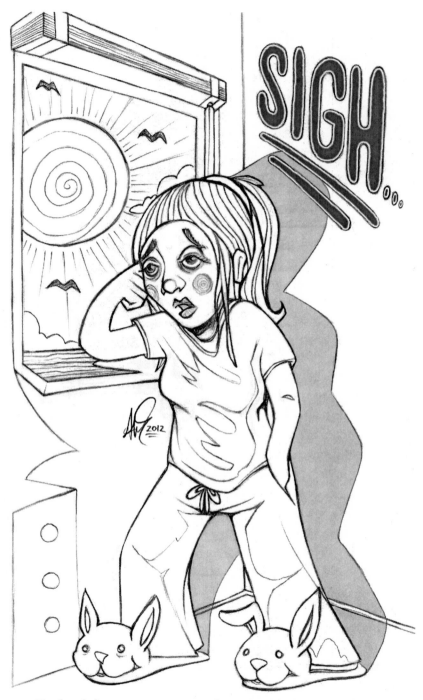

The female brain requires estrogen for serotonin activity. An estrogen imbalance can cause depression, poor sleep, and unprovoked anger.

hippocampus is where adrenal issues manifest in the way of an altered sleep-wake cycle (feeling too tired in the morning and too awake at bedtime, for instance) and impairment of short-term memory and learning. Certain nutritional compounds have been shown to be highly effective in restoring function to these areas and slowing hippocampal destruction.

PERIMENOPAUSE, MENOPAUSE, AND NEUROTRANSMITTER FUNCTION

So far I have talked about three ways to tame the inflammatory firestorm that accompanies an estrogen deficiency in perimenopause and menopause: correcting the estrogen deficiency through appropriate testing and bioidentical hormone replacement therapy, taming the inflammation, and managing the stress pathways.

As you may have guessed by now, when a woman is grappling with these multiple factors, her neurotransmitter function falters. She may have noticed her personality has changed, or depression has set in since perimenopause began. Granted, simply addressing a serotonin or dopamine deficiency alone would not be adequate for a woman in this position. But it can still be a necessary part of the puzzle, especially when it comes to providing symptom relief. It's important that a woman going through the steps to manage her estrogen deficiency keep her neurotransmitter function humming along as smoothly as possible.

Because the inflammation cascade will make it difficult to balance blood sugar, a perimenopausal woman is more likely to struggle with hypoglycemia or insulin resistance, even if she has corrected her diet. These blood sugar imbalances will disrupt the transport of precursors across the blood-brain barrier to make neurotransmitters.

Also, estrogen is very important for serotonin activity in the brain and an estrogen deficiency may compromise serotonin function. In this case symptoms may include depression, depression when there is lack of sunlight, loss of enthusiasm for favorite foods or activities, an inability to sleep well, unprovoked anger, or increased susceptibility to pain. If these symptoms are predominant, nutritional compounds to support serotonin activity can be extremely beneficial.

Although serotonin is the most likely to be hit, all the neurotransmitters can be affected by the ongoing inflammation of an estrogen deficiency. Poor dopamine activity can also be a predominant factor, with such symptoms as feelings of worthlessness or hopelessness, anger under stress, being easily distracted, short temper, and an inability to handle stress. This is the woman who snaps over little irritations, like getting the wrong order in a restaurant. In this case dopamine support may be warranted.

Anxiety is a common side effect of estrogen deficiency, and the blood sugar swings and chronic stress that accompany estrogen deficiency could compromise GABA function. Symptoms include feeling anxious or panicky for no reason, feelings of dread, feeling overwhelmed for no reason, guilt about decisions, disorganized attention, a restless mind, and worrying about things you had never thought of before. In this case GABA support can be helpful.

* *

Todd, 47, suffered from depression, unexplained episodes of sadness, chronic insomnia, and significant deterioration of his mental and cognitive abilities. He owned his own construction company but had to step down from running the business due to his poor brain function. He had spent his entire adult life under constant deadline pressure and managing the many problems that typically happen during construction and development. He tried to work out several times a week and eat well but had not been consistent with any regimen.

Todd had also completely lost his libido and his passion for life. He had consulted with many physicians and was prescribed various medications over the years, but he refused to take any medications unless faced with a life-threatening issue. A friend referred Todd to an anti-aging hormone clinic where he was diagnosed with low testosterone and placed on a testosterone cream. Within the first couple of weeks he experienced a huge spike in energy, major improvements in brain function, and overall improvement of physical and mental endurance. However, the testosterone therapy stopped working within a couple of weeks and he was back to how he originally felt.

He also now had more emotional ups and down than ever before and symptoms of prostate enlargement, including dribbling urine flow and frequent urination. His PSA was normal, and his urologist diagnosed him with benign prostate hypertrophy (enlargement) and told him to stop taking the testosterone cream, as it may be promoting the prostate hypertrophy.

When I evaluated Todd's previous lab work it was clear he did not receive comprehensive hormone testing. In addition to measuring his testosterone I also checked the other major hormones. His results showed his estrogen was five times greater than normal. Todd was aromatizing his testosterone. In other words, he was abnormally converting testosterone into estrogen through the aromatase enzyme. This explained why he did not do well with testosterone cream.

This situation is common in men today because insulin surges, a diet high in carbohydrates, and systemic inflammation promote the conversion of testosterone to estrogen in men (and estrogen to testosterone in women).

I immediately put Todd on the antioxidant resveratrol, which has been shown not only to dampen inflammation but also to suppress the aromatase enzyme. I also placed Todd on a sugar-free and anti-inflammatory diet. He was allowed to eat only vegetables, fruits, and meats and not allowed to eat any processed foods. He also took numerous anti-inflammatory supplements, including turmeric, green tea extract, and acai.

Todd lost about 20 pounds in two weeks and his hormone levels corrected themselves in that short period of time. His testosterone levels normalized, and his estrogen went down. He saw dramatic changes in his brain function and endurance as well as major changes in his overall energy.

Datis Kharrazian, DHSc, DC, MS

● ●

PAY SPECIAL ATTENTION TO ACETYLCHOLINE DURING PERIMENOPAUSE

Of special concern is acetylcholine activity. I look at this area like a hawk with my women patients who are in perimenopause or menopause. Symptoms of poor acetylcholine activity signal destruction in the hippocampus. Because of the inflammation accelerating brain degeneration, this is an area to which women in this predicament must pay close attention.

Symptoms include declining memory, difficulty learning, diminished comprehension, slower mental response, difficulty calculating numbers, difficulty recognizing objects and faces, constantly forgetting where you left things, and excessive urination. Also, circadian rhythm problems are another symptom—having trouble falling asleep, feeling too tired in the morning, or crashing around 4 or 5 p.m. These indicate an imbalanced sleep-wake cycle and hence poor hippocampus function.

First, it's important to eat sufficient foods that are rich in healthy fats, such as the fats from organic, pastured animals (eggs, butter, and meats), as well as other natural fats such as olive oil, coconut oil, nuts and seeds, and other unprocessed oils. These fats will supply the brain and body with the nutrients it needs to manufacture cells and hormones.

BONES, FAT, AND MENOPAUSE

The inflammatory process of an estrogen deficiency affects areas other than the brain. People don't think of osteoporosis as an inflammatory condition, but in fact it is. Studies show the cytokine surges associated with estrogen deficiency promote the breakdown of bone.

Studies also show even a small increase in belly fat during perimenopause can have a large impact on inflammatory cytokines. In estrogen-deficient menopausal women, estrogen replacement reduced this effect.

PROGESTERONE AND THE BRAIN

Although it's known as a female hormone, progesterone has a major influence on GABA receptor sites in both the male and female brain.[26][27][28] In the female brain it also exerts a profound influence on dopamine receptor sites and a progesterone deficiency in women can result in compromised GABA and dopamine activity.[29][30]

Progesterone has also been shown in studies to be a powerful modulator of the brain's microglia cells.[31][32][33] When an antigen or an injury activates these cells, they don't have a built-in off switch like the body's immune system does. Instead, the microglia cells rely on the dampening effects of other compounds, such as progesterone. In fact, progesterone's ability to dampen microglia activity is so profound research shows administering progesterone to a man or woman who has just suffered from a head injury or stroke helps with the repair process in the brain and remyelination of nerves (myelin is a protective nerve coating).[34] [35]

When a patient comes to me with a brain degeneration process, or with a recent history of a stroke or a head trauma, I always look at progesterone levels. If the trauma to the brain was recent I immediately supplement with progesterone due to its proven anti-inflammatory properties.

Again, this is not a license to go out and get on progesterone replacement therapy. A large part of my practice is devoted to "unwinding" the victims of such therapy, who have suffered considerable damage through the inappropriate and poorly monitored use of such hormones, even bioidentical ones. As an example, one study showed too much progesterone led to the decoupling of communication between the brain's hemispheres.[36]

That being said, progesterone can be highly therapeutic in certain instances. Studies on animals demonstrate the anti-inflammatory effects of progesterone on the brain. A 2004 study published in *Brain Research* showed rats with a prefrontal cortex injury treated with progesterone had significantly less swelling and accumulation of microglia cells, demonstrating a neuroprotective effect compared to those that did not receive progesterone.[37]

Another paper in the 2007 *Annals of Emergency Medicine* defined the use of progesterone for traumatic brain injuries in humans. In a randomized clinical trial, some subjects were given progesterone for three days after an acute traumatic brain injury and some were given a placebo. Of the group given progesterone, 13 percent died within 30 days after the injury, compared to 30 percent of the placebo group. This equates to a survival rate almost three times higher for individuals given progesterone immediately after a head trauma. The study showed the progesterone group also had better functional outcomes after 30 days compared to the placebo group.[38]

Studies like these demonstrate the health of your brain can determine how bad a head injury is, not necessarily the injury itself. One of the first things doctors look at when a person comes in with a head trauma or a stroke is how bad the damage is. They look at an MRI, or ask how hard the person's head was hit, but most likely they don't ask about a person's hormonal status or general brain health prior to the injury.

A very mild head injury can be devastating to someone whose brain health was fragile to start with. I have seen this myself when a friend of mine, a young woman with an autoimmune phospholipid disorder and existing brain inflammation, knocked her head while exiting an airport shuttle. It sent her health spiraling out of control, even though the injury itself was quite mild. For a person who is already hormonally imbalanced and whose brain microglia cells are already in a pro-inflammatory cascade, even the smallest trauma or stroke can have severe consequences neurologically.

TESTOSTERONE AND THE BRAIN

The frontal lobe of a man's brain is saturated with receptor sites for testosterone.[39] Low testosterone is a common problem these days, and it's clearly sabotaging the male brain. Symptoms include loss of cognitive function, memory problems, and the progression of dementia in Alzheimer's disease. Less advanced symptoms include depression, lack of drive or motivation, and general "grumpiness."[40 41 42]

Because testosterone influences dopamine activity, testosterone deficiency can increase the risk of Parkinson's disease in a man.[43] Testosterone also influences the activity of acetylcholine, our learning and memory neurotransmitter, and a deficiency can affect those areas as well, increasing the risk of dementia and Alzheimer's disease.[44] Research shows low testosterone increases the secretion of beta amyloid protein, a compound that "strangles" neurons, raising the risk of Alzheimer's disease.[45]

Sufficient testosterone has shown regenerative properties in the brain. A 2004 study published in the *Journal of Neuroscience Research* showed that of castrated rats with an injured sciatic nerve, those given testosterone had a 13 percent higher rate of regeneration in the first 11 days compared to the control group.[46]

I apologize but it's worth repeating, this is not a license to go out and get on testosterone replacement therapy. Testosterone creams—all hormone creams—can lead to excess levels, shut down receptor sites for that hormone, kill the communication loop between the hormone glands and the brain, and gravely disrupt other metabolic processes in the body and the brain. It is more important to look at *why* a hormone is deficient instead of just slapping on a hormone cream in what amounts to a risky form of Band-Aid therapy.

Unfortunately, addressing hormonal imbalances specifically is beyond the scope of this book, but I will mention some important concepts related to testosterone levels and men. Researchers have investigated the mechanisms of why men lose their testosterone levels, which is known medically as andropause. They discovered cells in the testis that produce testosterone, called leydig cells, are very susceptible to inflammation.[47][48] Basically, during states of chronic inflammation the leydig cells do not regenerate. They lose receptor site communication and the ability to produce testosterone. It appears andropause, identified as a pattern of low total testosterone and elevated LH, may be secondary to chronic systemic inflammation.

Besides systemic inflammation, I can tell you that when a patient walks into my clinic with a hormonal imbalance, it is most often the result of a blood sugar imbalance—hypoglycemia, insulin resistance, or diabetes. Insulin surges are like the domino at the front of a long line of metabolic dominos standing on end. Knock over that insulin domino and all the others come toppling down behind it. However, properly managing hormonal imbalances often requires a variety of lab panels and proper interpretation by a qualified health care practitioner beyond general suggestions that can be made in this book alone.

The most important concept to take away from this chapter is that if your brain is not working and you are suffering from hormone issues, there is an important connection between them.

● ●

Alma, 45, was diagnosed with hypothyroidism 10 years ago. Her doctor prescribed her a synthetic thyroid hormone that brought her lab range into normal, yet as the years wore on she felt increasingly worse. When her mom died four years ago, this sent her into a tailspin of depression and weight gain and acid reflux so bad she never went without her over-the-counter (OTC) anti-acid medication, which she took in abundance. She also suffered from headaches, migraines, digestive issues, fatigue and lethargy, and increasing irritability.

To make it through her days as a flight attendant, she kept herself going with caffeinated tea all day long and the "energy shots" so popular now. Although they kept her awake enough to get through her work day, they also gave her migraines, for which she regularly took a popular OTC migraine product. On her days off, her family knew not to call or stop by as she needed to spend all night and all day in bed sleeping to try and restore what little energy she had left. Her memory was noticeably slipping, and she found it increasingly difficult to concentrate.

On one flight she spied some nutritional supplements peeking out of my bag and started asking me questions. I am a practitioner trained in Dr. Kharrazian's protocols, and a month later Alma came to see me as a patient.

"She was the first doctor who did a blood test to measure something other than just one thyroid marker, TSH, and she discovered I have Hashimoto's, an autoimmune thyroid disease," said Alma. "When I started getting worse, my doctor wanted to put me on antidepressants, and I had been on birth control pills for 30 years for menstrual cramps, which I never should have been."

I told Alma to immediately remove gluten from her diet, as ample evidence shows a strong link between gluten intolerance, Hashimoto's, and neurological issues. Alma cried for two days at this news—this meant tossing the comfort foods that had solaced her after mother's death and through her worsening health. She also realized the OTC antacid medication she had been popping during the day and before bed every night to manage the extreme acid reflux she dealt with had gluten in it. The number of supplements she would be taking every day also dismayed her, although I assured her that would taper off over time.

Despite the initial shock, she followed my advice and was amazed to find she felt significantly better within three days of going on a gluten-free diet and taking the nutritional compounds, which included serotonin and dopamine support. "Dr. Labbe told me I would feel like a million bucks, and I was like, 'Yeah, right,'" says Alma. "She was right!"

Alma quickly lost seven pounds, her high blood pressure returned to normal, and her acid reflux and digestive issues disappeared. Best of all, however, was the return of her energy and saying goodbye to headaches and migraines. If she accidentally eats gluten, she now suffers severe diarrhea and stomach cramps, putting no doubt in her mind that she needs to avoid it.

"I have picked up a lot of overtime, and at the end of a 10-hour work day my coworkers are all exhausted, but I'm like the Energizer Bunny, ready to keep going," says Alma. "I don't need as much sleep and can get a lot done now. My memory is better—I don't feel myself grasping for words, and emotionally I'm back to my laid-back self. Recently my garage door broke, my phone broke, and I got locked out of the house all on the same day. Before I would have cried and been upset, but I can deal with things better now."

A month into her protocol and new diet, Alma says she feels like everything in life is falling into place, now that she's out from under the black cloud of depression and fatigue. She also learned she needed to lower her thyroid medication. "After 10 years of being on the same dose of thyroid medication, I needed to lower it after just one month of working with Dr. Labbe," says Alma. "Going gluten-free is a drastic diet, but I was very shocked how quickly I started to feel better."

Joni Labbe, DC, CCN, DCCN
San Diego, California
www.brain-dr.com

• •

HYPOTHYROIDISM AND THE BRAIN

Perhaps you have read or at least heard of my first book, *Why Do I Still Have Thyroid Symptoms When My Lab Tests Are Normal?* The thyroid's effect on the brain is profound and many people with hypothyroidism may find they also need brain support. Thyroid function affects brain inflammation, plasticity, neurotransmitter activity, and general brain function. The most common symptoms among those with low thyroid function are depression, fatigue, and brain fog.

Thyroid hormones play a vital role in dampening brain inflammation. They have a direct effect on microglia cells, the brain's immune cells that go into overdrive when presented with an infectious agent.

In fact, an unmanaged thyroid condition may accelerate brain degeneration, which is why it is so important to appropriately manage hypothyroidism and Hashimoto's, an autoimmune thyroid condition. And by manage I don't mean just taking thyroid hormone medication, although that is often necessary. Simply taking thyroid hormones does nothing to address a deteriorating thyroid condition caused by Hashimoto's, which is responsible for 90 percent of hypothyroid cases in the United States. Nor does it address other causes for the failure of thyroid function, such as chronic stress, high testosterone in women, or environmental toxicity.

Thyroid function is linked with all of the neurotransmitters. Good synapses for serotonin, dopamine, GABA, and acetylcholine all depend on healthy thyroid function. In fact, many of the neurological symptoms that accompany an unmanaged thyroid condition, such as depression or loss of memory, can be traced back to a breakdown in the neurotransmitter-thyroid connection.

Another cause of concern is that the autoimmune attacks that drive Hashimoto's increase the risk of autoimmune attacks in the brain. I frequently see evidence of autoimmune cerebellum attacks in my Hashimoto's patients. When a patient with Hashimoto's also presents with neurological symptoms, especially pertaining to balance, dizziness, or nausea, I always screen for an autoimmunity in the brain.

Hashimoto's encephalopathy (HE) is perhaps a worst-case scenario for people with Hashimoto's. Also known as autoimmune dementia, HE is an autoimmune inflammatory brain disorder that causes memory loss and other dementia-like symptoms. The same immune antibodies that destroy thyroid tissue, thyroid peroxidase (TPO) antibodies, also cause HE.

HE is suspected when an individual presents with both high TPO antibodies and symptoms of dementia or other neurological disorders, such as memory loss, decreased cognitive ability, tremors, seizures, impaired speech, confusion, partial paralysis, fine motor problems, poor coordination, and more. However, because 20 percent of the older population, especially women, may have TPO antibodies, and because myriad other factors can cause neurological symptoms, a practitioner should exercise caution in diagnosing HE.

A MISMANAGED THYROID CONDITION IS A MISMANAGED BRAIN CONDITION

When I learned the many connections between thyroid function and brain function, the gross mismanagement of hypothyroidism in the standard health care model seemed even more tragic. When patients are told to wait until their thyroid burns out, to treat their thyroid symptoms with antidepressants or beta-blockers, or that it all must be in their heads because their TSH (thyroid-stimulating hormone) levels are normal, the health care model is contributing the deteriorating brain health of millions of Americans.

Otherwise bright, motivated people struggle to accomplish the bare minimum each day, are filled with remorse because they can barely meet their children's needs, or burn through their life savings in search of a doctor who can help them. Some have given up and resigned themselves to a rapid decline in health while being kept afloat by disability and welfare. Others watch in despair as their children's mental development fails to keep up with their peers' because of a hypothyroid condition. Many succumb to the development of more autoimmune diseases because the underlying immune condition is not addressed.

As explained in my thyroid book, the underlying cause of poor thyroid function should always be addressed to prevent further decline in brain health.

CHAPTER SUMMARY

• Hormones significantly impact brain health. PMS, perimenopause, menopause, and high estrogen in women and low testosterone in men can compromise brain health and function.

• When hormones become imbalanced you lose neurotransmitter activity, which affects how you feel, function, and view your life. Hormonal imbalances also significantly impact brain inflammation and degeneration and considerably speed aging of the brain.

• Hormonal imbalances impact neurotransmitter activity in the following ways:
  • Estrogen impacts serotonin receptors in men and women
  • Progesterone impacts GABA receptors in men and women
  • Estrogen impacts dopamine receptors in women
  • Testosterone impacts dopamine receptors in men
  • Estrogen impacts acetylcholine receptors in women
  • Testosterone impacts acetylcholine receptors in men

- Thyroid hormones impact all neurotransmitter receptors in men and women

- Healthy hormone levels have been shown to facilitate neuron branching and plasticity, dampen brain inflammation, slow degeneration, and play a role in neuronal migration, the movement of neurons from one place to another to participate in activity and repair.

- All hormone production depends on adequate cholesterol.

- Hormone synthesis also requires DHEA. The majority of DHEA released into the body comes from the adrenal glands and many people suffer from low DHEA due to chronic stress. Supplementing with DHEA is only recommended for a short period of time and when lab testing shows chronic adrenal fatigue. Unnecessarily supplementing with DHEA can exacerbate the conversion of testosterone to estrogen in men and the production of testosterone in women.

- Pregnenolone is another substance necessary to make hormones. In pregnenolone steal, the body "steals" pregnenolone from cholesterol to make more cortisol as the adrenals fatigue, causing hormonal imbalances. This mechanism is a common underlying cause of PMS, infertility, male menopause, and PCOS.

- Studies have shown estrogen to be very protective of the brain. For postmenopausal women or perimenopausal women with chronically low estrogen, estrogen replacement therapy can be very protective of the brain. The need should first be determined with a clinical workup and appropriate testing, and the patient should be monitored regularly to ensure levels don't climb too high.

- Estrogen is linked to verbal and spatial memory, fine motor skills, and depressive illnesses. If estrogen declines too steeply or rapidly, one of the first things to pop up is depression and loss of some cognitive function, such as spatial memory, and fine motor skills. If the estrogen deficiency goes on long enough it could result in permanent degeneration to these areas of the brain and their related functions.

• Estrogen also helps neurons grow new dendritic spines so each neuron has a higher density of activity, which maintains plasticity. Estrogens also have a powerful dampening effect on microglia cells, the brain's immune cells, and sufficient estrogen helps prevent brain inflammation and degeneration.

• For the menopausal woman whose estrogen is too low, estrogen replacement therapy could be vital for brain health.

• Progesterone has a major influence on GABA receptor sites in both the male and female brain. In the female brain it also exerts a profound influence on dopamine receptor sites and a progesterone deficiency in women can result in compromised GABA and dopamine activity.

• Progesterone has been shown in studies to be a powerful modulator of the brain's microglia cells. Research shows administering progesterone to a man or woman who has just suffered from a head injury or stroke helps with the repair process in the brain and remyelination of nerves (myelin is a protective nerve coating).

• Because testosterone influences dopamine activity in men, testosterone deficiency can increase the risk of Parkinson's disease. Testosterone also influences the activity of acetylcholine and a deficiency can increase the risk of dementia and Alzheimer's disease.

• Thyroid hormones play a vital role in dampening brain inflammation and an unmanaged thyroid condition may accelerate brain degeneration. This is why it is so important to appropriately manage hypothyroidism and Hashimoto's, an autoimmune thyroid condition.

CHAPTER EIGHTEEN

ALTERNATIVE THERAPIES, BRAIN STIMULATION, AND BRAIN FUNCTION

• •

Joanne came into my office suffering from a multiple chemical sensitivity (MCS). MCS is a condition in which people react to chemicals. Before she came to see me she requested I not wear aftershave, cologne, or deodorant because the smells would give her a migraine, and she would not be able to get through an examination and history. She also asked to make sure there were no strong smells in my office that would make her sick.

When she came into my office she wore a filter mask. She told me when she travels she must wear the mask to avoid getting sick from the chemicals around her. What was interesting about Joanne's case is that her symptoms began after a car accident in which she suffered a concussion six years ago. The symptoms kicked in as soon as she left the hospital.

Most people with MCS usually develop it after an exposure to toxic chemicals and pollutants. The toxic exposure dysregulates their immune system and they lose what is called "chemical tolerance." In these cases, chemical exposures cause skin outbreaks, asthma, migraines, and other immune reactions.

Joanne's case, however, was different, as chemical exposures caused her excess tearing in her eyes, excess saliva production, visual auras, and excessive bowel movements. In other words, Joanne's reactions happened in her autonomic nervous system, not her immune system. Also, because the onset of MCS came after

her brain injury it was apparent Joanne's symptoms were neurological and not immunological.

When I examined Joanne I could see her pupils were dilating and
constricting abnormally in a lit room without stimulation from
a pen light. When I used a pen light to check her pupil responses
she started tearing and developed symptoms of nausea. When
I checked her resting pulse rate with an electronic pulse oximeter
it shifted from 72 to 110 beats per minute while she rested in a
seated position.

Numerous other findings indicated the car accident may have
damaged her brainstem's autonomic centers and that she was suffering from "autonomic dystonia," or dysfunction of the autonomic
nervous system. Unfortunately, there is no conventional treatment
for this.

Although neurons can be damaged it is still possible to stimulate and activate them so they branch into each other to develop
greater function. This is the basic concept of brain rehabilitation.
For example, after a person has a stroke he or she may be able
to rehabilitate the brain and regain function despite injury to the
neurons.

In Joanne's case we needed to support activity in her brainstem
but at a degree that did not cause her to crash. The examination
showed scent and light stimulation made her fall apart because
those neurons were not healthy. When neurons are not healthy
they do not have much endurance or stability. Over-stimulating
them causes them to fire inappropriately and creates such symptoms as increased heart rate, tearing, dizziness, fatigue, and other
autonomic reactions.

I initially placed Joanne on a nutritional program to support
her brain endurance using various mechanisms presented in this
book. Once her brain was chemically supported I began rehabilitating the integrity of her brainstem activity with some vestibular
(balance and spatial orientation) exercises, such as rocking in a
chair slowly and turning in a swivel chair. If she did them too fast
she became sick, so she worked slowly at her own pace.

As her neurons became healthier she could do the exercises
more aggressively. I also had her buy a box of essential oils and
slowly introduce scents she could barely tolerate by holding them
at arm's length. As time went on she would bring the scents in

closer and closer until she could bring them under her nose without getting symptoms.

Over the next few months Joanne was able to go outside without wearing her filter mask and could tolerate scents such as perfumes and gasoline fumes. Although she never made a full recovery, she improved significantly and completely changed her life around by learning how to stimulate her brain at an appropriate intensity to bring back its function.

I share Joanne's case with you because it illustrates how important stimulation to the brain is. Supplements and vitamins are no substitute for activating brain receptors. Brain injury causes loss of function specific to pathways that conduct those functions and the brain has phenomenal potential to change if it is chemically healthy and stimulated properly.

Unfortunately, the current model of neurology does very little to optimize brain health or provide therapy to rebuild compromised pathways. Neurologists are very good at diagnosing the condition but very poor at providing applications to regain health and function of the brain. As a matter of fact, among medical specialties, psychiatry and neurology have the poorest outcomes.

If your brain is injured and you have lost function such as coordination or the ability to do basic math, you can rehabilitate your own brain by finding ways to activate the pathways you have lost. Start with easy tasks and slowly build back up your neuron connections and function.

Brain rehabilitation can be simplified by saying "whatever you can't do is your rehabilitation program." Rehabilitating the brain is like building a muscle. You start with a weight you can handle and as time goes on you increase the weight. When you rehabilitate your brain, start very slowly with functions that are difficult but do not cause you to crash, and work your way up.

In addition to finding ways to stimulate your own brain, recent research now suggests a variety of therapies that have always been used in alternative healthcare may work because they activate the brain by stimulating various receptors.

Datis Kharrazian, DHSc, DC, MS

Music, yoga, massage, acupuncture, chiropractic spinal manipulation, and other therapies all stimulate the brain. When somebody treats you with a therapy such as aromatherapy or massage, they are stimulating receptors, such as joint receptors, muscle spindle receptors, smell receptors, or sound receptors. These receptors impact the brain and affect how you feel, your muscle tone, your digestive system, and more.

If you have ever had a massage or acupuncture, practiced yoga, listened to music, or meditated, chances are you experienced a positive effect on mood, muscle tone, pain tolerance, digestion, or your overall sense of well-being. Why is that exactly? Recent discoveries in neuroscience have allowed us to gain better insight into how different alternative healing modalities affect brain function, and thus overall health.

For instance, a 2005 article in the *Journal of Neuroscience* showed women with breast cancer who received massage therapy regularly experienced an increase in dopamine, our pleasure-and-reward brain chemical, as well as an increase in immune health.[1] They reported being less depressed and angry and having more vigor than the group who did not receive massages. We know massage stimulates muscles and their nerve receptors, which in turn impacts the brain's pathways that activate dopamine release. It is the dopamine release that makes you feel good and relaxed after a massage. Dopamine responses may also dampen stress responses in the brain, which can improve immune function.

Research using functional MRIs shows treating an area of the body with acupuncture creates a massive delivery of blood to the corresponding parts of the brain. This stimulates the production of serotonin, which is used in certain pathways to dampen pain. This explains acupuncture's successful track record in pain management.[2]

Treatments known to affect brain outcome include massage, acupuncture, spinal manipulation, hydrotherapy, aromatherapy, biofeedback, sound therapy, and yoga. All of these therapies work on the brain by acting on the nervous system. Both practitioners and patients have seen improvements in immune strength, mood, energy, digestion, hormone regulation, and more through the use of these therapies.[3 4 5 6 7 8 9 10 11 12 13 14 15 16 17 18 19 20]

"Chi," "energy," "chakras," "kundalini," and other terms are used in attempts to explain improvement in these areas, but neuroscience research has provided much evidence for a physiological explanation.

These therapies basically activate nervous system receptors, which increases brain firing and creates specific neurochemical changes.

For instance, if a woman's olfactory (smell) areas of the brain are not activating, she may respond profoundly to aromatherapy because it delivers more stimulation to that part of her brain. This increased activity in the olfactory areas in turn creates a neurochemical response that stimulates the rest of her brain. Her muscle tone improves and she feels lighter. Her autonomic functions such as digestion also improve, and she may feel happier and more energetic. She is so enthusiastic about how life-changing aromatherapy is that she talks her boyfriend into a session. However, his olfactory areas work great, so he doesn't receive the same awe-inspiring results she did. Instead, he is irritated because he feels he wasted his money.

It is not about whether aromatherapy is effective, but whether any therapy will positively impact areas of the brain in one person versus another at that specific point in their life. An everyday example can be as simple as evaluating your own response to listening to music, another sensory-based therapy. There are times when listening to music can totally change your mood, focus, motivation, and concentration—meaning it has impacted the activation of your brain. Other times listening to music has absolutely no effect.

It is not the music itself that determines your response, but the pre-existing state of your brain. Music stimulates your auditory (sound) pathways, which can then create profound neurochemical changes in several areas of the brain with varied responses at different times of your life.

● ●

Lisset, 40, consulted with me for her neuropathy, which had been rapidly progressing during the past year. Most days she used a walker but some days she needed a wheelchair. She was diagnosed with a condition called chronic inflammatory demyelinating polyneuropathy (CIDP). She sought care from highly accredited medical neurologists at different well regarded medical centers.

The doctors placed Lisset on anti-inflammatory medications and an anti-epileptic seizure medication, and she worked with a team of physical therapists on a weekly basis. However, her condition continued to worsen.

She seemed to be suffering with multiple sclerosis (MS) yet she had no MS antibodies, no white spots on a brain MRI, and no positive results from a recent spinal tap.

After reviewing the information I received in Dr. Kharrazian's metabolic courses, I felt that the first place I needed to evaluate was her gut and we did food sensitivity testing, blood tests to review her immune system, a comprehensive blood test to review other important metabolic systems, an expanded female hormone analysis, and a salivary adrenal panel to review her circadian rhythm. While we waited for the test results I started her on a strict anti-inflammatory elimination diet.

After the first two weeks of her diet she came into my office walking normally. She had lost about 10 pounds and had more strength in her legs and feet. She actually had a normal gait (walking) pattern and told me she had no more pain in her hands and feet. The night before she could actually feel her husband massaging her feet with lotion after she took a shower. Her neuropathy pain was completely gone and the numbness was about 50–60 percent better.

Her test results came back and showed she had autoimmune Hashimoto's hypothyroidism, iron anemia, and hypoglycemia. She also had a TH-1 dominance and positive intestinal transglutaminase antibodies indicating celiac disease. Hormone fluctuations at certain times of the month explained her loss of libido and her adrenal panel showed adrenal fatigue. We followed specific supplementation protocols to stabilize her blood sugars, anemia, and immune system.

After six months of functional neurological rehabilitation and an anti-inflammatory diet, her life with her husband and child were back to normal. On two occasions she suffered flare-ups that lasted a few days each and were caused by eating foods on her "do-not-eat" list.

She is now empowered with knowledge of how she can eat and supplement to support her health and is glad she has her life back.

Lonnie Herman, DC
Plantation, Florida
www.browardpaincenter.com

Have you ever listened to music and it just didn't sound good, or you tried to read a book but it was hard to focus? Let's say, you then decided to exercise. You may have noticed after exercising that suddenly music sounds so much better. You can hear the different pitches and your perception of the song is much greater than it was before you exercised. You may also notice that it's much easier to focus while reading. You are listening to the same music and reading the same book, but the firing of your brain changed before and after you exercised.

Exercise profoundly impacts your brain. It increases circulation and blood flow to your brain and causes massive surges of brain neurotransmitter activity. Did you know there is more scientific evidence for the treatment of depression with exercise than with antidepressants? I always jokingly say patients with depression should have to walk or run to the drugstore to pick up their prescription because once there they may feel they no longer need it. The only problem is many people with chronic depression cannot imagine getting out of bed, much less exercising, since their brain is firing so poorly. They don't find my joke funny.

Many everyday things we do, such as exercising, playing sports or recreational games, smelling and eating food, listening to music, and watching movies are actually therapies that stimulate our brain, keeping it healthy and activated. However, poor diets, hormonal imbalances, autoimmunity, brain inflammation, environmental pollutants, and other factors degenerate and neurochemically alter the brain. As a result, daily activities that would normally stimulate the brain have less of an ability to keep our brains working as they should.

Sensory-based stimulations of all kinds are important if you feel your brain is not working. Easy things you can do are to exercise, play a musical instrument, listen to music, get back to your favorite hobbies, take a yoga class, and more. You may also find support through massage, acupuncture, aromatherapy, biofeedback therapy, spinal manipulation, or anything else you feel enhances your well-being. Whether it's alternative therapies or just an entertaining hobby, such basic activities can be extremely positive ways to stimulate the brain.

There is one brain-based response that is so significant that all research studies must account for it in a well-designed study: the placebo effect. It is well known the mind influences physiology, which in the world of science is known as psycho-neuroendocrine-immunology. The placebo effect is a brain-based mechanism that signifies a healthy brain. If you do not have a healthy brain you cannot develop a placebo effect. Imagine trying to achieve a placebo effect with a group of patients with dementia or progressed brain degenerative disorders. It doesn't happen!

We all know the mind is powerful, but we sometimes forget the mind is really an expression of brain function. A person's brain health affects the outcome of therapy. For instance, a young, healthy person who exercises daily, eats a healthy diet with natural, unprocessed fats, enjoys her job, and is in rewarding relationships is likely to have a very positive response to music, acupuncture, chiropractic care, or a massage, and find these to be worthwhile ways to support her health.

But what about the person who is 50 or more pounds overweight, rarely spends time with others, clicks on the television as soon as he gets home from work, snacks on junk foods made with hydrogenated fats, and stirs from the sofa only long enough to microwave a TV dinner? This person may complain his chiropractor is no good because the adjustments never hold, that acupuncture does nothing for him, or that a massage is a waste of money.

His brain may be so neurochemically challenged that although the therapies deliver receptor activation, his brain is not able to create a neurophysiological response significant enough to affect his health. Or he may be so degenerated and prone to being overwhelmed that one of these sensory stimulating treatments may fatigue his brain and make him feel worse. For example, people who cannot handle loud noises, flashes of light, strong scents, or other stimuli typically have progressed neurodegeneration. Their brain is so unstable they cannot handle any activation from sensory receptors.

Also interesting is the person who is hypoglycemic and becomes shaky, light headed, and irritable if she goes too long without eating. She may get a great response to acupuncture or chiropractic therapy one day and a terrible response the next. Why? If she arrives for therapy hungry and hypoglycemic, her brain is low in glucose and oxygen, both vital to healthy function. As a result she cannot respond well to therapy.

If a person's brain is healthy, sensory-based treatments work better—neurotransmitters are active enough to relay communication between neurons, and the brain is not plagued with inflammation or degenerating due to poor gut health or blood sugar swings. As a result, input from therapies such as yoga, music, aromatherapy, acupuncture, or chiropractic will have more impact on brain function and consequently mood, digestion, hormone health, and immunity.

● ●

It is always shocking to me when physical therapists or functional neurologists developing rehabilitation programs for patients who have suffered a head injury, stroke, or other brain insult spend no time improving the chemistry and nutritional status of their patient's brain. They do not realize any attempt to rehabilitate a chemically challenged brain will lead to poor outcomes. It is like trying to develop muscle-strengthening exercises for a client who is dehydrated and depleted in muscle glycogen and energy. Not only will the exercise not help, but they may actually hurt the patient.

Another story that illustrates the importance of pre-existing brain chemistry health is an example of two Ph.D. students who enter the same graduate program at the same time and are the same age. One of the students eats a healthy diet that includes healthy fats. The other student is very fat-phobic—egg-white omelets are a regular breakfast, and she scrupulously avoids fats in every bite, unaware that fatty meats, egg yolks, cream, and nuts, are rich in choline.

Choline is a precursor of acetylcholine, the learning-and-memory neurotransmitter important for conversion of short-term memories to long-term memories. This is what allows us to learn new things. Dietary choline from fats is crucial for peak brain acetylcholine production. Acetylcholine has been shown effective in enhancing memory and cognition and photographic and verbal memory. It's common to see poor acetylcholine activity in people who are not eating any fats.

As the graduate program wears on, the fat-phobic student with poor acetylcholine production has to take notes over and over again and has trouble remembering what she has learned. Meanwhile her classmate whose acetylcholine activity is healthy has an easier time remembering and putting things together. The students' performances are not based on their IQ scores or their personality, but solely on the existing neurochemical makeup of

their brains. Acetylcholine sufficiency is essential for healthy memory and reducing your risk of dementia and Alzheimer's disease.
Datis Kharrazian, DHSc, DC, MS

• •

The take-away message is that you can maximize the potential of any brain-stimulating therapy, whether acupuncture or chiropractic, yoga, quilting, or playing your favorite sport, by attending to the overall health and wellness of your brain.

CHAPTER SUMMARY

• Music, yoga, massage, acupuncture, chiropractic spinal manipulation, and other therapies all stimulate receptors, such as joint receptors, muscle spindle receptors, smell receptors, or sound receptors. These receptors impact the brain and affect how you feel, your muscle tone, your digestive system, and more.

• It is not about whether a particular therapy is effective, but whether any therapy will positively impact areas of the brain in one person versus another at that specific point in their life.

• Sensory-based stimulations of all kinds are important if you feel your brain is not working. Easy things you can do are to exercise, play a musical instrument, listen to music, get back to your favorite hobbies, take a yoga class, and more. You may also find support through massage, acupuncture, aromatherapy, biofeedback therapy, spinal manipulation, or anything else you feel enhances your well-being. Whether it's alternative therapies or just an entertaining hobby, such basic activities can be extremely positive ways to stimulate the brain.

• One brain-based response is so significant that all research studies must account for it in a well-designed study: the placebo effect. The placebo effect is a brain-based mechanism that signifies a healthy brain. If you do not have a healthy brain you cannot develop a placebo effect. Imagine trying to achieve a placebo effect with a group of patients with dementia or progressed brain degenerative disorders. It doesn't happen.

• A person with a healthy brain is likely to have a very positive response to therapy compared to someone who is unhealthy—neurotransmitters are active and the brain is not plagued with inflammation or degenerating due to poor gut health or blood sugar swings. As a result, input from various therapies will have more impact on brain function and consequently mood, digestion, hormone health, and immunity.

CHAPTER NINETEEN
ESSENTIAL FATTY ACIDS

SYMPTOMS AND SIGNS ASSOCIATED WITH ESSENTIAL FATTY ACID DEFICIENCY

- Poor brain function
- Limited consumption of fatty fish, raw nuts and seeds, uncooked olive oil, or avocados
- Regular consumption of fried foods
- Painful joints; chronic pain and inflammation
- Regular consumption of processed foods with partially hydrogenated fats
- Dry or unhealthy skin
- Dandruff
- Hormone imbalances

• •

Allison, 37, was suffering from chronic depression. She had no desire or passion for life and could barely motivate herself to get out of bed every morning. She had tried various antidepressants but none of them helped her; instead they made her feel strange.

She described her depression as feeling like her brain was a cloudy day with no sunshine. In addition to chronic depression she also suffered from poor memory, hair loss, painful menstrual cramps, and severely dry and flaky skin. She had tried various hair products and skin lotions but nothing seemed to work. Her pre-

menstrual cramps were so severe she had to stay home from work and load up on over-the-counter painkillers. She suspected she might have a nutritional deficiency and took a daily vitamin and mineral product, but it did not help.

Her dietary history was quite revealing. She had a busy work schedule and ate fast foods for lunch and most dinners during the week. Allison loved French fries, chips, and anything salty and fried, and her diet was high in processed vegetable oils and fried foods. She also ate red meat and lots of cheese regularly. Like most Americans, Allison rarely ate fresh fish and did not eat nuts unless they were flavored or coated with chocolate. She found the taste of raw nuts too boring.

Allison was not getting any omega-3 oils in her diet. Omega-3 oils are called "essential fatty acids" (EFAs) because the body requires them from the diet for proper function. Many of Allison's chief complaints, including her poor brain function and chronic depression, stemmed from a lack of omega-3 fats, even though she was taking a vitamin and mineral supplement.

The EFAs found in raw seeds, nuts, and cold-water fish cannot be manufactured into a tablet or a powder-filled capsule. They must be consumed in the diet or supplemented with oil-filled capsules. Allison's multi-vitamin did not provide her with essential fatty acids.

Allison had various other issues associated with her health, but a change in her diet was necessary to impact her EFA issues. I placed Allison on a broad-spectrum essential fatty acid supplement as well as a product very high in DHA. DHA is the key ingredient in fish oils necessary for brain support. I also significantly restricted Allison's intake of fried foods and had her consume cold-water fishes, nuts, and seeds instead.

Within two months her menstrual cramps decreased by 80 percent, her hair and skin became healthier, and her symptoms of depression, memory, and general poor brain function improved dramatically. The dark, cloudy feeling in her brain dissipated, and she was able to finally lose weight. As she started to feel and look better she began to enjoy social events with others. A few simple dietary and lifestyle changes dramatically changed Allison's life for the better.

> *I share Allison's story with you because most American adults and children eat a diet high in processed vegetable oils and fried foods and low in EFAs. This diet can profoundly impact not only brain function and overall metabolism, but also how you look and feel. Despite the overconsumption of foods in the United States and the popularity of vitamins, many Americans are still deficient in ideal ratios of omega-3 EFAs.*
>
> *A diet insufficient in EFAs promotes neurodegenerative disease, cardiovascular disease, hormone imbalances, psychiatric disorders, chronic pain and inflammation, and impaired brain function.*[1]
>
> Datis Kharrazian, DHSc, DC, MS

Eating the appropriate fats is vital for good brain health. After all, 60 percent of the brain is made of fat and the fats you eat affect the composition of your brain. Fats found in processed foods, heated vegetable oil, processed vegetable oils, and hydrogenated fats can make the membranes of your nerve cells rigid and unresponsive, leading to improper neuron function, brain inflammation and degeneration, and symptoms of poor brain function.[2] But not all fats are bad. The fats found in certain foods are called "essential" because your body cannot synthesize them and they must be consumed in your diet. These fats are critical for healthy brain function.

If your brain is not working well you need to examine your dietary fat intake. Your diet must be high in the good fats that support your brain function and low in fats that impair brain function and promote brain decay. In order to improve your brain function you need to understand which fats are essential for your brain.

ESSENTIAL FATTY ACIDS BASICS
EFAs are critical for various functions of the body:
- Dampening inflammation
- Improving blood vessel health
- Supporting healthy skin growth
- Supporting healthy brain and nervous system function

The brain itself is made up of primarily fatty acids, or phospholipids (fats in their simplest form). EFAs are necessary for proper fluidity and flexibility of the neuron's membrane, which provides structure and a protective wall for the neuron. When the membrane's flexibility is healthy, it allows the appropriate fluids and nutrients to pass through the membrane and support the metabolic needs of the neuron.[3] It also communicates more effectively with other neurons through synapses.[4][5] Healthy communication between neurons in the brain means better brain function, mood, memory, and health.

If you eat high amounts of processed oils or partially hydrogenated fats found in boxed and bagged foods and at many restaurants, particularly fast food restaurants, the membranes of your neurons lose their fluidity and flexibility and become less efficient at their functions. If your brain is not working well, you need to evaluate your intake of fats.

UNDERSTANDING FATS IN YOUR DIET

Heat is the enemy of EFAs because it changes their structure so they are less nutritious. For example, olive oil that is not heated is more nutritionally supportive than heated olive oil used for cooking. Raw fish has more usable essential fatty acids than cooked fish, and foods such as fried fish sticks offer very little in the way of essential fatty acids. Nuts that are dry-roasted or treated with heat for flavoring end up losing their essential fatty acid levels.

Therefore, eating foods such as fish sticks, dry-roasted nuts, or foods fried in olive oil are not going to help your brain very much. You need to eat good-quality fresh fish that is not overcooked, use fresh olive oil on salads, and eat raw nuts and seeds to support your brain with proper essential fatty acids. Given how few essential fatty acids the average American eats, it is also a good idea to supplement with essential fatty acids such as fish oil to optimize brain health.

How much essential fatty acids should I eat?

It is really important to have a diet with the various forms of EFAs. The one Americans need to be the most cognizant of is omega-3 fatty acid, found in cold-water fish such as salmon, sardines, herring, mackerel, black cod, and bluefish. These sources contain the two most critical forms of omega-3 fatty acids, eicosapentaenoic acid (EPA) and docosahexaenoic acid (DHA). DHA is the fatty acid vital to brain function, taming brain inflammation, and preventing degeneration.

Vegetarian omega 3s contain alpha-linolenic acid (ALA), which the body may convert to EPA and DHA. Dietary sources include walnuts and flax seed. However, many people have trouble converting ALAs to beneficial forms of omega 3, particularly if insulin resistance is an issue. Eating a diet high in omega-6 fats may also hinder this conversion.

As you can see, the typical American diet does not contain many sources of omega-3 fatty acids, which explains why omega-3 deficiencies or imbalances are so rampant. On the other hand, foods high in omega-6 fatty acids are abundant. Although raw nuts and seeds have omega-6 fats, most people get them from processed vegetable oils used in packaged foods, such as chips, crackers, and other snack foods, as well as from fast foods.

Our hunter-gatherer ancestors ate about as many omega-6 fats as omega-3 for a one-to-one, or 1:1, ratio. Today the average American eats a ratio of as high as 25:1—way too many omega-6 fats compared to omega-3 fats. This is due largely to sunflower, cottonseed, soybean, sesame, and canola oils in processed foods.

This extreme imbalance between omega 6 and omega 3 creates a very inflammatory environment that plays a role in many chronic conditions, including heart disease, diabetes, autoimmune disease, and conditions that degenerate the brain. The way to prevent this inflammatory environment is to increase your consumption of omega-3 fats and lower consumption of omega-6. Researchers recommend a ratio of omega-6 to omega-3 that ranges from 1:1 to 4:1 for optimal health and prevention of disease.[6]

● ●

When animals are raised on grass they produce meat and eggs with a much higher concentration of omega 3 than animals confined and fed only grain or finished on grain. Eggs from pastured hens have an omega-3 content higher than factory-farmed eggs.[7] Grass-fed meat has two to four times more omega 3 than grain-fed meat. It is also higher in vitamins A and E, antioxidants, and conjugated linoleic acid, which has cancer fighting properties.[8]

One study showed subjects who ate grass-fed meats showed higher blood levels of omega 3 than those who ate grain-fed meats.[9] *Some cattle are raised on pasture but then finished on grain, which lowers the omega-3 profile, so it's important to look for pasture-finished meats. However, although grass-fed beef is a better option compared to grain-fed, don't be fooled into thinking it's a substitute for cold water fish. Salmon has 35 times more omega 3 than beef.*[10]

SUPPLEMENTS FOR ESSENTIAL FATTY ACIDS
How much fish oil should I take?

You can find a variety of EFA supplements, including flax seed oil, fish oil, olive oil, and evening primrose oil, but the oil that has the most impact on brain function is fish oil. How much fish oil you should take depends on your diet, but the dosage recommendations continue to increase with every new research paper published (probably because Americans continue to eat more poorly and become less healthy).

Most people do not have to worry about taking too much unless they are on blood thinners such as coumadin because fish oils thin your blood. In fact, the blood thinning effect is one of the mechanisms by which EFAs reduce the risk of heart attack and stroke.[11]

Also, some people who take very large doses of cod liver oil for extra vitamin D may find they are getting too much blood thinning effects from high amounts of EFAs. I have heard of this causing easy bruising, bleeding gums, and bleeding from every acupuncture needle inserted, with symptoms resolving by reducing the dose of total EFAs. But for most people, high doses of fish oil seem to offer great benefits. So how much should you take?

A paper published in the American Journal of Clinical Nutrition found in the United States healthy dietary intake of omega 3 is 3,500 mg for a person eating 2,000 calories per day.[12] So if you eat 3,000 calories you should take at least 5,250 mg of omega-3 oils daily. This is important to realize because the average EFA capsule is only 1,000 mg. That means if you are eating 3,000 calories a day (the typical healthy calorie intake in the United States is 2,000–3,000 calories a day) you should take at least 5 to 6 capsules of fish oil a day to support cardiovascular and brain health and reduce the risk of disease.

Not only are most people not consuming enough EFAs to support their heart and brain, but most also do not supplement with enough fish oil, especially if their diet is limited in essential fatty acids.

Understanding fish oil supplements

Fish oils contain EPA and DHA. Both are important for your health, but each has different functions in the body. Most fish oil supplements have a one-to-one ratio of DHA to EPA, both of which work to reduce inflammation and support the brain. However, it now appears EPA has more of an anti-inflammatory focus while DHA has the greatest effect on brain health.

If your goal is mainly to dampen inflammation, then regular fish oil or a fish oil with concentrated EPA is appropriate. However, if your goal is to positively impact the chemical status of your brain, then consider a fish oil with a high concentration of DHA.

I have found individuals with neurochemical imbalances such as depression, mood swings, bipolar reactions, or poor memory derive more benefit when ratios of DHA to EPA are greater than 1:1. I personally like to use ratios greater than 10:1 or 20:1 of DHA to EPA.

DHA best serves brain health

DHA is one of the major building blocks of the brain and is an essential nutrient for brain health and function of the neurons. DHA plays roles in improving the fluidity of neuron membranes, supporting growth of new neuronal dendrites, improving the ability of neurons to release neurotransmitters, and enhancing signaling between neurons.[13][14][15][16] DHA also has been shown to boost brain function, improve quality of life, reduce the incidence of neurodegenerative conditions, and improve both short-term and long-term memory.[17][18][19][20][21][22][23] In summary, DHA is used to enhance brain function, reduce brain inflammation, and decrease the incidence of neurodegenerative conditions.

The main problem with DHA-concentrated fish oils is they tend to be more expensive than regular fish oils. If you have all of the major symptoms of EFA deficiency listed in the beginning of this chapter you will probably need to begin with a more general fish oil, either alone or in conjunction with DHA. If you do not have EFA deficiency issues but want to support your brain, then you should consider a DHA-concentrated formula despite the slightly increased cost.

Also, if you suffer from chronic systemic inflammation—body aches, joint pain, and swelling—then you will be better off with regular fish oils that contain more EPA. EPA reduces inflammation both in the body and brain and may offer better brain support if inflammation is the primary issue.

To summarize, both EPA and DHA are beneficial for overall brain health, but there are times when a highly concentrated DHA supplement can dramatically improve brain function.

If overall inflammation is a problem, consider a fish oil with a 1:1 ratio of EPA to DHA. If inflammation (pain, swelling, body aches) is under control and you want to support your brain, use a highly concentrated DHA supplement.

Lastly, despite which supplement you use, limit your intake of fried foods, partially hydrogenated fats, and processed vegetable oils and eat more cold water fish, olive oil, avocados, and raw nuts and seeds. If possible, obtain your meat and eggs from animals raised on pasture and grass-finished. If your brain is not working well, it is very important to address intake of omega-3 and omega-6 fatty acids.

• •

My husband and I have 14-month-old twin girls who started taking a high-concentration of DHA four months ago. We've since become huge fans of this supplement, as the results were almost immediate. For example, one of our girls had a lazy eye that frequently veered to the right when she was looking directly at someone or something. A few days into taking DHA, her wandering eye corrected itself completely. When we miss a few days of DHA, her eye starts to wander again.

One daughter is as active as can be and is constantly moving. Prior to taking DHA, she had a short attention span and became frustrated easily. Since taking DHA, she will sit and play with a single toy for up to ten minutes. Instead of throwing a fit when she's frustrated with a toy, she persists in trying to figure it out. She now enjoys putting lids on containers, stacking objects, playing hide and seek (with people or objects), trying to put together toddler puzzles, and exploring cause-and-effect objects around the house.

Our other daughter was extremely slow to warm up to people. For example, when an unrecognizable person entered the room, she'd be so overcome with anxiety that she'd cry and cling to me while staring at the stranger in complete fear. While she is still on the shy side, her anxiety has almost disappeared. She now allows new people to hold her without expressing an ounce of fear. In fact, after taking DHA, the social awareness of both our daughters has improved tremendously. They are aware of other people and are very responsive to any interaction from someone else.

Our girls also began interacting, babbling, and laughing at each other within the first week of taking DHA. They are now developing language skills quickly. This past weekend we were surprised to hear difficult words like horsey, grandpa, car, and "roll it" come out of their mouths. We feel blessed that Dr. Geronimo recommended DHA for our daughters, as they are making progress faster than we thought possible. In the coming years, we will continue to start and end every day with DHA!

Dorothy and Derek B., parents of
   two patients of Dr. Geronimo
Rommel Geronimo, DC
San Diego, California
www.fecsd.com

• •

CHAPTER SUMMARY

• Sixty percent of the brain is made of fat and the fats you eat affect the composition of your brain. Fats found in processed foods, heated vegetable oil, processed vegetable oils, and hydrogenated fats can make the membranes of your nerve cells rigid and unresponsive, leading to improper neuron function, brain inflammation and degeneration, and symptoms of poor brain function.

• Essential fatty acids (EFAs) are termed "essential" because are body cannot make them—they must come from our diets. EFAs are critical for various functions of the body, including dampening inflammation, improving blood vessel health, supporting healthy skin growth, and supporting healthy brain and nervous system function.

• Omega-3 fatty acids are found in cold-water fish such as salmon, sardines, herring, mackerel, black cod, and bluefish. These are the fats most important to include in your diet, as most Americans are deficient.

• Vegetarian sources include walnuts and flax seed. However, many people have trouble converting these fats into omega-3 DHA and EPA, particularly if insulin resistance is an issue. Eating a diet high in omega-6 fats may also hinder this conversion.

• Our hunter-gatherer ancestors ate about as many omega-6 fats as omega-3 for a one-to-one, or 1:1, ratio. Today the average American eats a ratio of as high as 25:1—way too many omega-6 fats compared to omega-3 fats. This is due largely to sunflower, cottonseed, soybean, sesame, and canola oils in processed foods. This extreme imbalance creates a very inflammatory environment that plays a role in many chronic conditions, including heart disease, diabetes, autoimmune disease, and conditions that degenerate the brain.

• Researchers recommend a ratio of omega-6 to omega-3 that ranges from 1:1 to 4:1 for optimal health and prevention of disease.

• If you eat 3,000 calories you should take at least 5,250 mg of omega-3 oils daily. The average EFA capsule is only 1,000 milligrams, which means you should take 5 to 6 capsules of fish oil a day to support cardiovascular and brain health and reduce the risk of disease.

• EPA has more of an anti-inflammatory focus while DHA has the greatest effect on brain health. If your goal is mainly to dampen inflammation, then regular fish oil or a fish oil with concentrated EPA is appropriate. However, if your goal is to positively impact the chemical status of your brain, then consider a fish oil with a high concentration of DHA.

• I have found individuals with neurochemical imbalances such as depression, mood swings, bipolar reactions, or poor memory derive more benefit when ratios of DHA to EPA are greater than 1:1. I personally like to use ratios greater than 10:1 or 20:1 of DHA to EPA.

CHAPTER TWENTY

TOXINS AND THE BRAIN

● ●

Jack, 34, had just earned his law degree and gotten married. He was struggling, however, with erectile dysfunction, which was eroding his self-esteem and sense of masculinity. Jack tried Viagra and various herbs, but to no avail.

Desperate, Jack visited an alternative M.D., who ran some tests, found elevated levels of lead and mercury, and placed Jack on chelation therapy. Chelation therapy involves injections of chelating agents that bind with heavy metals in an attempt to remove them from the body. Immediately after beginning the therapy, Jack developed muscle wasting, loss of mental function, and general weakness.

His health deteriorated to the point he needed a cane to walk. After several weeks Jack discontinued chelation therapy. He regained function and was able to walk again without a cane. He then saw a neurologist, who performed a five-minute exam and sent him for a brain MRI, which came back normal. The neurologist concluded Jack was suffering from stress and needed to learn how to relax.

Because I had worked with some of Jack's family members, they referred him to me. His history revealed that in addition to erectile dysfunction, Jack experienced episodes of numbness in his face and legs. Jack's examination findings worried me. He was unable to feel parts of his arms, legs, and face when I stroked his skin with a metal pinwheel. When I scraped the bottom of his feet, he demonstrated what is called an "extensor toe sign"—a reflex in which the big toe extends. This is an abnormal reflex that potentially indicates a lesion in the spinal cord or brain.

I also found what are called "dysconjugate eye movements with saccades," which means when he looked quickly to a target his eyes would not move together as they should. Jack may have had a normal MRI, but his exam findings indicated a possible brain injury. It is important to remember that in early or mild cases of neuron damage, MRI scans are normal.

I ordered blood tests to evaluate Jack for antibodies to neurological tissue and environmental chemicals. His lab tests showed elevated antibodies to nerve sheaths, called "myelin," and elevated antibodies to mercury. It appeared Jack was suffering from neurological autoimmunity triggered by mercury.

In other words, his immune system was attacking the mercury in his body and, as a consequence, his own nerve sheaths. Myelin nerve sheaths protect and facilitate communication between neurons. When nerve sheaths are destroyed, nerve communication is lost and the brain cannot function normally.

These findings perhaps explained why chelation therapy caused Jack to fall apart. Chelating agents pull heavy metals from tissues and into the bloodstream, heightening their exposure to the immune system. Jack's immune system was most likely already overreacting to mercury, triggering his autoimmunity and his symptoms. Chelation simply intensified the reaction by pulling more mercury into the bloodstream. Had these mercury-induced autoimmune attacks continued, Jack most likely would have developed multiple sclerosis or some other type of demyelinating disease.

Jack had lost "chemical tolerance," as evidenced by elevated antibodies to mercury. When you have chemical tolerance it means your immune system does not react to environmental toxins in our everyday world, such as in cleaners, car exhaust, gas fumes, pesticides, paints, plastics, and body products. We all have toxins and heavy metals in our bodies, but if your immune system reacts to them it means you have lost chemical tolerance. Chelation therapy can exacerbate this reaction and the autoimmunity triggered by it, and it is not recommended for those who have lost chemical tolerance.

In Jack's case, we improved his chemical tolerance by supporting his blood-brain and intestinal barriers with the various supplements listed in previous chapters. I supported his regulatory T-cells with high doses of vitamin D and put him on compounds that support glutathione activity. Glutathione helps safely clear environmental compounds from the body while dampening the overzealous immune response. I also had him follow a diet and lifestyle to address his loss of chemical tolerance and supported his liver detoxification pathways. I will discuss these approaches in this chapter.

Many of Jack's symptoms began to improve during the next few months, including his erectile dysfunction, which was most likely caused by damage to the nerves used for an erection. He still struggles with autoimmune flare-ups from time to time, but overall he has learned how to control the episodes and improve his quality of life.

Both the conventional and alternative health care systems often overlook the issues Jack faced, but they are critical if a person is losing nervous system function due to environmental toxins. We are all exposed to high levels of environmental toxins and pollutants daily, but not all of us react to them adversely.

In this chapter we will review the concepts of immune chemical tolerance, liver metabolism of chemicals, and how they relate to the health of your brain and nervous system.

Datis Kharrazian, DHSc, DC, MS

Symptoms of loss of chemical tolerance

- Intolerance to smells
- Intolerance to jewelry
- Intolerance to shampoo, lotions, detergents, etc.
- Multiple food sensitivities
- Constant skin outbreaks

It's impossible to write a book about the brain without discussing the potential negative impact of environmental toxins, industrial chemicals, pollutants, and heavy metals on our brains and bodies. We are exposed to unprecedented levels of chemicals and heavy metals today, as well as hybridized, genetically modified, and industrially processed foods, all of which activate the immune system.

Only a minority of the synthetic compounds introduced to our environment has been researched individually, much less in conjunction with each other. The Environmental Protection Agency (EPA) doesn't require testing on chemicals introduced to market unless evidence of potential harm exists, which means testing seldom happens. The EPA approves about 90 percent of new chemicals. Only a quarter of more than 80,000 have been tested for toxicity.[1]

American children are born with increasingly high levels of chemical and toxin burdens. For example, a 2005 study of cord blood from newborns found almost 300 environmental compounds, including mercury and DDT.[2] Another study showed first-time mothers in the United States had levels of flame retardants in their breast milk 75 times higher than in similar European studies.[3] Yet the damage may not be obvious until we're older, as environmental toxins have been linked with such neurodegenerative conditions as Alzheimer's and Parkinson's disease.[4]

Additionally, pharmaceutical use today is shocking. Almost one-third of the U.S. population takes some type of medication and many people take multiple medications. This "polypharmacy" model of taking multiple drugs has diverse and potentially harmful consequences that go beyond adverse reactions and include death and disability.

The "Standard American Diet" (SAD) that most people follow includes not only excess sugar and refined carbohydrates but also industrially processed foods, chemical additives, GMO foods, and hybridized foods. This diet is very inflammatory.

This combination of chronic exposures to pollutants, toxins, multiple medications, and inflammatory foods has potentially contributed to the various inflammatory ailments clinicians face today. Many have theorized that today's skyrocketing incidences of autoimmunity, autism, neurodegenerative diseases, and other chronic inflammatory conditions result from our heavily industrialized, immune-reactive environment.[5][6][7]

In this chapter I will talk about some ways to help defend your body and brain against these daily assaults. Staying healthy in an industrial environment involves protecting the integrity of your antioxidant system, liver detoxification system, and immune barrier system (gut, blood-brain barrier, and lungs). By consciously tending to these systems you can help preserve your ability to maintain "chemical tolerance." Chemical tolerance means the immune system responds appropriately and does not overreact to toxins, pollutants, and dietary insults.

Of course, acute toxic exposures, such as a drug overdose, will lead to loss of health or even death. However, many people today can no longer tolerate relatively benign exposures such as perfumes, detergents, jewelry, or car exhaust because they have lost their chemical tolerance. Loss of chemical tolerance can significantly increase the risk not only for neurological autoimmunity, but also for systemic inflammation that can impact brain health.

LOSS OF CHEMICAL TOLERANCE: TOXICANT-INDUCED LOSS OF TOLERANCE

Over the years, hundreds of studies have explored the effects of environmental compounds on our health, turning up many disturbing findings. Toxins are linked with cancers, obesity, diabetes, heart disease, brain degeneration, neurological disorders, and other breakdowns in health. But these links can be difficult to identify for the average person. Unless there is an acute exposure, toxins do their work quietly and slowly over time.

Why are most people living relatively normal, healthy lives despite all these exposures while other people fall victim to toxin-induced illness? If you test random people in the United States, including the very healthy ones, chances are all of them will show contamination from heavy metals and environmental compounds. Being completely free of heavy metals and environmental chemicals these days is impossible. Anthropological studies show even mummies were contaminated by heavy metals.[8]

Instead, what we see is some people have an immune reaction to these environmental compounds while others don't. In fact, one person can have fairly high levels of toxicity and be symptom-free while another person has low levels of contamination yet reacts severely. The issue isn't how many toxins are in your system but whether your immune system reacts to them. This is the mechanism behind chemical intolerance, multiple chemical sensitivities, and toxin-induced brain degeneration mechanisms that are becoming so common today.

In the literature, this is called "toxicant-induced loss of tolerance," or TILT. (Researchers use the term "toxicant" instead of toxin). When people suffer from TILT, they aren't necessarily sick from heavy metals and chemicals. Instead, they are sick from reacting to them.[9]

Losing a tolerance to environmental chemicals

The loss of chemical tolerance is a phenomenon both researchers and clinicians have identified in more than a dozen countries and across diverse groups of people.[10] These are the people who cannot tolerate common chemicals without symptoms. Gas fumes, scented body products, laundry detergents, fabric softeners, new carpeting, the new car smell, and so on trigger their symptoms. For others, like Jack in the opening story, although a heavy metal or chemical is triggering autoimmunity and inflammation, it's not clear without testing or symptoms from chelation that one is reacting to a toxin.

For people with loss of chemical tolerance, trivial exposures can trigger a long list of conditions, including asthma, migraines, depression, fibromyalgia, fatigue, Gulf War syndrome, brain fog, memory loss, incontinence, neurological dysfunction, rashes, and so on. These people increasingly isolate themselves from the world and other people. They can't tolerate many indoor places, other people's scented body products, or clothes laundered in scented detergents. Even the smell of dryer sheets coming from a neighbor's vent during a walk makes them sick. It's common for them to feel increasingly angry at other people, and understandably so. When a scented product triggers a migraine, incontinence, or symptoms of multiple sclerosis, the person wearing it can seem cruel and selfish.

This isn't a condition just for adults. At a school function for my daughter I came across one child who had to put a blanket down before sitting on the carpet or he would break out in a rash. Another child could not play on the black top at recess or he became ill. These were five-year-olds, meaning the loss of tolerance is starting very early, perhaps even before birth due to the mother's own immune or chemical burden problems.

This bodes poorly for both children and adults as the mechanisms that cause loss of chemical tolerance are the same ones that cause loss of tolerance to one's own body tissue, setting the stage for autoimmunity.

What causes loss of chemical tolerance?

So why do some people develop a chemical intolerance and others don't? Several mechanisms are at work.

Poor glutathione activity.

Depletion of glutathione, the body's master antioxidant, is a primary cause of loss of chemical tolerance. Everyday levels of an environmental compound do not become an immune trigger unless the body's glutathione levels are depleted.[11]

Breakdown of immune barriers.

Glutathione depletion is also a major contributing factor to leaky gut, a leaky blood-brain barrier, and even leaky lungs. As I discussed in previous chapters, many other dietary and lifestyle factors can break down these immune barriers, increasing the risk for both loss of chemical tolerance and autoimmunity.[12]

Poor regulatory T-cell function.

Regulatory T-cells are immune cells that regulate and balance the immune system and prevent autoimmunity or loss of chemical tolerance.[13] They are key in preventing a TH-1 or TH-2 dominance, which I talked about in Chapter Eleven. Glutathione depletion causes loss of regulatory T-cell function, as do vitamin D deficiency and omega-3 fatty acid deficiency.

Chronic inflammation.

Chronic inflammation is very common today and contributes to glutathione depletion, loss of immune barrier integrity, and poor regulatory T-cell function. Chronic inflammation is a major predisposing factor in loss of chemical tolerance. Some common symptoms of chronic inflammation include bloating, skin rashes or eruptions, joint pain, brain fog, depression, anxiety, chronic pain, chronic fatigue, and autoimmune flare-ups.[14]

The evolution of loss of chemical tolerance

Loss of chemical tolerance appears to evolve in two stages. The first stage is characterized by a breakdown in the body's natural tolerance to chemicals and heavy metals. In the second stage, an ordinary exposure to an environmental compound suddenly triggers an immune response, whether it's traffic exhaust, fragrances, a drug, or other chemical.[15]

I know of one woman in her 30s who had long suffered mild sensitivities to chemicals but it suddenly became severe when she stayed with a relative in a small apartment, which was heavily scented from commercial laundry products. She became dizzy as soon as she walked in the home. While staying the night she experienced the most severe vertigo of her life. By the time she made it home by plane (which was likely sprayed with an insecticide), she struggled with severe fatigue for the next two months and was largely confined to her bed. She went on to develop symptoms of MS, including loss of strength and motor function in her arms and legs when exposed to scented products or industrial fumes. Today she must largely stay at home and eat a very strict diet to avoid a flare-up. As a mother of four in her 30s, this has been an incredible hardship. There have been many days when she simply cannot function.

This is an example of an immune response leading to a profound breakdown of immune function. Many of these people go on to develop multiple chemical sensitivities (MCS), severe allergies, multiple food intolerances, and autoimmunity.[16] Loss of chemical tolerance increasingly shrinks not only their world but also their diet as they react to a growing list of foods. Managing their cases may be difficult as many herbs and supplements also trigger reactions. Not only do they struggle with multiple and sometimes debilitating symptoms, but we also see changes in their immune panels that reflect inflammation and imbalances.

I had one patient with lupus so severe her immune system was attacking almost her entire body. She was one of the worst autoimmune cases I have ever seen. She had worked as a florist and regularly mixed buckets of pesticides with her bare hands. Her employees didn't wear gloves either but she became severely sick while they didn't.

Another patient had gone to help her parents clean and update their home. She was exposed to multiple chemicals in cleaning solutions, paints, and other products, after which she developed symptoms of Parkinson's disease.

Prior to the exposures, these women likely suffered from glutathione depletion, leaky immune barriers, and other health imbalances that predisposed them to developing loss of chemical tolerance and autoimmunity. It wasn't the amount of toxins in their system that triggered them so much as their loss of tolerance to chemicals.

When we suffer from leaky gut, chronic inflammation, hormonal imbalances, chronic stress, and so on, we are just one major stress event away from falling apart. It can be an IRS audit, a divorce, a lawsuit, a car accident, or other trauma. It's important to maintain your immune health and shore up your defenses so you are better able to withstand the chemical assaults and occasional crises life delivers.

Loss of chemical tolerance underlies many chronic illnesses today

More and more people today are showing up in their practitioners' offices with health problems triggered by environmental compounds. So what do many of these practitioners do? They test for heavy metals and environmental chemicals, which always come back positive, and then chelate the patient using chemicals such as DMSA, DMPS, or EDTA.

Or they put the patient on an intense liver detoxification program. If a patient has adverse reactions this is simply dismissed as a detox reaction. But the truth is chelating someone with neurological autoimmunity and loss of chemical tolerance can be devastating and permanently destroy brain and nerve tissue.

Why? Because research has clearly found that chelation pulls heavy metals out of body tissue and redistributes them so they make their way into the brain, promoting toxicity, inflammation, neurodegeneration, and sometimes serious side effects.[17][18][19] In these cases chelation promotes immune activation from chemical intolerance—it's like giving a person with celiac disease gluten. Studies since 1999 have repeatedly shown chelation pushes toxins into the brain, yet it continues as a popular practice.[20]

I learned about chelation the hard way before I knew any better, and these experiences almost drove me to quit. Twice I had referred patients with multiple sclerosis for chelation, worsening their symptoms in both cases. Unlike other cells in the body, your body doesn't grow new nerve cells to replace destroyed ones, and neurological damage can be permanent. I am emphatic about the dangers of chelation because I want to spare other practitioners and patients from the same experiences.

When it's safe and appropriate to chelate

Does this mean I'm anti-chelation? No, I am not anti-chelation any more than I am anti-iodine (which you know about if you read my thyroid book). Just as iodine is not safe for most people with Hashimoto's because it stimulates autoimmunity, chelation is not safe for people with loss of chemical tolerance who have exaggerated immune responses to chemicals.

However, there are times when chelation is appropriate, such as in the case of an acute exposure to toxic chemicals or heavy toxicity. A serum heavy metal test, which most chelation enthusiasts disdain, can help determine toxicity levels in the case of acute exposure.

Also, in some cases when a neurodegenerative disease is severe and progressed, it is assumed these toxic metals have already reached the brain and removing them might be advantageous. However, for a relatively healthy person who isn't suspected of having heavy metal toxicity in the brain, yet who fails the GABA challenge or shows intestinal permeability, chelation can unnecessarily expose the brain to heavy metals.

But chelation must not be undertaken until the person demonstrates the immune barrier integrity and glutathione status is restored, which I will talk about more in this chapter.

A person needs to be healthy enough to tolerate the adverse reactions chelation may produce and always calculate the clinical risk-to-benefit ratio. Make no mistake, there are associated risks and reactions with chelation therapy, such as redistribution of the metals into the brain. [21 22 23 24]

How toxins and heavy metals can imbalance the immune system

It may sound like toxins are innocent when it comes to loss of chemical tolerance. Not so. Even with healthy immunity, exposure to toxic compounds burdens our bodies. Manufacturers are not required to test the safety of new synthetic chemicals and government regulations are lax. The majority of people continue to pretend they don't exist, despite the studies linking toxic compounds to many modern ailments today. So although glutathione status, immune barrier integrity, and regulatory T-cell function are important, unfortunately environmental toxicity is a constant stressor, increasing the risk of brain disorders for us all.

Although loss of chemical tolerance signifies a breakdown of the body's self-defense mechanisms, environmental chemicals are partly to blame for this breakdown.

For instance, low concentrations of mercury have been shown to disrupt immune function and influence the risk of autoimmunity.[25] Polychlorinated biphenyls (PCBs) have been banned but are still found in the environment and have been shown to break down the blood-brain barrier and gut barrier.[26][27] Chronic exposure to arsenic in drinking water breaks down the lung barrier.[28] Chronic toxic exposure can deplete the glutathione system. These are just a few examples of the ways environmental chemicals attack our self-defense systems, making us more vulnerable to loss of chemical tolerance.

TESTING FOR LOSS OF CHEMICAL TOLERANCE

How do you know if you suffer from loss of chemical tolerance? We can test for loss of chemical tolerance by measuring antibodies to environmental chemicals. Positive antibodies indicate an overzealous immune reaction to environmental chemicals and thus loss of chemical tolerance.

Do not confuse testing for antibodies with tests that measure the quantity of chemicals and heavy metals as shown in urine, hair, stool, or with a DMPS challenge. When it comes to loss of chemical tolerance, the immune system's tolerance to these compounds is the key factor, not the quantities of the compounds in the body. This explains why some people cannot tolerate even trace exposures without reacting.

Standard lab tests for heavy metals

Most labs measure levels of environmental chemicals in the body using serum, urine, hair, or stool, and each type of testing has its limitations. Blood serum testing for acute toxic exposures is the most commonly accepted test in conventional toxicology. However, this test is criticized for being inaccurate for non-acute exposures or for its inability to measure levels of toxins stored in tissues.

The reproducibility and accuracy of hair testing is controversial and has been shown to be inaccurate when samples are submitted to various laboratories.[29] I personally do not find hair testing to be accurate or reliable enough for clinical use. Urine and stool tests also raise concerns in terms of reliability and reproducibility.

Other tests involve a "challenge" with a chelating agent such as dimercaptosuccinic acid (DMSA), 2-3 dimercapto-1-propanesulfonic acid (DMPS), or ethylenediaminetetraacetic acid (EDTA). A challenge test typically involves a baseline urine measurement for heavy metals and then a second urine test after a challenge with a chelating agent. If the challenge test shows higher levels of heavy metals it is theorized the individual has high amounts of toxins in their tissues.

Which test you're given depends on your health care provider's bias and training, and there is much controversy in this field. Regardless of the test, I personally find measuring for the quantity of an isolated heavy metal or environmental toxin is a limited diagnostic marker compared to assessing an individual's immune tolerance of environmental chemicals.

We can screen for elevated antibodies to environmental compounds with the Chemical Immune Reactivity Screen from Cyrex Laboratories. Elevated chemical antibodies indicate an exaggerated immune response to the chemicals, which can trigger neurological autoimmunity or degeneration of the brain as a consequence of systemic inflammation.

Ideally, we should not have high levels of antibodies to common environmental chemicals found in plastic bottles, upholstery, carpeting, dry cleaning, cosmetics, etc. Elevated antibodies indicate loss of chemical tolerance and a risk for abnormal immune reactions to everyday environmental chemicals.[30]

Cyrex Array 11 Chemical Immune Reactivity Screen

Aflatoxin antibodies

These antibodies indicate immune reactivity to a toxic metabolite from fungi called mycotoxins. These toxins tend to be found on stored grains and are a common source of exposure in the U.S. food supply.

Formaldehyde antibodies

These antibodies indicate immune reactivity to chemicals found in commonly used plastic products such as kitchen utensils, toys, adhesives, etc.

Trimellitic and phthalic anhydride antibodies

These antibodies indicate immune reactivity to chemicals used in the production of plasticizers and are found in PVC pipes, fiberglass products, paint resins, perfumes, insect repellents, etc.

Isocyanate antibodies

These antibodies indicate immune reactivity to chemicals in polymers and polyurethane products used in various foams and insulators found in bedding, window frames, shoe padding, etc.

Benzene antibodies

These antibodies indicate immune reactivity to petrochemicals from gasoline, with exposure typically coming from the burning of gasoline.

Bisphenol-A antibodies

These antibodies indicate immune reactivity to chemicals found in commonly used plastic products such as plastic water bottles and plastic bags.

Tetrabromobisphenol-A antibodies

These antibodies indicate immune reactivity to chemicals in fire retardants used on most new furniture, mattresses, and carpets.

Tetrachloroethylene antibodies

These antibodies indicate immune reactivity to a chemical found typically in dry cleaning and upholstery products.

Mercury and heavy metals antibodies

These antibodies indicate immune reactivity to metal compounds found in lead pipes, paints, and dental amalgams.

HOW CAN WE PROTECT OURSELVES FROM LOSS OF CHEMICAL TOLERANCE?

The most obvious question is, "How can I prevent this and what can I do once it has already happened?"

When most people think of toxicity they think of a liver detox that typically involves liver support. For most environmental compounds, the liver is the wrong target as it cannot detoxify heavy metals and many synthetic chemicals. However, liver detoxification still plays a role in brain health and chemical tolerance, which I will discuss later in this chapter.

We can improve chemical intolerance and protect the brain by supporting the immune barriers, immune regulation, and inflammation.

The various systems we want to support include:
- Glutathione levels and recycling
- Immune barrier health (gut, blood-brain barrier, and lungs)
- Immune balancing through regulatory T-cell support
- Inflammation in the body and brain

● ●

TOP 10 US GOVERNMENT PRIORITY LIST OF HAZARDOUS SUBSTANCES

These compounds are prevalent in our environment. It's important to note that none of these can be effectively detoxified by the liver. Their ability to create health problems depends on the integrity of your immune system. It is almost certain that you have these chemicals in your body, but the real question is does your immune system react to them inappropriately.

Arsenic
Mercury
Vinyl Chloride
Polychlorinated biphenyls
Benzene
Polycyclic aromatic hydrocarbons
Cadmium
Benzopyrene

Fluoranthene

Benzofluoranthene

● ●

GLUTATHIONE UNDERPINS LOSS OF CHEMICAL TOLERANCE SUPPORT

One of the most vital approaches to improve chemical tolerance is to support glutathione levels and your glutathione recycling system. Glutathione is the body's most powerful antioxidant and is integral to a healthy defense system. Ideally, the body maintains sufficient glutathione levels. However, extreme or chronic stress depletes it.

These stressors can include poor diets, diets lacking in sulfur, relentless traffic, smoking or second-hand smoke, over exercising, alcohol consumption…in other words, normal daily life for many people.

On top of this, autoimmune disease and exposure to toxic environmental compounds further deplete the precious supplies of glutathione. In fact, it is difficult to develop chemical intolerance or autoimmunity if the glutathione system is robust. [31] [32] [33] We can, however, use what researchers have learned to boost glutathione status nutritionally and theoretically better manage loss of chemical tolerance.

Glutathione's job is to take the bullet

Glutathione is like the bodyguard or Secret Service agent whose loyalty is so deep that she will jump in front of a bullet to save the life of the one she protects. When there is enough of the proper form of glutathione in the body to "take the bullet," no free radical response occurs. But when glutathione levels drop too low, this triggers a destructive inflammatory process.

When the body is low in glutathione, an environmental compound such as plastics, pesticides, perfumes, or gasoline fumes is more likely to cause an immune reaction. This eventually leads to loss of chemical tolerance and exaggerated immune responses to environmental compounds. It is in this scenario that heavy metal chelation can have disastrous consequences. As chelation releases heavy metals into a glutathione-depleted system, these freed metals can flare autoimmune diseases and inflammation.

I have seen plenty of people fall apart from chelation therapy. They are told they are detoxing but the reality is they are flaring up because glutathione wasn't there to absorb the damage and body tissue took the hit instead. It's vital to ensure the glutathione system is healthy before undertaking chelation (and that the gut, brain, and respiratory tract immune barriers aren't permeable or damaged).

Glutathione is a safe chelator

Glutathione doesn't just protect cells by acting as an antioxidant. It is also a safe chelator in itself, meaning it can bind to environmental compounds and help remove them from the body. Nutrients that support glutathione levels and recycling (which I explain below) have been shown to chelate and excrete heavy metals from the body without displacing them into other tissues, such as the brain.[34] Although glutathione does not have the same chelating and binding ability as commonly used chelating agents such as DMSA, DMPS, and EDTA, it is a very attractive form of therapy because it chelates without redistributing metals into other tissues.

Glutathione also binds to metals to form complex structures that are less toxic and immune reactive than unbound metals. These factors make glutathione a preferred source of support for those that have lost their chemical tolerance. Also, glutathione support is available as a dietary supplement over the counter, unlike DMSA, DMPS, and EDTA, which require a prescription.

Glutathione recycling explained

Supporting glutathione recycling is a little different than just boosting glutathione levels. Glutathione recycling does what the name implies, it recycles existing glutathione for reuse. What's important about supporting glutathione recycling is that it helps raise levels inside the cells (intracellular).

More common forms of glutathione delivery, such as a liposomal cream or intravenous (IV) glutathione, do not raise levels of glutathione inside the cells, only outside. Intracellular glutathione is important because it is the main antioxidant for mitochondria, the little factories inside each cell that convert nutrients into energy. This is crucial because the degenerative process of an autoimmune disease destroys the mitochondria in affected cells, such as thyroid tissue in autoimmune Hashimoto's or nerve sheath tissue in brain degenerative disorders.

There are two main forms of glutathione in the body: reduced glutathione and oxidized glutathione. The form that protects mitochondria is called "reduced glutathione."

Reduced glutathione is the bodyguard that "takes the hit" from free radicals that damage cells. Free radicals are molecules that are unstable because they have unpaired electrons and are looking for electrons to steal in order to become stable. They steal electrons from the mitochondria, thus destroying them and causing inflammation and degeneration.

However, with plenty of intracellular reduced glutathione, the glutathione sacrifices its electrons to the free radicals to protect the mitochondria. As a result, the reduced glutathione ends up with an unpaired electron and becomes unstable, at which point it becomes oxidized glutathione, which is technically a free radical itself.

The unstable oxidized glutathione then pairs with available glutathione with the help of an enzyme called glutathione reductase, returning back to its reduced glutathione state so it's ready for action once again. The body's ability to constantly recycle oxidized glutathione back to reduced glutathione is critical for managing loss of chemical tolerance and autoimmunity.

Two enzymes come into consideration when we look at how to support glutathione recycling nutritionally:

Glutathione peroxidase

Glutathione peroxidase triggers the reaction of reduced glutathione to oxidized glutathione, which is when glutathione "takes the hit" to spare the cell.

Glutathione reductase

Glutathione reductase triggers the conversion of oxidized glutathione back to useable reduced glutathione.

Studies show various botanicals, nutritional compounds, and their cofactors activate glutathione reductase and the synthesis of reduced glutathione. By boosting glutathione reductase and supplementing glutathione levels, we can help quench inflammation and, even better, prevent the onset of inflammation or an autoimmune flare-up in the first place.

Studies have also shown that efficient glutathione recycling helps boost regulatory T-cells, which promotes immune balance and helps prevent immune system hyperreactivity. Proper glutathione activity also regulates cell proliferation and immunity, and helps tissues recover from damage.[35 36 37 38 39 40 41]

Maintaining sufficient glutathione levels and glutathione recycling helps buffer the body from the many stressors hurled at us each day and can reduce our chances of developing chemical intolerance or autoimmunity, or help nutritionally support those conditions.

Supporting glutathione recycling

So how do we support glutathione recycling? The first thing is to reduce the stressors that deplete this vital system. Balancing blood sugar, addressing food intolerances, restoring gut health, balancing hormones, supporting brain health, and so on are some foundational approaches. Of course, lifestyle changes that include getting enough sleep, paring down an over-active schedule, and getting regular physical activity (but not overtraining) are also important. However, nutritional support also may be necessary. Below I cover the basic botanicals and nutritional compounds researchers have found support glutathione recycling pathways.

N-acetylcysteine (NAC)

NAC is a key compound to glutathione activity. It is rapidly metabolized into intracellular glutathione.[42 43]

Alpha-lipoic acid (ALA)

ALA directly recycles and extends the metabolic life spans of vitamin C, glutathione, and coenzyme Q10, and it indirectly renews vitamin E, all of which are necessary for glutathione recycling.[44 45]

L-glutamine

Research has shown that l-glutamine is important for the generation of glutathione. It is transported into the cell, converted to glutamate, and readily available to intracellular glutathione synthesis.[46 47 48]

Selenium

Selenium is a trace element nutrient that serves as the essential cofactor for the enzyme glutathione peroxidase, which converts GSH to GSSG so glutathione can "take the hit" by free radicals to spare cells.[49][50][51]

Cordyceps

Cordyceps has been shown to activate both glutathione and peroxidase synthesis in the body and protect cells by engaging the glutathione enzyme cycle. Cordyceps increases glutathione levels in the cells by 300 percent within minutes.[52][53]

Gotu kola (Centella Asiatica)

Research has clearly demonstrated that oral intake of gotu kola rapidly and dramatically increases the activity and amount of glutathione peroxidase and the quantity of glutathione.[54]

Milk thistle (Silybum marianum)

Milk thistle has been shown to significantly increase glutathione, increase superoxide dismutase (another powerful antioxidant) activity, and positively influence the ratios of reduced and oxidized glutathione.[55][56]

Dosing

Using these compounds together creates a synergistic effect, making them more effective at activating the glutathione peroxidase and reductase enzymes. Start with modest amounts and increase the doses until a positive effect is noticed.

For people with severe leaky gut issues, I suggest they take these compounds as long as they are working on repairing intestinal permeability—glutathione has been shown to protect and regenerate the gut barrier, as well as the brain and lung barriers.[57]

It's important to use these compounds in conjunction with approaches that boost overall glutathione levels (below). This way the glutathione you take is assured to stay in your body longer and get inside your cells where it can do its best work.

Other practitioners and I have witnessed positive outcomes in patients who build up their glutathione recycling system. As a result they begin to regain their tolerance to the chemicals around them, they have fewer autoimmune flare-ups, and they recover faster from their flare-ups when they do happen.

Boosting glutathione levels with S-acetyl-glutathione

While you support glutathione recycling, you also want to boost overall glutathione levels. In the thyroid book, I recommend a liposomal glutathione cream because oral glutathione is difficult to absorb. Glutathione IVs are also popular.

Now we have access to a new form of glutathione known as S-acetyl-glutathione, which the gastrointestinal tract can efficiently absorb.[58 59 60 61 62] Oral doses can start at 300 mg per day and go up to several thousand milligrams if necessary with certain inflammatory conditions. However, it is not cheap and the amount used may depend on what you can afford.

I suggest using about 1000 mg a day in most cases, although I suggest much higher doses in certain inflammatory, progressed neuro-degenerative, or autoimmune conditions. I still recommend liposomal glutathione cream for use in localized areas, such as an area of pain or inflammation. Examples include over an inflamed joint or over the thyroid of someone with an autoimmune thyroid condition.

MANAGE LOSS OF CHEMICAL TOLERANCE WITH GUT, BLOOD-BRAIN, AND LUNG BARRIER HEALTH

The gut, brain, and lung barriers take a beating from environmental toxins, especially if the glutathione system is depleted. Research shows environmental toxins degrade these immune barriers. Once degraded, a leaky gut, brain or lungs allow toxins into the bloodstream and the brain, where they can inflict damage.[63]

This is where the information on gut repair in Chapter Nine comes into play.

One way to shore up your defenses against environmental toxins is to dampen gut inflammation and repair a leaky gut. This includes screening for food intolerances, following an anti-inflammatory diet, and supporting gut health with the nutrients described in Chapter Nine. Some chemically intolerant people may need to follow an anti-inflammatory diet long term or even lifelong to manage their chemical intolerance. Following the gut repair protocol will also help restore the lining of the blood-brain barrier and the lungs.

As previously mentioned, glutathione is vital to gut repair, as low glutathione leads to leaky gut.[64][65] Because the blood-brain barrier functions similarly to the gut barrier, glutathione is also vital for repairing the blood-brain barrier and protecting the brain.

NITRIC OXIDE MODULATION FOR LOSS OF CHEMICAL TOLERANCE

Nitric oxide modulation, which I discuss in Chapter Seven, is another important tool to manage loss of chemical tolerance. Healthy nitric oxide function supports tissue healing, a healthy anti-inflammatory response, and a balanced immune response.

The beneficial form of nitric oxide, eNOS, helps repair the immune barriers,[66] boost blood flow, and dampen inflammation.[67][68] Promoting eNOS also inhibits iNOS, the form of nitric oxide that promotes inflammation, tissue damage, and leaky gut.[69][70]

Bursts of high-intensity aerobic exercise activate eNOS, as do a variety of nutritional and botanical compounds, including vinpocetine, Ginkgo biloba, ATP, huperzine A, xanthinol niacinate, alpha GPC, L-acetyl carnitine, butcher's broom, and feverfew.

I recommend my patients get their heart rate up within the first hour of waking, even if it's only for one to five minutes. Doing this will jump start eNOS for the day and help dampen inflammation, improve blood flow, and repair the immune barriers, all of which help restore chemical tolerance and dampen autoimmunity.

ASSESSING GUT, BRAIN, AND LUNG BARRIER INTEGRITY

Because leaky gut symptoms aren't always easy to identify, it's best to monitor your progress with an immune barrier integrity test. For some people symptoms are obvious, as they have multiple food sensitivities. Others eat a diet heavy in gluten, dairy, and processed and junk foods and claim they have no symptoms. Often these people are so chronically bloated and inflamed they no longer realize the impact of their diet on their health. It isn't until they follow the restricted anti-inflammatory diet for a month or so that they realize how badly those foods affect them upon reintroduction.

The Cyrex Labs Intestinal Antigenic Permeability Screen measures the degree of gut permeability. Because the mechanisms for gut integrity are similar to those for blood-brain barrier and lung integrity, we can use this test to gauge overall immune barrier health. The blood-brain barrier has zonulin and occludin hormones identical to those in the gut lining.

As discussed in Chapter Nine, this test measures zonulin and occludin antibodies to assess tight junction damage, actomyosin antibodies to assess damage to the cells of the lining, and bacterial LPS antibodies to assess overgrowth of harmful bacteria and whether LPS are causing systemic inflammation.

Note: You should never consider chelation therapy until the intestinal permeability test is normal.

Additionally, I use the GABA challenge to assess blood-brain barrier integrity. Symptoms of a leaky blood-brain barrier can include brain fog or a headache or neurological symptoms after eating certain foods or being exposed to environmental chemicals. When I see people fail the GABA challenge, show neurological symptoms, and have positive antibodies on the gut permeability test, I assume they have loss of blood-brain barrier integrity.

I use a simple breathing test to assess the lung barrier. I ask my patients to take three breaths as deeply as possible. If they start coughing during this exercise I view that as positive for a breach in the lung barrier. The deep breaths pull respiratory particles into the lining of the lungs. If it's leaky this causes an inflammatory response with coughing. This is common in smokers or people such as firefighters who have been exposed to toxic smoke. Other symptoms of poor lung barrier integrity include coughing all the time or difficulty breathing with exertion.

SUPPORT VITAMIN D

When managing loss of chemical tolerance, you should always address vitamin D levels. Research shows vitamin D plays a critical role in the development of general tolerance, immune system defense, immune balance (regulatory T-cells), and immune barrier integrity.[71][72] On a 25-hydroxy vitamin D test, I like to see a level no lower than 50 ng/mL.

SUPPORT INFLAMMATION IN THE BODY AND THE BRAIN TO MANAGE LOSS OF CHEMICAL TOLERANCE

As you learned in Chapters Nine and Ten, inflammation in the gut, the body, and the brain can severely impact brain health. This also holds true when loss of chemical tolerance is causing neurological problems. Inflammation can exacerbate loss of chemical tolerance and autoimmunity, making it an important target for managing these conditions.

There is no unique inflammation protocol here beyond what I have already discussed throughout this chapter and the book. Strategies include:

- Repairing leaky gut
- Supporting glutathione levels and recycling
- Supporting nitric oxide modulation
- Supporting vitamin D levels
- Nutritional compounds to support brain inflammation (Chapter Ten)
- High doses of emulsified resveratrol and curcumin to dampen NF-kappaB and TH-17 pathways (Chapter Eleven). In studies researchers use doses as high as 400 mg a day of resveratrol and 800 mg a day of curcumin. However, you may need a different dose.

* *

I first saw Dr. Herbold more than 20 years ago. I had just moved to the area and was looking for a chiropractor to help with what I thought was a pinched nerve in my shoulder causing my arm to go numb. He was able to help me with that and relieved the numbness.

Then, some years later, I began to experience numbness below both knees. The medical doctors I saw were perplexed. Eventually the numbness advanced to above my knees and then up into my waist on one side and up to my chest on the other. They ran a number of tests on me, all of which came back negative, but they went on to diagnose me with multiple sclerosis.

Once a week I received a shot of a low-dose chemotherapy drug that made me sick with flu-like symptoms. I had to have my blood tested regularly, as the drug is hard on the liver. During the spring and fall of that year the MS flared a couple of times and I ended up in the hospital flat on my back and unable to move. I was given intravenous steroid therapy. Then my blood tests started showing the drug was affecting my liver and I went off it. I don't remember it working well enough to be worth damaging my liver.

That was when I asked Dr. Herbold what I could do, and he put me on a new diet and supplement protocol. It took me a long time to comply with the diet, but now I eat a gluten-free, dairy-free, and sugar-free diet. I was a carb addict, and he helped me overcome that.

For the next 10 years that worked, and although I still had flare-ups in the spring and fall, I didn't need IV steroids, just prednisone tablets. Then when I started going through menopause, my spring and fall flare-ups intensified again for a while. I began daily injections of a drug for MS, and there are no major side effects.

Between that and continuing with my diet and supplementation, things have leveled out. Supporting my glutathione and nitric oxide systems has been incredibly important. Inflammatory and vitamin D support have also been critical. I am "vertical," which is great!

I was diagnosed with MS the same year as two other women I work with who are about the same age. I drive a school bus, and back in those days in the winter they would start up all the school buses for more than an hour before we drove our routes so the buses could warm up. We said it was like being in a gas exhaust chamber, the smoke was so thick. It was very uncomfortable.

The law changed and they're not allowed to do that anymore, but I wonder about all that exhaust and the three of us getting MS. The other two women went the conventional route with treatment. I would say I am in a much different place than they are, thanks to my diet and my clinical nutrition work with Dr. Herbold.

Leanne, 52, patient of Dr. Herbold
Richard Herbold, DC, DACNB
Clifton Park, New York
capitaldistrictvitalitycenter.com

• •

THE ROLE OF THE LIVER IN LOSS OF CHEMICAL TOLERANCE

Symptoms of poor liver detoxification

- Acne and unhealthy skin
- Bloating
- Swelling
- Hormone imbalances
- Weight gain
- Poor bowel function

So far I have talked about environmental toxins without mentioning the liver. Although the liver cannot metabolize heavy metals and many environmental compounds, liver health still plays a role in chemical tolerance. If liver function becomes compromised it can increase your toxic load and your chemical intolerance. Likewise, toxic exposures and inflammation can hinder liver metabolic function.

The common term for how the liver works is "liver detoxification." However, I want you to know this is not the term researchers use. If you decide to research the subject yourself on PubMed, an online repository of peer-reviewed studies, you should instead use the terms "hepatic biotransformation," "detoxication," or "metabolomics."

A tremendous amount of research goes into this topic, largely to study why some people have adverse reactions to drugs and environmental toxins. In the field of "pharmacogenomics" researchers use gene testing to predict adverse drug reactions based on genetic variations and abnormalities in liver clearance metabolism.

Liver detoxification basics

In a nutshell, liver detoxification involves making fat-soluble compounds water-soluble so they can be eliminated in urine, feces, or sweat. Examples of compounds the liver metabolizes are hormones, drugs, and "xenobiotics," chemicals that are foreign to the body but still pass through liver detoxification pathways. An example of a xenobiotic is xenoestrogen, a synthetic chemical that mimics estrogen and is found in many plastics, pesticides, insecticides, food additives, and other compounds.

When a fat-soluble compound comes into the liver it first enters the "Phase I pathway." The Phase I pathway changes the structure of the compound for the sole purpose of having molecules attach to it in the Phase II pathway to prepare it for elimination.

Phase II has several different pathways that metabolize the compounds in different ways: methylation, glucuronidation, sulfation, acetylation, and glutathione conjugation. Once molecules are added to the compound in Phase II it is heavy and stable enough to be eliminated from the body safely.

In Phase III the metabolized compounds are end products ready for elimination. This phase depends on a sufficiently alkaline diet (a diet rich in produce with little to no processed foods) and healthy bile synthesis and gallbladder function, especially for fecal elimination. Naturally, healthy bowel function and lack of constipation is important for this phase as well.

When liver detox pathways don't work

When a compound goes through Phase I it becomes more immune reactive and pro-inflammatory. Theoretically this is not a problem as Phase II is there to sweep in and stabilize these immune reactive compounds.

However, inherited genetic traits may cause variations or defects in how these pathways work, which is one reason medications affect people differently. Just because you have a genetic predisposition does not necessarily mean that gene will express itself, but factors such as diet or lifestyle can trigger these genes. The detoxification pathways have also been shown to gradually lose integrity as we age.[73]

When a person's liver Phase II pathway is hindered, two different possibilities exist. One is that an already inflammatory compound, such as an environmental toxin, is made more inflammatory in Phase I. Because a hindered Phase II pathway is not capable of completing the job, this more toxic compound goes back into circulation, where it may activate the immune system and inflammation.

Because the liver cannot metabolize it, this new toxic metabolite is now officially a toxicant, which I explained in the first part of this chapter. Increased toxicants due to failures in detoxification increase your chemical load and your risk of developing inflammatory conditions such as loss of chemical tolerance and autoimmunity.[74][75][76]

The second possibility is that formerly inactive (inactive means it does not react with the immune system) compounds are metabolized into immune reactive compounds. For instance, if the liver fails to detoxify a xenoestrogen, which resembles natural hormones in the body, it can attach to hormone receptor sites and disrupt metabolism. Even the body's own estrogen can be transformed into a more toxic version that competes with healthy forms of estrogen for receptor sites.

The average person doesn't know his or her liver detoxification metabolism is inefficient. Instead one may complain of chronic immune issues, such as a never-ending sinus infection, weight gain, allergies, loss of chemical tolerance, migraines with PMS (because impaired Phase II pathways prevent the liver from clearing toxic forms of hormones during the surges that occur at different times during the cycle), intolerances to certain groups of foods, and so on. Of course, other factors also play a role in these symptoms, but liver detoxification should be considered.

(Sometimes these genetic variations, called single nucleotide polymorphisms [SNPs], can be beneficial. For example, some people have a genetic SNP variation that makes them immune to malaria or HIV. Although it's possible to test for some of these genetic SNPs, there are simply too many to screen for them all.)

Another factor to consider is that just because you have a particular genetic makeup, or "genotype," this doesn't mean your genes will necessarily be expressed. Diet, environment, and life events can affect the expression of your genes.

How your genes are expressed is called a "phenotype." For instance, someone who smokes and drinks regularly, eats processed foods daily, and works in a chemical plant may not have the best expression of their genotype compared to someone who eats a healthy diet, exercises regularly, and does not endure heavy toxic exposures.

For example, about 20 percent of the population are slow methylators—methylation is a Phase II pathway which attaches a single carbon group to the chemical compound. Consider a slow methylator who takes birth control pills (which deplete methyl donors), diuretics (which deplete the magnesium, the main cofactor for this pathway), and is a junk-food vegetarian. If she's exposed to an environmental compound that requires methylation, her liver may not be up to the task. Because methylation defects have been associated with breast cancer, this woman may be at an increased risk.

The effect of poor liver detoxification on the brain

In the literature, researchers are linking these detoxification breakdowns with serious neurological diseases such as Alzheimer's or Parkinson's.[77 78 79 80 81 82 83] For instance, in one case study researchers investigated why a man developed a sudden onset of late-stage Parkinson's symptoms after exposure to particular pesticide. A genetic profile of his liver detoxification pathways revealed a defect in the pathways that metabolized this particular pesticide.[84] Because aging also impacts liver detoxification, older people taking multiple drugs may react to their medications.[85]

The effect of environmental compounds on the brain and nervous system is particularly devastating because tissue in the nervous system does not undergo further cell division throughout your lifespan. Environmental toxicity affects all of the body.

However, cells in the skin, the gut, the liver, and other tissues can regenerate after death. Neurons don't, which explains why neurological symptoms are so pronounced. This explains why neurological diseases such as Alzheimer's and Parkinson's have been linked with poor Phase II detoxification pathway function.

A great example that perhaps illustrates the effect of toxins when liver detox systems are impaired is the 2012 incident in LeRoy, New York. Sixteen people, most of them high school girls, developed Tourette's-like neurological disorders around the same time. The area was home to spills of arsenic and trichloroethylene (TCE) in the 1970s, which may have been released by heavy rains and flooding. It is also an area for natural gas fracking. The official diagnosis? Mass hysteria.

Our world overlooks the effect of environmental compounds on health, but it is very real. It's like when people refused to believe the connection between germs and infection because they couldn't see the germs. We cannot see these environmental compounds, but the research shows without question they negatively impact our health. Although we are all coping with exposure, the integrity of our body's defense system is an important factor to health.

Nutrients to support healthy liver detoxification

Different nutritional and botanical compounds support all three of the liver's detoxification pathways. I use all of these, as they work well together and we can't be sure which pathway is compromised.

Phase I and Phase II support

The compounds that support these pathways are milk thistle seed extract, dandelion root extract, gotu kola extract, panax ginseng, L-glutathione, glycine, N-acetylcysteine, and DL-methionine. In addition to supporting Phase I and Phase II, these compounds also support blood flow and cell growth in the liver.[86][87][88][89][90][91][92][93][94][95][96][97][98][99][100][101][102][103][104][105][106][107]

Phase II methylation support

Methylation is a Phase II detox pathway also important for healthy brain function. Nutrients that support methylation include choline, trimethylglycine, MSM, beet root, and betaine HCl. These nutrients also support homocysteine metabolism (for an anti-inflammatory effect) and healthy bile synthesis and metabolism.[108][109][110][111][112][113][114][115][116]

Bile support

These nutrients support healthy bile synthesis and elimination, to help remove metabolized toxins from the body. They include dandelion root extract, milk thistle seed extract, ginger root, phosphatidylcholine, and taurine.[117][118][119][120][121][122][123][124][125][126][127][128][129][130][131][132][133]

Detoxification and glutathione support

These nutrients not only support liver detoxification, they also support glutathione levels and recycling, which I talked about earlier in the chapter. They include N-acetylcysteine, cordyceps extract, gotu kola extract, milk thistle seed extract, L-glutamine, and alpha lipoic acid.

How the brain affects liver detoxification

Poor brain function can affect liver detoxification. Earlier in the book I talked about how brain degeneration and declining brain function can impact autonomic function and cause such symptoms as poor digestion, dry eyes, incontinence, high blood pressure, and so on. Poor brain function can also impact the liver and its ability to detoxify the body.[134][135]

In some cases, doing exercises that stimulate the vagus nerve, the nerve that relays communication between the brain and the organs, can help neurologically activate or reboot liver function. This includes vigorous gargling, singing loudly, or engaging the gag reflex, techniques I describe in more detail in Chapter Nine. Symptoms of insufficient vagal tone include poor intestinal motility (constipation), poor digestive enzyme production (bloating, indigestion), floating stool or undigested food in stool, and symptoms of poor liver detoxification.

Poor neurotransmitter activity can also play a role in liver function. The liver requires dopamine, our "pleasure and reward" neurotransmitter, to detoxify properly.[136][137][138] When I see symptoms of poor liver detoxification I also look for symptoms of poor dopamine activity. Sometimes supporting dopamine can make a huge impact on liver function.

Symptoms of low dopamine activity (Chapter Sixteen) include depressed thoughts, poor motivation, becoming easily angered, slow movements and thoughts, and poor ability to either start or finish tasks.

In general, when liver detoxification presents as a health problem, it is always worth investigating brain health. Simply throwing a bunch of supplements at the liver may have limited and frustrating results when brain function is failing. Instead, it may be more worthwhile to improve brain health by looking for the following symptoms and addressing them per the information throughout this book, including:

• Brain inflammation

• Poor oxygenation (blood flow) to the brain

• Loss of brain function

• DHA deficiency

• Low serotonin, dopamine, acetylcholine, or GABA activity

The brain has its own detoxification system

The Phase I pathway of liver detoxification uses a diverse family of enzymes called cytochrome P450 (CYP450). As it turns out, the brain also contains CYP450 enzymes for its own detoxification.[139] These enzymes are responsible for breaking down toxins in the brain for elimination. Unfortunately, brain inflammation and poor brain health can hinder the function of these CYP450 enzymes. In fact, poor brain detoxification has been linked with a variety of neurological and psychiatric disorders.[140][141][142]

The compounds we use to support liver detoxification are not really effective for brain detoxification because they cannot cross the blood-brain barrier. The key to supporting healthy brain detoxification is to prevent and manage inflammation in the brain, as discussed in Chapter Ten. Nutrients that have been shown to quench brain inflammation include apigenin, luteolin, baicalein, resveratrol, rutin, catechin, and curcumin.

HOW LIVER DETOXIFICATION AFFECTS LOSS OF CHEMICAL TOLERANCE

When liver detoxification fails, toxicity increases—compounds the liver fails to metabolize go back into circulation in a more toxic form. A serious fallout from this cycle I haven't talked about yet is the activation of NF-kappaB. [143 144 145 146 147 148]

NF-kappaB is a protein inside of cells that acts as a switch to turn inflammation on and off in the body. It responds to whatever may be conceived as a threat to the cell, including environmental toxins or toxic metabolites the liver failed to detoxify. I talked about NF-kappaB in previous chapters in regards to inflammation and autoimmunity because it is a powerful force, capable of igniting relentless inflammatory cascades that play a role in degeneration, autoimmunity, cancer, and loss of chemical tolerance.

NF-kappaB's role in poor liver detoxification helps create a dangerous web that may ultimately lead to loss of chemical tolerance. When the liver fails to properly metabolize environmental toxins and other compounds, they become more toxic, which activates NF-kappaB's inflammatory cascade. The trouble is that the activation of NF-kappaB not only causes more failure in the liver's detox pathways, but it also depletes the vital glutathione system needed to shield the body from toxicants the liver can't metabolize. As these systems continue to fail, this further triggers NF-kappaB in a self-perpetuating cycle of toxicity and inflammation that ultimately may lead to loss of chemical tolerance, autoimmunity, and neurodegeneration.

You see this in people whose condition fails to improve or worsens despite eating a perfect diet and following all the "healing" rules, because they are trapped in this self-perpetuating web. For some people taking medications, this vicious inflammatory cycle can impair the body's ability to break down the drug for elimination, which impacts the effectiveness of the drug or can cause side effects or adverse reactions. Not only does their toxic load increase, but also the chronic inflammation degrades the barriers of the gut, brain and lungs, further increasing inflammation and loss of chemical tolerance.[149] [150]

If it sounds dire, it is. Just ask someone coping with loss of chemical tolerance and toxin-induced neurological symptoms. These include children, mothers with children to care for, men with families to support, college students, and so on. Many get to where they cannot eat but only a small list of foods and cannot tolerate many public areas or other people's homes, much less the workplace, because of carpet fumes, mildew, paint fumes, scented body products, scented laundry detergents, and so on. Otherwise they suffer neurological consequences that can be debilitating, such as loss of brain function, severe fatigue, symptoms that mimic MS, Parkinson's or other diseases, and, of course, poor mood.

An extreme example of the damaging effects of loss of chemical tolerance is Victor Yushchenko, the Ukranian candidate who was poisoned with dioxin in an assassination attempt during the 2005 presidential campaigns. Yuschenko went from dashingly handsome to quite disfigured from a toxic dose of dioxin, looking as if he had aged more than 20 years in just three weeks. He continues to suffer from symptoms today.

We can assume the dioxin poisoning obliterated his detox pathways and his glutathione systems and drove NF-kappaB inflammation through the roof. The interesting thing about Yushchenko, however, is that he did not die, a testament to robust liver detoxification and glutathione systems before the poisoning. The level of dioxin in his blood would have killed most of us. However Yushchenko was blessed with "good-defense" genes. This explains why some people live to be over 100 while drinking and smoking every day.

Supporting the liver to manage loss of chemical tolerance

Many practitioners default to a standard liver detox or heavy metal chelation when they see these patients, but as you now know, these approaches alone may be ineffective or, in the case with chelation, even contraindicated. I don't promise an easy way out, but the literature has shown us strategies that can help slowly unravel this inflammatory web.

The most effective compounds we've seen for dampening NF-kappaB are high doses of emulsified resveratrol and curcumin given in combination. Although each is a powerful anti-inflammatory compound alone, given together their effect is four-fold greater, and when emulsified they are even more powerful. Studies show both compounds are effective in protecting the body from damage due to environmental toxins and for dampening NF-kappaB activation and inflammation.[151][152][153][154][155][156][157]

You have to take high enough amounts of each of these in order to notice an effect. In studies subjects were given up to 400 mg of resveratrol and 800 mg of curcumin daily. However, the necessary dose is different for everyone, so don't assume that is the correct dose for you.

You must also address the factors that lead to loss of chemical tolerance, which I covered in the first part of this chapter. This includes supporting regulatory T-cells with vitamin D, fish oil, and glutathione; supporting leaky gut; and supporting glutathione levels and recycling.

Another important strategy, especially when symptoms of poor liver detoxification are present, is to support the Phase I, II, and III pathways with the nutrients listed earlier. Don't forget, the brain also has Phase I detox enzymes, which can be impaired by brain inflammation.

Managing chemical intolerance—and brain health—in a nutshell

It can be overwhelming to support all of these at the same time, not to mention costly. Where to begin unraveling this web can take some professional discernment or trial and error.

That said, here is an ultra-condensed version of how to manage loss of chemical tolerance. If you have read the entire book you will notice that this provides a good foundation not only for loss of chemical tolerance but for general inflammatory conditions that contribute to loss of brain function. If you're brain is not working, this is a good place to start.

Basics to managing loss of chemical tolerance

Step one: Dampen NF-kappaB inflammatory cascades with therapeutic amounts of emulsified resveratrol and curcumin initially. In studies subjects were given up to 400 mg of resveratrol and 800 mg daily of curcumin, however the necessary dose is different for everyone and most people do better with much higher doses, so don't assume that is the correct dose for you. You may need to experiment with the proper dose for yourself.

I also add therapeutic doses of vitamin D, as most people with this degree of inflammation are deficient. Therapeutic doses can be a minimum of 5,000 IU a day to 10,000 IU or sometimes more, depending on serum 25-hydroxy vitamin D levels and the severity of the condition.

Begin preparing for the anti-inflammatory diet (Chapter Nine) in week two by putting together menus and shopping lists. The diet is quite different from what most people are used to, so plenty of advance planning is essential.

Step two: Continue with the resveratrol, curcumin, and vitamin D. At this point you will embark on the anti-inflammatory diet. If possible, add in nutrients to support gut repair, gut detoxification, and healthy gut flora. How long you stay on the diet depends largely on the severity of your condition. I recommend at least 30–60 days on the diet to allow for significant recovery. Many people stay on it longer, some for life, as it offers the most relief.

Step three: After inflammation has calmed down on the diet, add in nutrients to support liver detoxification pathways. Again, when you do this depends on the severity of your condition. Signs that your inflammation is calming down can include less bloating, calming of your chemical intolerance or autoimmune symptoms, weight loss (if necessary), less chronic pain, reduced skin rashes or eruptions, and improved mood and energy. Because of possible genetic variations in liver detoxification, some people find they function better staying on the liver support.

Throughout this protocol I also prefer to use nutrients to support the glutathione system and nitric oxide regulation if finances allow.

This is a broad overview to the steps involved. I realize it would be easier to tell you how much of which specific products to take instead of having you look at long lists of ingredients, but I don't want to promote any specific product or be accused of being a salesman—that is not what motivates me in this work. Although it requires more work on your part, showing you the ingredients and their actions empowers you with information when purchasing supplements from the store or from your practitioner.

Knowing how your supplements support you is important to your wellness program. Don't just take whatever your practitioner gives you without question. Otherwise you have no idea what is happening or why, or how to troubleshoot if things don't go as planned.

Providing additional brain support

In addition to this basic protocol above, you may need to bring in additional brain support along the way, as discussed throughout the book. This can include nutritional compounds to dampen brain inflammation, support brain oxygenation, or support neurotransmitter activity. However, dampening overall inflammation, repairing leaky gut, and following the anti-inflammatory diet are foundations that give you the most mileage for your efforts.

CHAPTER SUMMARY

• We are exposed to unprecedented levels of chemicals and heavy metals today, as well as hybridized, genetically modified, and industrially processed foods, all of which activate the immune system. Only a minority of the synthetic compounds introduced to our environment has been researched individually for safety, much less in conjunction with one another.

• Additionally, almost one-third of the U.S. population takes some type of medication and many people take multiple medications. This "polypharmacy" model of taking multiple drugs has diverse and potentially harmful consequences that go beyond adverse reactions and include death and disability.

• Many have theorized that today's skyrocketing incidences of autoimmunity, autism, neurodegenerative diseases, and other chronic inflammatory conditions result from our heavily industrialized, immune-reactive environment.

• One person can have fairly high levels of toxicity and be symptom-free while another person has low levels of contamination yet reacts severely. The issue isn't how many toxins are in your system but whether your immune system reacts to them. This is the mechanism behind chemical intolerance, multiple chemical sensitivities, and toxin-induced brain degeneration mechanisms that are becoming so common today.

• In the literature, this is called "toxicant-induced loss of tolerance," or TILT. When people suffer from TILT, they aren't necessarily sick from heavy metals and chemicals. Instead, they are sick from reacting to them.

• So why do some people develop a chemical intolerance and others don't? Several mechanisms are at work:
  • Poor glutathione activity
  • Breakdown of immune barriers
  • Poor regulatory T-cell function
  • Chronic inflammation

• Loss of chemical tolerance appears to evolve in two stages. The first stage is characterized by a breakdown in the body's natural tolerance to chemicals and heavy metals. In the second stage, an ordinary exposure to an environmental compound suddenly triggers an immune response.

• Although loss of chemical tolerance is a breakdown of the body's self-defense mechanisms, environmental chemicals are partly to blame for this breakdown. A number of compounds have been shown to degrade the immune barriers.

• We can improve chemical intolerance and protect the brain by supporting the immune barriers, immune regulation, and inflammation. The various systems we want to support include:
  • Glutathione levels and recycling
  • Immune barrier health (gut, blood-brain barrier, and lungs)
  • Immune balancing through regulatory T-cell support
  • Inflammation in the body and brain

• Liver detoxification still plays a role in brain health and chemical tolerance. Symptoms of poor liver detoxification:
  • Acne and unhealthy skin

- Bloating
- Swelling
- Hormone imbalances
- Weight gain
- Poor bowel function

- If liver function becomes compromised it can increase your toxic load and your chemical intolerance. Likewise, toxic exposures and the inflammation can then hinder liver metabolic function.

- Nutrients to support healthy liver detoxification:
  - Phase I and Phase II support
  - Phase II methylation support
  - Bile support
  - Detoxification and glutathione support

- When liver detoxification fails, toxicity increases—compounds the liver fails to metabolize go back into circulation in a more toxic form. A serious fallout from this cycle is the activation of NF-kappaB.

- The most effective compounds we've seen for dampening NF-kappaB are high doses of emulsified resveratrol and curcumin given in combination.

Chapter Twenty One
THE BRAIN HEALTH REFERENCE GUIDE

In this section I will go over the bare-bone basics of what you need to know to get your brain back online.

One of the most common complaints I received after the thyroid book came out was that it was too hard to understand or too difficult to implement. The truth is this material is complex and difficult to understand. I have done my best to distill extremely intricate immune and neurological mechanisms into information people can apply, but I agree it may not be easy to grasp at first, even for practitioners (which is why the good practitioners study the material regularly instead of just showing up at seminars). Throw in poor brain function and it can be downright overwhelming.

Although working with a qualified practitioner is frequently necessary, you must realize the bulk of the work falls on your shoulders. Hippocrates said, "Let food be thy medicine and medicine be thy food." When it comes to addressing your brain health, your first and most important step—and probably your most difficult—is changing your diet.

Take charge of your brain by taking charge of your diet

If you want your brain to work you have to change your diet. This can make it more difficult to eat out, eat at friends' houses, grab easy snacks, or eat dirt-cheap. If you are going to complain endlessly, then this program is probably not right for you. Your negative attitude will raise stress levels and inflammatory cytokines. Also, if you are working with a practitioner, he or she will not be able to give you the best care if you derail your progress by eating foods that trigger an inflammatory reaction. If you have an eating disorder, I realize that can make this difficult. That is a topic for a different book, but every effort counts, and it may be worth getting professional help or group support.

That's the bad news. The good news is many, many people experience profound improvement on a stricter diet and love following it. Many also experience devastating rebounds through cheats or accidental exposures, which helps compliance. The other good news is, thanks to the Internet, you can find support and friendship from online tribes of people on the same path.

GO GLUTEN-FREE (CHAPTER EIGHT)

At the very least you should adopt a strict gluten-free diet. No food is a more potent trigger of neurological problems and autoimmunity than gluten.

Standard lab testing for gluten is not reliable, as most labs only test for antibodies to alpha gliadin and intestinal transglutaminase (TG2). A more complete screen, such as Cyrex Labs' Wheat/Gluten Proteome Sensitivity and Autoimmunity Panel Array 3, includes:

- alpha gliadin
- omega gliadin
- gamma gliadin
- deamidated gliadin
- wheat germ agglutinin (WGA)
- gluteomorphin
- prodynorphin
- transglutaminase-2 (TG2)
- transglutaminase-3 (TG3)
- transglutaminase-6 (TG6)

If your brain is not working, a gluten-free diet is your first step toward better brain health.

THE LEAKY GUT DIET (CHAPTER NINE)

In many cases, going gluten-free alone is not enough. Many people, particularly those with autoimmune and neurological issues, have sensitivities to other foods due to cross-reactivity and leaky gut. This is the diet I recommend to people experiencing brain health issues. This diet allows the immune system to rest and the gut to repair, which profoundly impacts brain health as discussed in Chapter Nine.

Length of time on diet

You may only need to follow this diet for a few days to a week after accidental exposure or a slip. Or you may need to follow it for a month or more to repair leaky gut. You can confirm whether you have repaired your leaky gut by using the Cyrex Intestinal Antigenic Permeability Screen. However, many people with autoimmune reactions or brain health issues make this diet or some variation of it a way of life for optimal function.

How often you eat—keeping blood sugar stable is key

A key aspect to this diet is keeping your blood sugar stable. This means you should eat often enough that you do not become hungry or feel your energy crash, which will trigger stress and inflammation. As your blood sugar becomes more stable you may find you can go longer between eating.

Keeping overall carbohydrate consumption low compared to the standard American diet (SAD) is vital to stabilizing blood sugar. The amount of carbohydrates a person needs varies entirely upon the person, his or her lifestyle, and health issues.

Foods to avoid

You avoid these foods because they have been shown to trigger inflammation and stress in many people, which will exacerbate your autoimmune condition, inflammation, and poor brain health.

- ALL sugars and sweeteners, even honey, agave, maple syrup, coconut sugar, date sugar, etc. Do not be deceived by "low-glycemic" sweeteners; they are still high in sugar
- High-glycemic fruits: watermelon, mango, pineapple, raisins, grapes, canned fruits, dates, dried fruits, etc.
- Tomatoes, potatoes, or mushrooms
- Grains: wheat, oats, rice, barley, buckwheat, corn, quinoa, etc.

- Dairy: milk, cream, cheese, butter, whey. Ghee is OK for many people, but it depends on the individual
- Eggs or foods that contain eggs (such as mayonnaise)
- Soy: soy milk, soy sauce, tofu, tempeh, soy protein, etc.
- Alcohol
- Lectins— a major promoter of leaky gut—found in nuts, beans, soy, potatoes, tomato, eggplant, peppers, peanut oil, peanut butter and soy oil, among others
- Instant coffee: Many brands of instant coffee are contaminated with gluten
- Processed foods
- Canned foods

Foods to eat

You need to give yourself more time to shop and prepare so you always have something on hand to eat or when you go out. For resources visit my website.

- Most vegetables (except tomato, potatoes, and mushrooms): asparagus, spinach, lettuce, broccoli, beets, cauliflower, carrots, celery, artichokes, garlic, onions, zucchini, squash, rhubarb, cucumbers, turnips and watercress, among others.
- Fermented foods: sauerkraut, kimchi, pickled ginger, fermented cucumbers, coconut yogurt, kombucha, etc. You will probably need to make your own or buy one of the few brands that are genuinely fermented and free of sugars or additives.
- Meats: fish, chicken, beef, lamb, organ meats, etc. Best choices are grass-fed and pastured meats from a local farm. Second best is organic. Avoid factory-farmed meats that contain antibiotics and hormones. For a source of good meat near you, contact your local Weston A. Price chapter leader.
- Low-glycemic fruits: apricots, plums, apples, peaches, pears, cherries and berries, to name a few.
- Coconut: coconut oil, coconut butter, coconut milk, coconut cream
- Herbal teas
- Olives and olive oil

Food sensitivity panel

You may also choose to do a food sensitivity panel to confirm whether certain foods are causing an immune reaction. The Cyrex Labs Gluten-Associated Sensitivity and Cross Reactive Foods Array 4 tests for these various food reactions.

SUPPLEMENTS TO SUPPORT THE LEAKY GUT DIET (CHAPTER NINE)

This diet is very therapeutic in itself. However, you may want to further support this diet with various nutritional and botanical compounds to tame inflammation and facilitate repair of the gut lining.

Nutrients to support the gut lining

- L-glutamine
- Deglycyrrhizinated licorice
- Aloe leaf extract
- Tillandsia
- Marshmallow extract
- MSM
- Gamma oryzanol
- Slippery elm bark
- German chamomile
- Marigold flower extract

Probiotics

Probiotics can be an important part of modulating the gut's immune system and restoring a healthy balance of gut flora.

- Saccharomyces boulardii
- Lactobacillus sporogenes
- DDS-1 Lactobacilli acidophilus
- Arabinogalactan

Detoxing yeast, bacteria, and parasites

Sometimes eradicating yeast and bacterial overgrowths and parasites is a necessary part of restoring gut health. However, it's also necessary to tread gently in this territory. Too aggressive of a detox makes some people very ill with symptoms of nausea, vomiting, diarrhea, or other effects. Always start slowly and with small doses when taking gut detoxifying compounds.

Yeast and bacterial overgrowth
- Undecylenic acid
- Caprylic acid
- Uva ursi
- Cat's claw
- Pau d'arco

Parasites
- Wormwood extract
- Olive leaf extract
- Garlic extract
- Black walnut extract

H. pylori and bacterial overgrowth
- Berberine
- Yerba mansa
- Oregano extract

STIMULATE THE VAGUS NERVE (CHAPTER NINE)

We know the health of the gut profoundly impacts brain health and function. Likewise, poor brain function can impact gut function by impairing activity of the vagus nerve, which handles communication between the brain and gut. Symptoms of poor vagal function include poor intestinal motility (constipation), poor digestive enzyme production (bloating, indigestion), floating stool or undigested food in stool, and symptoms of poor liver detoxification. You can improve the plasticity and function of the vagus nerve with some simple exercises:

- Gargling: Drink several large glasses of water per day and gargle each sip until you finish the glass of water. You should gargle long enough and deep enough to make it a bit challenging. Do this exercise for several weeks to help strengthen the vagal pathways.
- Sing loudly: Sing as loud as you can when it's appropriate. This works the muscles in the back of the throat to activate the vagus.
- Gag: Lay a tongue blade on the back of your tongue and push down to activate a gag reflex.

Gag reflexes with the tongue depressors are like doing push-ups for the vagus while gargling and singing loudly are like doing sprints. You need to perform them for several weeks to produce change, just as you would with weight training.

Use a coffee enema for poor motility and to improve vagal plasticity

In patients with brain degeneration and regular constipation, I encourage them to perform daily coffee enemas. Purchase an enema bag with an anal insert tube and a lubricant such as KY Jelly. Make organic coffee and cool it to room temperature (avoid instant coffee as it may be contaminated with gluten). Fill the enema bag with coffee and lubricate the anal tip of the tube. You will then need to lie on your right side. It is best to perform this in the bathtub in case you spill anything. Insert the tube into your anus and raise the bag with your hand so it is higher than your head. The higher you raise the bag the faster the bag will empty.

Once the coffee has drained from the bag into your intestines try to hold the contents in your bowel for five to 10 minutes. You will have urges to have a bowel movement, but hold the contents as long as you can.

STABILIZE BLOOD SUGAR (CHAPTER FIVE)

Balancing blood sugar is vitally important to brain health. Symptoms of both low blood sugar and high blood sugar are signs your brain may be suffering from damage caused by a blood sugar imbalance.

SYMPTOMS OF BLOOD SUGAR IMBALANCES

Reactive hypoglycemia symptoms (low blood sugar spikes):
- Increased energy after meals
- Craving for sweets between meals
- Irritability if meals are missed
- Dependency on coffee and sugar for energy
- Becoming lightheaded if meals are missed
- Eating to relieve fatigue
- Feeling shaky, jittery, or tremulous
- Feeling agitated and nervous
- Becoming easily upset
- Poor memory, forgetfulness
- Blurred vision

Insulin resistance symptoms (high blood sugar spikes):
- Fatigue after meals
- General fatigue
- Constant hunger
- Craving for sweets not relieved by eating them
- Must have sweets after meals
- Waist girth equal to or larger than hip girth
- Frequent urination
- Increased appetite and thirst
- Difficulty losing weight
- Migrating aches and pains

Stabilizing blood sugar

- Eat a breakfast of high quality protein and fats.

- If you have hypoglycemia, eat a small amount of protein and/or healthy fat every two to three hours.

- Find your carbohydrate tolerance and stick to it. If you feel sleepy or crave sugar after you eat, you have eaten too many carbohydrates. You can also use a glucometer to check your fasting blood glucose, which ideally should be in the mid- to high-80s, and at least between 80–100.

- Never eat high-carb foods without some fiber, fat, or protein. These will slow down the rate at which the glucose is absorbed into the bloodstream and help prevent "insulin shock."

- Do not eat sweets or starchy foods before bed. This is one of the worst things the hypoglycemic person can do. Your blood sugar will crash during the night, long before your next meal is due. Chances are your adrenals will kick into action, creating restless sleep or that 3 a.m. wake up with anxiety.

- Avoid all fruit juices and carrot juice. These can be more sugary than soda, and will quickly have you crashing.

- Avoid or limit caffeine.

- Eat a well-balanced diet consisting mostly of vegetables, and quality meats and fats.

- Eliminate food allergens and intolerances.

Nutrients to support blood sugar balance

Your diet is the most profound way to stabilize blood sugar. However, certain nutritional compounds can help stabilize hypoglycemia or insulin resistance.

Nutrients to support a healthy response to hypoglycemia (low blood sugar)

- Chromium
- Bovine adrenal gland
- Choline bitartrate
- Bovine liver gland

- Bovine pancreas gland
- Inositol
- L-carnitine
- CoQ10
- Rubidium chelate
- Vanadium aspartate

Nutrients to support a healthy response to insulin resistance (high blood sugar)
- Gymnema sylvestre
- Banaba leaf extract
- Maitake mushroom
- Bitter melon
- Opuntia streptacantha Lemaire
- Guar gum
- Pectin
- Chromium
- Vanadium
- Alpha lipoic acid
- Vitamin E (tocopherols)
- Magnesium
- Biotin
- Zinc
- Inositol
- Niacin
- L-carnitine

Sometimes a person will swing back and forth between insulin resistance and hypoglycemia. In these cases I recommend taking nutritional compounds for insulin resistance with meals, and nutritional compounds for hypoglycemia between meals.

It's important to work with a qualified health care practitioner so you take the right nutrients and botanicals in the right amounts. Taking the wrong nutrients for your blood sugar condition has the potential to make your condition worse.

DAMPEN STRESS (CHAPTER SIX)

If you suffer from the symptoms below, stress may be negatively impacting your brain health:

- Always having projects and things that need to be done
- Never having time for yourself
- Not getting enough sleep or rest
- Not having enough time or motivation to get regular exercise
- Not accomplishing your life's purpose

Reducing inflammation and dampening the stress response are a couple of ways to address the effects of stress on brain health. This means reducing dietary stressors with the leaky gut diet, managing lifestyle stressors, and addressing health imbalances that contribute to stress.

Nutritional compounds to help manage stress
- Phosphatidylserine: Dampens the influence of stress on the brain. You can take it orally, but I prefer liposomal methods of phosphatidylserine delivered through the skin.
- Herbal adrenal adaptogens: Powerful support when chronic stress is a problem. These herbs work on the stress pathways on the brain, particularly in the hippocampus. You can use them individually, but they have a greater synergistic effect when used in combination.
- Panax ginseng extract
- Ashwagandha
- Holy basil extract
- Rhodiola rosea
- Eleuthero

IMPROVE BRAIN CIRCULATION AND OXYGEN (CHAPTER SEVEN)

One of the most vital nutrients for the brain is oxygen. If you suffer from any of the symptoms below your brain may not be getting optimal amounts of oxygen:

- Low brain endurance and poor focus and concentration
- Must exercise or drink coffee to improve brain function
- Cold hands and feet
- Poor nail health or fungal growth on toes
- Must wear socks at night
- White nail beds instead of bright pink
- Cold tip of nose

Chronic stress, anemia, smoking, low blood pressure, high blood pressure, poor lung function, poor cardiovascular function, and any mechanism that impairs blood vessels, such as diabetes, can impair the flow of blood to the brain.

Nutritional compounds for brain oxygenation

Although these herbal compounds have been shown to dilate cerebral arteries, they do not increase blood pressure; in fact they can do the opposite.

- Feverfew extract
- Butcher's broom extract
- Ginkgo biloba
- Huperzine
- Vinpocetine

Nitric oxide

Nitric oxide is a chemical-signaling molecule in the body involved with communication in the nervous, immune, and vascular systems. eNOS and nNOS are anti-inflammatory forms of nitric oxide while iNOS is inflammatory and associated with tissue damage from autoimmune disease.

Raising your heart rate through high-intensity aerobic exercise for at least five minutes in the morning is one way to release anti-inflammatory eNOS. Use good judgment to work within your limits and not harm yourself.

Nutritional compounds that support nitric oxide modulation
- ATP (Adenosine 5'-triphosphate)
- Huperzine A
- Xanthinol niacinate
- Alpha-Glycerylphosphorylcholine (Alpha GPC)
- Vinpocetine
- N-acetyl L-carnitine

Blood pressure
Both low and high blood pressure can impact the amount of oxygen delivered to your brain. Your blood pressure should be around 120/80. If the first or second number is higher or lower by 10 points, then your blood pressure is abnormal. The greater the amount of deviation from 120/80 the worse it is.

Low blood pressure
For patients with low blood pressure I recommend glycyrrhiza, a natural compound from licorice that increases the hormone aldosterone, which helps you retain your sodium and can help raise low blood pressure. Many people can also raise their blood pressure to normal by salting their food, supplementing with licorice root, and managing hypoglycemia.

High blood pressure
If you have high blood pressure you must cut salt from your diet, exercise routinely, and reduce your stress. You can also take natural compounds such as magnesium and potassium to help bring your blood pressure down. Supporting nitric oxide modulation may also help reduce your blood pressure.

DAMPEN BRAIN INFLAMMATION (CHAPTER TEN)

Inflammation in the brain doesn't cause pain, so most people aren't aware it may be an issue for them. However, it accelerates brain degeneration and is associated with the following symptoms:

- Brain fog
- Unclear thoughts
- Low brain endurance
- Slow and varied mental speeds
- Loss of brain function after trauma
- Brain fatigue and poor mental focus after meals
- Brain fatigue promoted by systemic inflammation
- Brain fatigue promoted by chemicals, scents, and pollutants

Brain inflammation is considered a model for chronic depression and other mood disorders. Because the brain's immune cells, microglia, have no off switch, inflammation in the brain can continue long after the insult. Factors that cause brain inflammation include:

- Diabetes and high-carbohydrate diets, which lead to the production of glycosylated end products that activate the microglia cells
- Lack of oxygen from poor circulation, lack of exercise, chronic stress response, heart failure, lung disorder, anemia
- Previous head trauma
- Neurological autoimmune reaction
- Dietary gluten for those who are gluten intolerant
- Low brain antioxidant status
- Alcohol and drug abuse
- Environmental pollutants
- Systemic inflammation
- Inflammatory bowel conditions
- Compromised blood-brain barrier

Leaky brain challenge

You can perform the Leaky Brain Challenge to determine whether your blood-brain barrier is permeable.

Take 800–1,000 mg of GABA and give yourself a two-to-three hour window to see whether it affects you. It is best to take GABA between 6 p.m. and 9 p.m., so you can sleep it off if it sedates you. If GABA causes relaxation, calming, and sedation, don't keep taking it regularly or you risk shutting your GABA receptor sites and a retest won't be accurate.

If the GABA causes anxiety, irritability, or panic this also indicates a permeable blood-brain barrier (for reasons explained in the neurotransmitter section). Eating some protein may help alleviate these symptoms.

Feeling no change after taking GABA is a good sign your blood-brain barrier is intact. GABA should produce no symptoms, as GABA "bounces off" a healthy blood-brain barrier.

Taming brain inflammation

The most important steps to reducing brain inflammation are to address food intolerances, blood sugar imbalances, gut infections and inflammation, unmanaged autoimmune disease, poor brain oxygenation, chronic stress, hormonal imbalances and deficiencies, and more.

While addressing these factors you can use flavonoids that have been shown to dampen the microglia cells and brain inflammation. They include:

- Apigenin
- Luteolin
- Baicalein
- Resveratrol
- Rutin
- Catechin
- Curcumin

MANAGE NEUROLOGICAL AUTOIMMUNITY (CHAPTER ELEVEN)

A common area of autoimmune attack is the brain and the nervous system, which can create diverse symptoms, including weakness, poor brain function, dizziness, burning sensations in the hands and feet, obsessive compulsive disorder, and more. Things to look for include:

• Brain and neurological symptoms with a history or family history of autoimmune disease

• Brain and neurological symptoms at an early age not associated with age-related brain degeneration

• History of celiac disease or gluten sensitivity

• Brain and neurological symptoms and signs with a relapsing and remitting pattern associated with stress, poor sleep, or immune activation

The main clues a person may be suffering from neuroautoimmunity are a history of another autoimmune disease, gluten sensitivity or celiac disease, and symptoms of neurological dysfunction that appear early in life. This includes children and adults under the age of 50, the earliest symptom being autism.

Three stages of autoimmunity

• *Silent autoimmunity:* The immune system is attacking body tissue but does not result in any significant loss of tissue or even symptoms. We can identify silent autoimmunity through elevated tissue antibodies in the blood.

• *Autoimmune reactivity:* The autoimmune reactions have progressed to the point that enough tissue has been destroyed so that signs, symptoms, or loss of function are noticeable. However, the condition is not so advanced as to be labeled an autoimmune disease.

• *Autoimmune disease:* Symptoms and loss of tissue are significant. The loss of tissue is also advanced enough to be identified with imaging studies and other tests, such as nerve conduction studies.

Many people stay in the autoimmune reactivity stage for years without a diagnosis. Some may never develop enough destruction of their nervous system to be diagnosed, yet suffer significant signs and symptoms that impair quality of life. Many eventually progress to various neurological diseases.

Testing for neurological autoimmunity

We identify autoimmunity by screening for antibodies against the proteins of various nerve cell structures. Many labs offer tests for neurological tissue antibodies, but I have found that Cyrex Labs does the most complete and sensitive evaluation. Their neurological autoimmunity panel includes:

- *Myelin basic protein antibodies:* autoimmune reactions to the outer covering of nerve cells

- *Asialoganglioside antibodies:* autoimmune reactions to sugar and protein chain clusters on the surface of nerve cells

- *Alpha and beta tubulin antibodies:* autoimmune reactions to proteins found in neurons

- *Synapsin antibodies:* autoimmune reactions to chemical proteins found within nerve cells that regulate nerve cell communication called a synapse

- *Glutamic acid decarboxylase (GAD) antibodies:* autoimmune reactions to the enzyme in the body that produces the inhibitory neurotransmitter GABA

- *Cerebellum antibodies:* autoimmune reactions to a specific part of the brain called the cerebellum involved with balance and muscle movement calibration

GAD autoimmunity

GAD autoimmunity is the most common neuroautoimmunity and creates the most specific symptoms because it prevents production of GABA, which is responsible for calming the nervous system. Elevated GAD antibodies are linked to OCD, motion sickness, vertigo, autism, and "stiff man syndrome."

In addition to avoiding gluten, people with positive GAD antibodies should also avoid foods high in artificial glutamates.

An autoimmune reaction to GAD is more common among those with a gluten intolerance or celiac disease. Gluten intolerance and celiac disease should always be considered in the case of persistent symptoms of poor GABA activity.

How high are your neurological antibodies?

Antibody levels typically are not clinically significant because antibodies themselves do not destroy tissue. However, researchers have found neurological antibodies themselves are destructive. This is unique in immunology because it means the antibody count indicates the degree of destruction that may be occurring.

Managing neurological autoimmunity

Although there is no cure for autoimmunity it can be modulated, or "tamed" with proper lifestyle, dietary, and nutritional strategies.

You may need to make significant changes to preserve your brain health, such as changing your job, relationship, where you live, or some other important part of life. It is important for you to pay attention to what triggers and dampens your autoimmunity.

Strategies to dampen autoimmunity

Increase opioids: Natural opioids activate TH-3 cells, which helps dampen autoimmunity. A positive mental attitude, love, appreciation for life, positive self-esteem, and healthy levels of exercise are ways to increase opioids. On the other hand, a negative attitude, violence, poor relationships, and internal mental stress are examples of ways to promote IL-6, which activates TH-17 and promotes autoimmunity.

Stabilize blood glucose levels: If you have autoimmunity you cannot let your blood glucose spike or drop sharply. Blood sugar spikes and drops raise IL-6 and TH-17, promoting autoimmunity.

Avoid gluten: Gluten is a potent trigger for neurological autoimmunity for many people.

Improve gut-brain axis: The health of the brain depends on gut health. Addressing gut inflammation and the gut-brain axis can help manage neurological autoimmunity.

Nutritional compounds to dampen neurological autoimmunity

Vitamin D: Vitamin D has been shown to increase TH-3 activity, thus dampening autoimmunity. Typical doses of vitamin D for autoimmunity can be anywhere from 5,000 to 10,000 IU per day.

Test your vitamin D levels with a serum 25-hydroxy vitamin D test. Most people with autoimmunity have low levels of vitamin D when tested. Your level should be around 50 ng/mL. Levels above 100 ng/mL may indicate a vitamin D overload.

Glutathione: Glutathione preserves and protects neurons against inflammation, supports TH-3 responses, supports regeneration of the blood-brain barrier and the intestinal barrier, and is a natural chelator that can bind to environmental compounds such as heavy metals and pollutants.

Glutathione recycling recycles existing glutathione for reuse and raises glutathione levels inside the cells. Compounds that have been shown to support this mechanism include:

- Cordyceps
- N-acetylcysteine
- Gotu kola
- Milk thistle
- L-glutamine
- Alpha lipoic acid

These are all TH-1 and TH-2 neutral and because they support TH-3, they have the potential to dampen an overactive TH-1 or TH-2 response in autoimmunity.

To boost overall levels of glutathione I use S-acetyl-glutathione, a form that can be absorbed orally. Oral doses can start at 300 mg and per day and go up to several thousand milligrams. However, it is not cheap and the amount used may depend on what you can afford. I suggest using about 1000 mg a day in most cases, although I suggest much higher doses in certain conditions. I still recommend liposomal glutathione cream for use in localized areas, such as over an inflamed joint or over the thyroid of someone with an autoimmune thyroid condition.

Resveratrol and curcumin: Curcumin and resveratrol dampen the two major inflammatory pathways in autoimmunity, TH-17 and NF-kappaB. You have to take high enough amounts of each of these in order to notice an effect. In studies subjects were given up to 400 mg of resveratrol and 800 mg of curcumin daily, however the necessary dose is different for everyone, so don't assume that is the correct dose for you.

Compounds to support gut repair and brain inflammation: You may also want to take compounds to support intestinal permeability and dampen brain inflammation, explained in Chapter Nine, the gut-brain axis chapter.

Supplements to avoid: Be sure to avoid supplements made with immune-reactive ingredients (often used as fillers), whole-food supplements that may contain gluten, stimulate the TH-1 or TH-2 systems. Botanicals that stimulate TH-1 include echinacea, astragalus, lemon balm (*melissa officinalis*), and maitake mushrooms. Botanicals that stimulate TH-2 include pine bark extract, grape seed extract, green tea extract, acai berry extract, and Pycnogenol.® These are antioxidant compounds with immune activating properties; however, most flavonoids and nutritional antioxidants do not stimulate immunity.

NEUROTRANSMITTER SUPPORT (CHAPTER TWELVE)

Although neurotransmitter support can often promote brain health, it should not be viewed as a one-size-fits-all approach that will work for everyone or every condition.

Dosing neurotransmitter support

Supporting neurotransmitter activity is dependent on symptoms, not body size. Gradually increase your dose until you notice an improvement. Once you no longer feel any improvement, go back the previous dose at which you felt improvement. How often you take support also varies with the individual.

What if you crash and burn on neurotransmitter support?

If supporting neurotransmitter activity causes intense fatigue or other symptoms it may mean the neurons are too close to threshold. In these cases, use even less while addressing such issues as brain inflammation and oxygenation.

SUPPORT ACETYLCHOLINE (CHAPTER THIRTEEN)

Symptoms of impaired acetylcholine activity include:

- Loss of visual and photographic memory
- Loss of verbal memory
- Memory lapses
- Impaired creativity
- Diminished comprehension
- Difficulty calculating numbers
- Difficulty recognizing objects and faces
- Slowness of mental responsiveness
- Difficulty with directions and spatial orientation

Foods that impact acetylcholine activity are high in natural fats, particularly animal fats (processed vegetable oils are not beneficial to acetylcholine activity).

Foods rich in choline include:

- Liver and organ meats
- Egg yolk
- Beef
- Tofu
- Nuts
- Cream
- Milk with fat (not non-fat or skim milk)
- Fatty cheeses

Nutritional compounds that support acetylcholine activity:
- Alpha-GPC
- Huperzine A (from a standardized extract of *Huperzi serrate*)
- N-acetyl L-carnitine hydrocholride
- Pantothenic acid (as calcium pentothenate)

SUPPORT SEROTONIN ACTIVITY (CHAPTER FOURTEEN)

Symptoms of impaired serotonin activity:
- Loss of pleasure in hobbies and interests
- Feelings of inner rage and anger
- Feelings of depression
- Difficulty finding joy from life pleasures
- Depression when it is cloudy or when there is lack of sunlight
- Loss of enthusiasm for favorite activities
- Not enjoying favorite foods
- Not enjoying friendships and relationships
- Unable to fall into deep restful sleep

Estrogen and serotonin

Estrogen increases serotonin activity in the brain. With symptoms of high serotonin, excess estrogen should be considered. Likewise, low estrogen levels can cause symptoms of low serotonin activity and deficiency.

Nutritional compounds that support serotonin activity:

The following botanicals to increase receptor site sensitivity, ensure the breakdown of used serotonin, and provide necessary cofactors for serotonin production:
- 5-HTP
- Tryptophan
- St. John's wort
- SAMe
- P-5-P

- Niacinamide
- Magnesium citrate
- Methyl B12
- Folic acid

A serotonin-healthy diet

Although certain foods are rich in tryptophan, most Americans, with the exception perhaps of poorly practicing vegans or junk-food vegetarians, eat enough protein-rich foods to supply precursors for all their amino acids, including serotonin. The bigger issue is general brain health, stress, and blood sugar imbalances, which affect how well the brain is able to uptake and use serotonin precursors.

SUPPORT GABA (CHAPTER FIFTEEN)

Symptoms associated with GABA imbalances:

- Feelings of anxiousness or panic for no reason
- Feelings of dread
- Feelings of inner tension and inner excitability
- Feelings of being overwhelmed for no reason
- Restless mind
- Difficulty turning your mind off when you want to relax
- Disorganized attention
- Worry about things you never had thought of before

Nutritional compounds that support GABA activity:

- Valerian root
- Lithium orotate
- Passion flower extract
- L-theanine
- Taurine
- P-5-P, magnesium, zinc, manganese

Autoimmune GABA disorder

Gluten intolerance, celiac disease, and autoimmune diseases can trigger an autoimmune reaction against the enzyme GAD, which is responsible for making GABA. People with a GAD autoimmunity are also more prone to gluten ataxia, a form of gluten intolerance that manifests in the brain. As with Type I diabetes, positive GAD antibodies are an early screening tool for gluten ataxia.

People with positive GAD antibodies should avoid eating gluten and foods high in artificial glutamates, such as MSG. Many people with GAD autoimmunity can react to foods high in glutamates with extreme anxiety, nervousness, migraines, and more.

This mechanism should be considered when people have an autoimmune disease and symptoms of poor GABA activity, especially if those symptoms have been happening for a long time.

Genetic GABA conversion disorder—alpha-ketoglutaric acid challenge

Some people have a genetic disorder that impacts the production of GABA, thus causing increased anxiety. This is a consideration for someone who has had lifelong GABA deficiency symptoms or a history of anxiety in the family.

How do you know if a GABA deficiency is genetic? Take 3,000 to 4,000 mg of alpha-ketoglutaric acid. For someone with no genetic GABA abnormality, taking this supplement will not produce much in the way of symptoms, perhaps a slight energy increase. For the person with the genetic disorder, however, this surge of glutamates combined with the genetic inability to convert them to GABA will cause symptoms of excitability, nervousness, anxiety, and other GABA-deficiency symptoms. For this person, taking GABA support on a regular, lifelong basis may be helpful.

SUPPORT DOPAMINE (CHAPTER SIXTEEN)

Symptoms of low dopamine:

- Inability to self-motivate
- Inability to start or finish tasks
- Feelings of worthlessness
- Feelings of hopelessness

- Lose temper for minor reasons
- Inability to handle stress
- Anger and aggression while under stress
- Desire to isolate oneself from others
- Unexplained lack of concern for family and friends

Nutritional compounds that support dopamine activity

- Mucuna pruriens
- Beta-phenylethylamine (PEA)
- Blueberry extract, selenium, alpha lipoic acid, N-acetylcysteine
- D, L-Phenylalanine (DLPA)
- N-acetyl L-tyrosine
- Vitamin B6—P-5-P

Dopamine and hormones

A common presentation of low dopamine is heavy menstrual cycles in women or low testosterone in men, as well as low libido, erectile dysfunction, and an inability to gain muscle mass. Depression may also be a symptom. Dopamine stimulates luteinizing hormone (LH), a hormone that triggers the release of progesterone in women and testosterone in men. When I see low LH and low progesterone in women and low testosterone in men I always look for dopamine symptoms.

Dopamine and compliance with a protocol

A dopamine-deficient person tends to be non-compliant, which is problematic when there is a need to transition into a new diet or lifestyle change. Although underlying issues most likely drive a dopamine deficiency, I may start with dopamine support right away with these patients to boost their motivation so they can follow through with the rest of the protocol. I ask the spouse or another family member to create a strict schedule of when they need to take their dopamine nutritional compounds, leaving as little as possible to their own direction.

ADDRESS HORMONAL IMBALANCES
(CHAPTER SEVENTEEN)

Symptoms of hormone imbalance in men (any age):

- Low libido
- Fluctuations in mood, brain function, and focus
- Loss of muscle mass
- Sweating attacks (hot flashes in men)

Symptoms of hormone imbalance in perimenopause:

- Alternating menstrual cycle lengths
- Hot flushes and spontaneous sweating
- Fluctuations in mood, brain function, and focus

Symptoms of hormone imbalance in menopause:

- Vaginal dryness, itching, or pain
- Deterioration in mood, brain function, and focus
- Loss of bone density
- Mental fogginess after perimenopause

When hormones become imbalanced you lose neurotransmitter activity, which affects how you feel, function, and view your life. Hormonal imbalances significantly impact brain inflammation and degeneration and considerably speed aging of the brain.

Hormones and neurotransmitters

Poor neurotransmitter activity may stem from a hormonal imbalance. For instance, simply upping nutritional compounds to boost serotonin activity won't go the distance in an estrogen-deficient woman.

- Estrogen impacts serotonin receptors in men and women
- Progesterone impacts GABA receptors in men and women
- Estrogen impacts dopamine receptors in women
- Testosterone impacts dopamine receptors in men
- Estrogen impacts acetylcholine receptors in women
- Testosterone impacts acetylcholine receptors in men

- Thyroid hormones impact all neurotransmitter receptors in men and women

Hormones and brain function and inflammation

Healthy hormone levels have been shown to facilitate neuron branching and plasticity, dampen brain inflammation, slow degeneration, and play a role in neuronal migration, the movement of neurons from one place to another to participate in activity and repair.

Blood sugar and hormones

Hormone replacement therapy can create dangerously high levels of hormones that can cause a host of other problems, such as receptor site resistance and poor communication between the brain and the hormone glands. It's better to first address the root cause of the hormonal imbalances, which the majority of the time is a blood sugar imbalance from a high carbohydrate diet.

High estrogen in men

A high-carbohydrate diet creates insulin surges that increase the enzyme aromatase in men. Found in body fat, aromatase converts testosterone to estradiol, a form of estrogen. The excess estradiol causes insulin resistance in a vicious cycle. Testosterone creams can increase the production of estrogen. These men may develop breasts or hips, cry easily, and experience changes in their motivation, drive, and personality.

High testosterone in women

In women insulin surges from high-carb diets increase the enzyme 17,20 lyase, which increases testosterone production. Excess testosterone causes insulin resistance in a vicious cycle. Common symptoms include PCOS, excess facial hair, and thinning hair on the scalp. The high testosterone also knocks estrogen and progesterone levels out of balance, affecting neurotransmitter activity in the brain and as a result drive, motivation, and personality.

Cholesterol and hormones

Hormone production depends on adequate cholesterol. This is a concern today as the trend in cardiology is to push cholesterol levels below 100. In functional medicine we believe cholesterol under 150 is too low for healthy hormone, brain, and immune function. Clinically we see depression and poor cognition and memory develop in patients with low cholesterol.

Adrenal stress and hormones

Microglia cells use DHEA to make testosterone and estrogen. DHEA is made throughout the body, including by the adrenal glands, the liver, the testes, and the ovaries. However, the majority of DHEA comes from the adrenal glands. Many people suffer from low DHEA due to chronic stress. Although DHEA is necessary, supplementing with DHEA is only recommended for a short period of time and when lab testing shows chronic adrenal fatigue. Unnecessarily supplementing with DHEA can exacerbate the conversion of testosterone to estrogen in men and the production of testosterone in women.

Pregnenolone steal

Pregnenolone is a substance the endocrine system and the brain use to make hormones. In pregnenolone steal, the body "steals" pregnenolone from cholesterol to make more cortisol instead of sex hormones because the adrenals are fatiguing. This mechanism commonly underlies PMS, infertility, male menopause, and PCOS. A blood sugar imbalance is the most common cause of pregnenolone steal.

Low cholesterol, chronic stress, blood sugar imbalances, low DHEA, and pregnenolone steal are factors that impact hormone balance. Functions that suffer as a consequence include neuronal transmission, myelination (the protective coating glia cells offer to neurons), synaptic activity, neuronal repair, and neuronal migration (the movement of neurons to areas where they're needed for activity or repair).

Estrogen and the brain

Studies have shown estrogen to be very protective of the brain. Estrogen that declines too steeply or rapidly can cause depression and loss of some cognitive function, such as spatial memory, and fine motor skills. These factors are behind many menopausal symptoms, including irritability, brain fog, forgetfulness, depression, fatigue, anxiety, stress, insomnia, and a worsening of existing conditions.

Hormone replacement therapy has risks and I believe the underlying mechanism of the imbalance or deficiency should be investigated first. Also, estrogen replacement therapy has not been shown to be protective of the brain in menstruating women. However, for postmenopausal women or women going through menopause who have steep dips in estrogen or chronically low estrogen, hormone replacement therapy can be very protective of the brain.

Progesterone and the brain

Progesterone deficiency in women can result in compromised GABA and dopamine activity. Progesterone also dampens microglia cells. Administering progesterone to a man or woman who has just suffered from a head injury or stroke helps with the repair process in the brain and remyelination of nerves (myelin is a protective nerve coating).

Testosterone and the brain

Testosterone is essential for healthy function of the male brain. Symptoms of testosterone deficiency include loss of cognitive function, memory problems, and the progression of dementia in Alzheimer's disease. Less advanced symptoms include depression, lack of drive or motivation, and general "grumpiness."

Because testosterone influences dopamine activity, testosterone deficiency can increase the risk of Parkinson's disease in a man. Testosterone also influences the activity of acetylcholine and a deficiency can increase the risk of dementia and Alzheimer's disease. Research shows low testosterone increases the secretion of beta amyloid protein, which contributes to Alzheimer's disease.

Hypothyroidism and the brain

The most common symptoms among those with low thyroid function are depression, fatigue, and brain fog. Thyroid function affects brain plasticity, neurotransmitter activity, and general brain function. Thyroid hormones also play a vital role in dampening brain inflammation.

Good synapses for serotonin, dopamine, GABA, and acetylcholine all depend on healthy thyroid function. In fact, many of the neurological symptoms that accompany an unmanaged thyroid condition, such as depression or loss of memory, can be traced back to a breakdown in the neurotransmitter-thyroid connection.

Hashimoto's encephalopathy (HE) is perhaps a worst-case scenario for people with Hashimoto's. Also known as autoimmune dementia, HE is an autoimmune inflammatory brain disorder that causes memory loss and other dementia-like symptoms. HE is suspected when an individual presents with both high TPO antibodies and symptoms of dementia or other neurological disorders. However, because 20 percent of the older population, especially women, may have TPO antibodies, and because myriad other factors can cause neurological symptoms, a practitioner should exercise caution in diagnosing HE.

An unmanaged thyroid condition may accelerate brain degeneration, which is why it is important to appropriately manage hypothyroidism and Hashimoto's, an autoimmune thyroid condition. Simply taking thyroid hormones does nothing to address a deteriorating thyroid condition caused by Hashimoto's, which is responsible for 90 percent of hypothyroid cases in the United States. Nor does it address other causes for the failure of thyroid function, such as chronic stress, high testosterone in women, or environmental toxicity. As explained in my thyroid book, the underlying cause of poor thyroid function should always be addressed to prevent further decline in brain health.

HOW TO GET MORE OUT OF ACUPUNCTURE, CHIROPRACTIC CARE, MASSAGE, AND OTHER FORMS OF BODY WORK AND ALTERNATIVE CARE (CHAPTER EIGHTEEN)

Music, yoga, massage, acupuncture, chiropractic spinal manipulation, aromatherapy, and other therapies stimulate the brain. Both practitioners and patients have seen improvements in immune strength, mood, energy, digestion, hormone regulation, and more through the use of various therapies.

But whether any therapy will positively impact the brain depends on its pre-existing state. Poor diets, hormonal imbalances, autoimmunity, brain inflammation, environmental pollutants, and other factors degenerate the brain and alter its chemistry. As a result, such therapies may not work well because the brain cannot respond significantly enough to affect health. Or the brain may be so degenerated and prone to being overwhelmed that one of these sensory stimulating treatments may fatigue the brain and make the person feel worse.

ESSENTIAL FATTY ACIDS FOR GOOD BRAIN HEALTH (CHAPTER NINETEEN)

Symptoms and signs associated with essential fatty acid deficiency:

- Poor brain function
- Limited consumption of fatty fish, raw nuts and seeds, uncooked olive oil, or avocados
- Regular consumption of fried foods
- Painful joints; chronic pain and inflammation
- Regular consumption of processed foods with partially hydrogenated fats
- Dry or unhealthy skin
- Dandruff
- Hormone imbalances

Processed vegetable oils and hydrogenated fats can make the membranes of your nerve cells rigid and unresponsive, leading to improper neuron function, brain inflammation and degeneration, and symptoms of poor brain function.

Essential fatty acids (EFAs), on the other hand, are critical for healthy brain function.

Recommended omega-6 to omega-3 ratio

Our hunter-gatherer ancestors ate about a 1:1 ratio of omega-6 to omega-3 fats. Today the average American eats a ratio of as high as 25:1 due largely to sunflower, cottonseed, soybean, sesame, and canola oils in processed foods. This imbalance creates a very inflammatory environment that plays a role in many chronic conditions. Researchers recommend a ratio of omega-6 to omega-3 that ranges from 1:1 to 4:1.

How much EFAs to take

Healthy dietary intake of omega 3 is 3,500 mg for a person eating 2,000 calories per day. If you eat 3,000 calories you should take at least 5,250 mg of omega-3 oils daily. The average EFA capsule is only 1,000 mg. That means if you are eating 3,000 calories a day you should take at least 5 to 6 capsules of fish oil a day to support cardiovascular and brain health and reduce the risk of disease.

EPA and DHA

If your goal is mainly to dampen inflammation, then regular fish oil or a fish oil with concentrated EPA is appropriate. However, if your goal is to positively impact the chemical status of your brain, then consider a fish oil with a high concentration of DHA.

I have found individuals with neurochemical imbalances such as depression, mood swings, bipolar reactions, or poor memory derive more benefit when ratios of DHA to EPA are greater than 1:1. I personally like to use ratios greater than 10:1 or 20:1 of DHA to EPA.

TOXINS AND THE BRAIN (CHAPTER TWENTY)

Symptoms of loss of chemical tolerance:

- Intolerance to smells
- Intolerance to jewelry
- Intolerance to shampoo, lotions, detergents, etc.
- Multiple food sensitivities
- Constant skin outbreaks

The issue isn't how many toxins are in your system but whether your immune system reacts to them. This is the mechanism behind chemical intolerance, multiple chemical sensitivities, and toxin-induced brain degeneration mechanisms that are becoming so common today.

Factors that cause loss of chemical tolerance include:
- Poor glutathione activity
- Breakdown of immune barriers
- Poor regulatory T-cell function
- Chronic inflammation

When we suffer from leaky gut, chronic inflammation, hormonal imbalances, chronic stress, and so on, we are just one major stress event away from falling apart. It can be an IRS audit, a divorce, a lawsuit, a car accident, or other trauma. It's important to maintain your immune health and shore up your defenses so you are better able to withstand the chemical assaults and occasional crises life delivers.

Do not chelate if you have loss of chemical tolerance

Research has shown chelation pulls heavy metals out of body tissue and redistributes them so they make their way into the brain, promoting toxicity, inflammation, neurodegeneration, and sometimes serious side effects. Chelation must not be undertaken until a person demonstrates immune barrier integrity and glutathione status is restored.

Testing for loss of chemical tolerance

We can test for loss of chemical tolerance by measuring antibodies to environmental chemicals. Positive antibodies indicate an overzealous immune reaction to environmental chemicals and thus loss of chemical tolerance. Do not confuse testing for antibodies to chemicals with tests that measure the quantity of chemicals and heavy metals as shown in urine, hair, stool, or with a DMPS challenge.

Cyrex Array 11 Chemical Immune Reactivity Screen:
- Aflatoxin antibodies
- Formaldehyde antibodies
- Trimellitic and phthalic anhydride antibodies
- Isocyanate antibodies
- Benzene antibodies
- Bisphenol-A antibodies

- Tetrabromobisphenol-A antibodies
- Tetrachloroethylene antibodies
- Mercury and heavy metals antibodies

Managing loss of chemical tolerance

We can improve chemical tolerance and protect the brain by supporting the immune barriers, immune regulation, and inflammation. All of these systems are talked about throughout the book.

- Glutathione levels and recycling
- Immune barrier health (gut, blood-brain barrier, and lungs)
- Immune balancing through regulatory T-cell support
- Inflammation in the body and brain

The liver's role in chemical tolerance

Although the liver cannot metabolize heavy metals or many environmental compounds, it still plays a role in chemical tolerance. If liver function becomes compromised it can increase your toxic load and your chemical intolerance. Likewise, toxic exposures and inflammation can hinder liver metabolic function.

Symptoms of poor liver detoxification:

- Acne and unhealthy skin
- Bloating
- Swelling
- Hormone imbalances
- Weight gain
- Poor bowel function

When a person's liver Phase II pathway is hindered, two different possibilities exist. One is that an already inflammatory compound, such as an environmental toxin, is made more inflammatory in Phase I. Because a hindered Phase II pathway is not capable of completing the job, this more toxic compound goes back into circulation, where it may activate the immune system and inflammation. The second possibility is that formerly inactive (inactive means it does not react with the immune system) compounds are metabolized into immune reactive compounds.

Nutrients to support healthy liver detoxification

Phase I and Phase II support: The compounds that support these pathways are milk thistle seed extract, dandelion root extract, gotu kola extract, panax ginseng, L-glutathione, glycine, N-acetylcysteine, and DL-methionine. In addition to supporting Phase I and Phase II, these compounds also support blood flow and cell growth in the liver.

Phase II methylation support: Methylation is a Phase II detox pathway also important for healthy brain function. Nutrients that support methylation include choline, trimethylglycine, MSM, beet root, and betaine HCl. These nutrients also support homocysteine metabolism (for an anti-inflammatory effect) and healthy bile synthesis and metabolism.

Bile support: These nutrients support healthy bile synthesis and elimination, to help remove metabolized toxins from the body. They include dandelion root extract, milk thistle seed extract, ginger root, phosphatidylcholine, and taurine.

Detoxification and glutathione support: These nutrients not only support liver detoxification, they also support glutathione levels and recycling, which I talked about earlier in the chapter. They include N-acetylcysteine, cordyceps extract, gotu kola extract, milk thistle seed extract, L-glutamine, and alpha lipoic acid.

When brain function affects liver function

For people with poor vagal tone, doing exercises that stimulate the vagus nerve can help neurologically activate or reboot liver function. This includes vigorous gargling, singing loudly, or engaging the gag reflex, techniques I describe in more detail in Chapter Nine. Symptoms of insufficient vagal tone include poor intestinal motility (constipation), poor digestive enzyme production (bloating, indigestion), floating stool or undigested food in stool, and symptoms of poor liver detoxification.

The liver also requires dopamine to detoxify properly. Sometimes supporting dopamine can make a huge impact on liver function. Symptoms of low dopamine activity (Chapter Sixteen) include depressed thoughts, poor motivation, becoming easily angered, slow movements and thoughts, and poor ability to either start or finish tasks.

IN CONCLUSION: THE BRAIN HEALTH ATTITUDE AND APPROACH

This book is not about "fixing" or "curing" your brain or chronic health problems. Please be wary of health care practitioners who make such claims. It is also not a definitive source of information—research is continually evolving.

We have learned many new things about how to manage chronic conditions since my thyroid book was published in early 2010, and will surely learn much more in the years to come. My books are merely stopping points along the way, adding to an ever-growing pool of health awareness. This book is also not anti-medicine. Do not doggedly refuse medical treatment that could improve your quality of life or prevent a worsening of your health.

Instead, this book is about is exploring the underlying causes of why your brain isn't working, why you have a chronic health problem, or why you don't feel as good as you once did. Far too many people—thousands—have contacted us to say their doctors brush them off, tell them they have depression, or say their lab tests and exams are normal and they're fine. All of these patients are clearly suffering and not functioning well. Just because medicine does not have a diagnosis or a cure for your condition does not mean it doesn't exist!

Many important topics were not included in this book, and your investigations may need to delve into those areas. However, I endeavored to share new information, the result of years of exhaustive research and clinical application, that has helped many patients with "mysterious" and chronic conditions. Although we have many success stories, there are also those patients for whom little could be done. We have much yet to learn. However, I have found when a person knows *why* they are losing function or having symptoms, this can provide an enormous sense of relief. The mind needs something to wrap itself around in order to make sense of the chaos.

It is my sincerest hope the information in this book has helped you or a loved one feel and function better or at least make sense of your condition. You are not crazy, making it up, or suffering from an anti-depressant deficiency. We are experiencing a critical lack of awareness and care for the explosion of chronic neurological and autoimmune cases—the "mystery" conditions—in our population today. Medicine is in desperate need of a revolution to address this population and it can only come from one place: you. Our health care model needs an educated and empowered populace to govern their own health and expect more from their doctors, an advance that will benefit both patients and doctors.

It is my sincerest hope I have helped you become one of those people, and that you in turn will help practitioners like myself continue to learn and grow so we can serve you better.

CHAPTER REFERENCES

INTRODUCTION

[1] Rice C, Schendel D, Cunniff C, Doernberg N. Public health monitoring of developmental disabilities with a focus on the autism spectrum disorders. Am J Med Genet C Semin Med Genet. 2004 Feb 15;125C(1):22-7.

[2] Autism and Developmental Disabilities Monitoring Network Surveillance Year 2008 Principal Investigators; Centers for Disease Control and Prevention. Prevalence of autism spectrum disorders—Autism and Developmental Disabilities Monitoring Network, 14 sites, United States, 2008.

[3] Costello EJ, Mustillo S, Erkanli A, Keeler G, Angold A. Prevalence and development of psychiatric disorders in childhood and adolescence. Arch Gen Psychiatry. 2003 Aug;60(8):837-44.

[4] Mayeux R, Stern Y. Epidemiology of Alzheimer disease. Cold Spring Harb Perspect Med. 2012 Aug 1;2(8).

[5] Kessler RC, Petukhova M, Sampson NA, Zaslavsky AM, Wittchen HU. Twelve-month and lifetime prevalence and lifetime morbid risk of anxiety and mood disorders in the United States. Int J Methods Psychiatr Res. 2012 Aug 1.

CHAPTER TWO: BRAIN PLASTICITY AND HOPE

[1] Iacono D, Markesbery WR, Gross M, Pletnikova O, Rudow G, Zandi P, Troncoso JC. The Nun study: clinically silent AD, neuronal hypertrophy, and linguistic skills in early life. Neurology. 2009 Sep 1;73(9):665-73.

[2] Gosche KM, Mortimer JA, Smith CD, Markesbery WR, Snowdon DA. An automated technique for measuring hippocampal volumes from MR imaging studies. AJNR Am J Neuroradiol. 2001 Oct;22(9):1686-9.

[3] Mortimer JA. The nun study: risk factors for pathology and clinical-pathologic correlations. Curr Alzheimer Res. 2012 Jul 1;9(6):621-7.

[4] Mercier C, Léonard G. Interactions between Pain and the Motor Cortex: Insights from Research on Phantom Limb Pain and Complex Regional Pain Syndrome. Physiother Can. 2011 Summer;63(3):305-14.

[5] Kang SJ, Liu MG, Chen T, Ko HG, Baek GC, Lee HR, Lee K, Collingridge GL, Kaang BK, Zhuo M. Plasticity of Metabotropic Glutamate Receptor-Dependent Long-Term Depression in the Anterior Cingulate Cortex after Amputation. J Neurosci. 2012 Aug 15;32(33):11318-11329.

[6] Mahan AL, Ressler KJ. Fear conditioning, synaptic plasticity and the amygdala: implications for posttraumatic stress disorder. Trends Neurosci. 2012 Jan;35(1):24-35. Epub 2011 Jul 26.

[7] Reagan LP, Grillo CA, Piroli GG. The As and Ds of stress: metabolic, morphological and behavioral consequences. Eur J Pharmacol. 2008 May 6;585(1):64-75. Epub 2008 Feb 26.

[8] Feldman DE. The spike-timing dependence of plasticity. Neuron. 2012 Aug 23;75(4):556-71.

[9] Atkins CM, Selcher JC, Petraitis JJ, Trzaskos JM, Sweatt JD. The MAPK cascade is required for mammalian associative learning. Nat Neurosci. 1998 Nov;1(7):602-9.

[10] Lutz A, Greischar LL, Rawlings NB, Ricard M, Davidson RJ. Long-term meditators self-induce high-amplitude gamma synchrony during mental practice. Proc Natl Acad Sci U S A. 2004 Nov 16;101(46):16369-73.

CHAPTER FOUR: THE NEEDS OF THE NEURON

[1] Accardi G, Caruso C, Colonna-Romano G, Camarda C, Monastero R, Candore G. Can Alzheimer disease be a form of type 3 diabetes? Rejuvenation Res. 2012 Apr;15(2):217-21.

CHAPTER FIVE: BLOOD SUGAR IMBALANCES

[1] Shanmugasundaram ERB, et al. Use of Gynema sylvestre leaf extract in the control of blood glucose in insulin-dependent diabetes mellitus. J Ethanopharmacol 1990; 30: 281-294.

[2] Shanmugasundaram ERB, et al. Use of Gynema sylvestre leaf extract in the control of blood glucose in insulin-dependent diabetes mellitus. J Ethanopharmacol 1990; 30: 281-294.

[3] Persaud SJ, Al-Majed H, Raman A, Jones PM. Gymnema sylvestre stimulates insulin release in vitro by increased membrane permeability. J Endocrinol 1999; 163(2):207-12.

[4] Shanmugasundaram ERB, et al. Possible regeneration of the islet of Langerhans in streptozoticin-diabetic rats given Gynema sylvestre leaf extracts. J Ethnopharmacol 1990 30; 265-279.

[5] Shanmugasundaram KR, et al. Enzyme changes and glucose utilization in diabetic rabbits: the effect of Gymnema sylvestre, R.Br. J Ethnopharmacol 1983;7(2):205-34.

[6] Kaskaran K, et al. Antidiabetic effect of a leaf extract from Gymnema sylvestre in non-insulin dependent diabetes mellitus patients. J Ethnopharmacol 1990; 30: 295-305.

[7] Khare AK, Tondon RN, Tewari JP. Hypoglycemic activity of an indigenous drug (Gymnema sylvestre, 'Gurmar') in normal and diabetic persons. Indian J Physiol Pharmacol 1983;27(3):257-8.

[8] Kakudat T, Sakane L, Takihara T, Ozaki Y, Takeuchi H, and Kuroyanagi M. Hypoglycemic effects of extracts from Lagerstroema speciosa L. leaves in genetically diabetic KK-AY mice. Biosci Biotechno Biochem, 1996; 60:204-208.

9   Murakami C, Myoga K, Kasai R, Othani K, Kurowkasca T, Ishibashi S, Dayrit F, Padolina WG, and Yamaski K. Screening of plant constituents for effect on glucose transport activity in Erlich ascites tumor cells. Chem Pharm Bull (Tokyo), 1993;41:2129-2131.

10   Kubo K, Aoki H, and Nanba H. Anti-diabetic activity present in the fruit body of Grifola frondosa (Maitake). Biol Pharm Bull,1994; 17:1106-1110.

11   Manohar V, Talpur N, Echard BW, Leiberman S, and Preusss HG. Effects of water soluble extract of maitake mushroom on circulating glucose/insulin concentrations in KK mice. Diabetes, Obesity nd Metabolism, 2001.

12   Mizuno T and Zhuang C. Maitake, Grigola frondosa; pharmacologic effects. Food Reviews Int, 1995;11:135-149.

13   Therapeutic Research Faculty. Maitake. In: Natural Medicnes. Comprehensive Database. Stockton, CA, 2001; pp 699-700.

14   Marles,RJ, Farnsworth,NR: Plants as sources of antidiabetic agents. Economic and Medical Plant Research 6:149-187, 1993

15   Marles,RJ, Farnsworth,NR: Antidiabetic plants and their active constituents. Phytomed 2:137-189, 1995

16   Grover,JK, Yadav,S, Vats,V: Medicinal plants of India with anti-diabetic potential. J Ethnopharmacol. 81:81-100, 2002

17   Shapiro,K, Gong,WC: Natural products used for diabetes. J Am Pharm Assoc (Wash.) 42:217-226, 2002

18   Yeh,GY, Eisenberg,DM, Kaptchuk,TJ, Phillips,RS: Systematic review of herbs and dietary supplements for glycemic control in diabetes. Diabetes Care 26:1277-1294, 2003

19   Basch,E, Gabardi,S, Ulbricht,C: Bitter melon (Momordica charantia): a review of efficacy and safety. Am J Health Syst Pharm 60:356-359, 2003

20   Nag,B, Medicherla,S, Sharma,SD: Orally active fraction of momordica charantia, active peptides thereof, and their use in the treatment of diabetes. US Patent 6,391,854:1-14, 2002

21   Basch,E, Gabardi,S, Ulbricht,C: Bitter melon (Momordica charantia): a review of efficacy and safety. Am J Health Syst Pharm 60:356-359, 2003

22   Therapeutic Research Faculty. Prickly Pear Cactus. In : Natural Medicines. Comprehensive Database. Stockton, CA, 2001; pp 858-859.

23   Frait-Munari AC, Gordillo Be, Altamirano P, and Ariza CR. Hypoglycemic effect of Opuntia streptacantha Lemiare in NIDDM. Diabetes Care, 1988; 11:63-66.

24   Gin H, Orgerie MB & Aubertin J: The influence of guar gum on absorption of metformin from the gut in healthy volunteers. Horm metabol Res 1989; 21:81-83.

25   Groop PH, Aro A, Stenman S et al: Long-term effects of guar gum in subjects with non-insulin-dependent diabetes mellitus. Am J Clin Nutr 1993; 58(4):513-518.

26   Grupta A & Singh V: Study of effect of guar gum on long term glycemic control in patients of diabetes mellitus. JAPI 1988; 36(3):204-207.

27 Uusitupa M, Siitonen O, Savolainen K et al: Metabolic and nutritional effects of long-term use of guar gum in the treatment of noninsulin-dependent diabetes of poor metabolic control. Am J Clin Nutr 1989; 49:345-351.

28 Jenkins DJA, Hockaday TDR, Haworth R et al: Treatment of diabetes with guar gum. Lancet 1977; 2(8149): 779-780.

29 Kirsten R, Domning B, Nelson K et al: Long-term blood cholesterol-lowering effects of a dietary fiber supplement. Am J Prev Med 1999; 17(1):18-23.

30 Landin K, Holm G, Tengborn L et al: Guar gum improves insulin sensitivity, blood lipids, blood pressure, and fibrinolysis in healthy men. Am J Clin nutr 1992; 5696):1061-1065.

31 Simons LA, Gyst S, Balasubramania S et al: Long-term treatment of hypercholesterolemia with a new palatable formulation of guar gum. Atherosclerosis 1982; 45:101-108.

32 Biesenbach G, Grafinger P, Janko P, Kaiser W, Stuby U, Moser E. The lipid lowering effect of a new guar-pectin fiber mixture in type II diabetic patients with hypercholesterolemia. Leber Magen Darm. 1993 Sep;23(5):204, 207-9.

33 Gardner DF, Schwartz L, Krista M, Merimee TJ. Dietary pectin and glycemic control in diabetes. Diabetes Care. 1984 Mar-Apr;7(2):143-6.

34 Raven-Haren G, Dragsted LO, Buch-Anderson T, et al. Intake of whole apples or clear apple juice has contrasting effects on plasma lipids in healthy volunteers. Eur J Nutr. 2012, Dec. 28. Epub ahead of print.

35 Striffler JS, Polansky MM, Anderson RA. Overproduction of insulin in the chromium-deficient rat. Metabolism 1999;48:1063-1068.

36 Striffler JS, Polansky MM, et al. Chromium improves insulin response to glucose in rats. Metabolism 1995;44:1314-1320.

37 Anderson RA, Polansky MM, Bryden NA, Canary JJ. Supplemental-chromium effects on glucose, insulin, glucagon, and urinary chromium losses in subjects consuming controlled low-chromium diets. Am J Clin Nutr 1991:54:909-916.

38 Offenbacher EG, Pi-Sunyer FX. Beneficial effect of chromium-rich yeast on glucose tolerance and blood lipids in elderly subjects. Diabetes 1980; 29:919-925.

39 Riales R, Albrink MJ. Effect of chromium chloride supplementation on glucose tolerance and serum lipids including high-density lipoprotein of adult men. Am J Clin Nutr 1981;34:2670-2678.

40 Evans GW, Browman TD. Chromium picolinate increases membrane and rate of insulin internalization. J Inorg Bio 1992;46:243-250.

41 Roeback, Jr. JR, Hla KM, Chambless, et al. Effects of chromium supplementation on serum high density lipoprotein cholesterol levels in men taking beta-blockers. Ann Intern Med. 1991:115:917-924.

42 Anderson R, Cheng N, Bryden, et al. Beneficial effects of chromium for people with type II diabetes. Diabetes. 1996;45:124A.

43 Anderson RA, Cheng N, Bryden NA, et al. Elevated intakes of supplemental chromium improve glucose and insulin variables in individuals with type 2 diabetes. Diabetes 1997;46:1786-1791.

[44] Levine R, Streeten D, Doisy R. Effect of oral chromium supplementation on the glucose tolerance of elderly human subjects. Metabolism 1968; 17:114-125.

[45] French RJ, Jones PJ. Role of vanadium in nutrition: metabolism, essential and dietary considerations. Life Sciences. 1992;52:339-346.

[46] Shechter, Li Meyerovitch, et al. Insulin-like actions of vanadate are mediated in an insulin receptor independent manner via non-receptor protein tyrosine kinases and protein phosphotyrisine phosphates. Mol Cell Biochem. 1995;153(1-2):39-47.

[47] Halberstm M, Cohen N, Shlimovish P, et al. Oral vanadyl sulfate improves insulin sensitivity NIDDM but not in obese nondiabetic subjects. Diabetes. 1996;45:659-665.

[48] Boden G, Chen X, Ruiz J, et al. Effects of vanadyl sulfate on carbohydrate and lipid metabolism in patients with non-insulin dependent diabetes mellitus. Metabolism. 1996;45:1130-1135.

[49] Cohen N,Halberstam M, Shlimovih P, et al. Oral vanadyl sulfate improves hepatic and peripheral insulin insensitivity in patients with non-insulin dependent diabetes mellitus. J Clin Invest. 1995;95:2501-2509.

[50] Goldfine AB, Simonson DC, Folli F, et al. Metabolic effects of sodium metavandate in humans with insulin-dependent and noninsulin-dependent diabetes mellitus in vivo and vitro studies. J Clin Enco and Meta. 1995;80(11);3311-3319.

[51] Shang H, Osada K, Maebashi M, et al. A high biotin diet improves the impaired glucose tolerance of long-term spontaneously hyperglycemic rats with non-insulin dependent diabetes mellitus. J Nutr Sci Vitamin 1996;42:517-526.

[52] Jacob S, Henriksen EJ, Schiemann AL, et al. Enhancment of glucose disposal in patients with Type 2 diabetes by alpha-lipoic acid. Arzneim-Rosch Drug Res 1995;45(2):872-874.

[53] Jacob S, Streeper RS, Fogt DL, et al. The antioxidant alpha-lipoic acid enhances insulin-stimulated glucose metabolism in insulin resistant rate skeletal muscle. Diabetes 1996;45:1024-1029.

[54] Streeper RS, Henriksen EJ, Jacob S, et al. Differential effects of lipoic acid stereoisomers on glucose metabolism in insulin resistant skeletal muscle. Am J Physiol 1997;273:E185-E191.

[55] Konard T, Vicini P, Kuster K, et al. Alpha-lipoic acid treatment decreases serum lactate and pyruvate concentrations and improves glucose effectiveness in lean and obese patients with type 2 diabetes. Diabetes Care 1999;22(2):280-287.

[56] Rudich A, Tirosh A, Potashinik R, Khamaisi M, Bashan N. Lipoic acid protects against oxidative stress induced impairment in insulin stimulation of protein kinase B and glucose transport in 3T3-L1 adipocytes. Diabeologia 1999;42:949-957.

[57] Kawabata T and Packer L. Alpha-lipoate can protect against glycation of serum albumin, bu nto low density lipoprotein. Biochem Biophys Res Comm 1994;203:99-104.

58 Jacob S, Ruus P, Hermann R, et al. Improvement of insulin-stimulated glucose-disposal in type 2 diabets after repeated patenteral administration of thioctic acid. Exp Clin Endocrinol Diabetes 1996;104:284-288.

59 Jacob S, Ruus, Herman R, et al. Oral administration of RAC-alpha-lipoic acid modulates insulin sensitivity in patients with type-2 diabetes: a placebo-controlled pilot trial. Free Radic Biol Med 1999;27:309-314.

60 Nagamstsu M, et al. Lipoic acid improves nerve blood flow, reduces oxidative stress, and improves distal nerve conduction in experimental diabetic neuropathy. Diabetes Care 1995;18:1160-1167.

61 Paolisso G, D'Amore A, Galzenano D. Daily vitamin E supplementations improve metabolic control but not insulin secretion in elderly type II diabetic patients. Diabetes Care 1993;16:1433-1437.

62 Salonen JT, Jyyssonen K, Tuomainen TP. Increased risk of non-insulin diabetes mellitus at low plasma vitamin E concentrations. A four year follow-up study in men. Br Med J 1995;311:1124-1127.

63 Barbagallo M, Dominquez LJ, Tagliamonte MR, et al. Effects of vitamin E and glutathione on glucose metabolism: role of magnesium. Hypertension 1999;34:1002-1006.

64 Paolisso G, D'Amore A, Guigliano D, et al. Pharmacologic doses of vitamin E improves insulin action in healthy subjectsand in non-insulin-dependent diabetic patients. Am J Clin Nutr 1993;57:650-656.

65 Paolisso G, Gambardella A, Giugilano D, et al. Chronic intake of pharmacological doses of vitamin E might be useful in the therapy of elderly patients with coronary heart disease. Am J Clin Nutr 1995;81:848-852.

66 Jain SK, McVie R, Jaramillo JJ, et al. Effect of modest vitamin E supplementation on blood glycated hemoglobin and triglyceride levels and red cell indices in type I diabetic patients. J Amer Col Nutr 1996; 15(5);458-461.

67 Paolisso G, Ravussin E. Intercellular magnesium and insulin resistance; results in Pima Indians and Caucasians. J Endocrinol Metab 1995;80:1382-1385.

68 Paolisso G, Sgambato S, Pizza G, et al. Improved insulin response and action by chronic mangnesium administration in aged NIDDM subjects. Diabetes Care 1989:12;265-269.

69 Paolisso G, Sgambato S, Gambardell A, et al. Daily magnesium supplements improve glucose handeling in elderly subjects. Am J Clin Nutr 1992;55:1161-1167.

70 Nadler JL, Buchanan T, Natarajan R, et al. Magnesium deficiency produces insulin resistance and increased thromboxne synthesis. Hypertension 1993;21:1024-1029.

71 Humphries S, Kushner H, Falkner B. Low dietary magnesium is associated with insulin resistance in a sampling of young, nondiabetic Black Americans. Am J Hypertens 1999;12:747-756.

72 Dominguez LJ, Barbagallo M, Sowers JR, Resnick LM. Magnesium responsiveness to insulin and insulin-like growth factor I in erthrocytes from normotensive and hypertensive subjects. J Clin Endocrinol Metab 1998;83:4402-4407.

[73] Reddi A, DeAngelis B, Frank O, et al. Biotin Supplementation improves glucose and insulin tolerances in genetically diabetic KK mice. Life Science 1998;42:1323-1330.

[74] Kutosikos D, Fourtounas C, Kepetanaki A, et al. Oral glucose tolerance test after high-dose i.v. bioitin administration in normoglucemic hemodialysis paitents. Ren Fail 1996;18:131-137.

[75] Shang H, Osada K, Maebashi M, et al. A high biotin diet improves the impaired glucose tolerance of long-term spontaneously hyperglycemic rats with non-insulin-dependent diabetes mellitus. J Nutr Sci Vitamin 1996;42:517-526.

[76] Maebashi M, Makino Y, Furukawa Y, et al. Therapeutic evaluation of the effect of biotin on hyperglycemia in patients with non-insulin dependent diabetes mellitus. J Clin Biochem Nutr 1993;14:211-218.

[77] Hegazi SM. Effects of zinc supplementation on serum glucose, insulin, glucagons, glucose-6-phosphate, and mineral levels in diabetics. J Clin Biochem Nutr 1992;12:209-215.

[78] Mooradian AD, Morley JE. Micronutrient status in diabetes mellitus. Am J Clin Nutr 1987;45:877-895.

[79] Chen MD, Lin PY, Lin Wh. Investigation of relationship between zinc and obesity. Kao Hsiung I Hsueh Tsa Chih 1991;7:628-634.

[80] Singh RB, Niaz MA, Rastogi SS, et al. Current zinc intake and risk of diabetes and coronary artery diseasse and factors associated with insulin resistance in rural and urban populations of North India. J Am Col Nutr 1998;17:564-570.

[81] Leslie RDG, Elliot RB. Early environmental events as a cause of IDDM. Diabetes 1994;43:843-850.

[82] Urberg M, Zemel MB. Evidence of synergism between chromium and nicotinic acid in the control of glucose tolerance in elderly humans. Metabolism 1987;36:574-576.

[83] Pocoit F, Reimers JI, Anderson HU. Nicotimaminde – biological action and therapeutic potential in diabetes prevention. Diabetologia 1993;36:574-576.

[84] Clearly JP. Vitamin B3 in the treatment of diabetes mellitus: case reports and review of the literature. J Nutr Med 1990;1:217-225.

[85] Pozzilli P, Andreani D. The potential role of nicotinimide in the secondary prevention of IDDM. Diabetes Metabol Rev 1993;9:219-230.

[86] Anderson HU, Jorgensen KH, Egeberg J. Nicotinamide prevents interleukin-1 effects on accumulated insulin release and nitric oxide production in rat islets of langerhans. Diabetes 1994;43:770-777.

[87] Heller W, Mushi HE, Gaebel G, et al. Effect of L-carnitine on post-stress metabolism in surgical paitents. Infusiosther Klin Ernahr 1986;13:268-276.

[88] Gunal AI, Celiker H, Donder E, Gunal SY. The effect of L-carnitine on insulin resistance in hemodialysed patients with chronic renal failure. J Nephrol 1999;12:38-40.

[89] Mingrone G, Greco AV, Capristo E, et al. L-carnitine improves glucose disposal in type 2 diabetic patients. J Am Coll Nutr 1999;18:77-82.

90 Greco AV, et al. Effect of propionyl-L-carnitine in the treatment of angiopathy: Controlled double blind trial versus placebo. Drugs Exp Clin Res 1992;18:69-80.

91 Abdel-Aziz MT, Abdou MS, Soliman K, et al. Effects of L-carnitine on blood lipid patterns in diabetic patients. Nutr Rep Int 1984;29:1071-1079.

CHAPTER SIX: STRESS AND THE BRAIN

1 Tavanti M, Battaglini M, Borgogni F, Bossini L, Calossi S, Marino D, Vatti G, Pieraccini F, Federico A, Castrogiovanni P, De Stefano N. Evidence of diffuse damage in frontal and occipital cortex in the brain of patients with post-traumatic stress disorder. Neurol Sci. 2012 Feb;33(1):59-68.

2 Esposito P, Gheorghe D, Kandere K, Pang X, Connolly R, Jacobson S, Theoharides TC. Acute stress increases permeability of the blood-brain-barrier through activation of brain mast cells. Brain Res. 2001 Jan 5;888(1):117-127.

3 Yates KF, Sweat V, Yau PL, Turchiano MM, Convit A. Impact of metabolic syndrome on cognition and brain: a selected review of the literature. Arterioscler Thromb Vasc Biol. 2012 Sep;32(9):2060-7.

4 Zhang L, Zhou R, Li X, Ursano RJ, Li H. Stress-induced change of mitochondria membrane potential regulated by genomic and non-genomic GR signaling: a possible mechanism for hippocampus atrophy in PTSD. Med Hypotheses. 2006;66(6):1205-8.

5 Hatfield CF, Herbert J, van Someren EJ, Hodges JR, Hastings MH. Disrupted daily activity/rest cycles in relation to daily cortisol rhythms of home-dwelling patients with early Alzheimer's dementia. Brain. 2004 May;127(Pt 5):1061-74.

6 Onen F, Onen SH. [Sleep rhythm disturbances in Alzheimer's disease]. Rev Med Interne. 2003 Mar;24(3):165-71.

7 Kessler RC, Berglund PA, Coulouvrat C, Hajak G, Roth T, Shahly V, Shillington AC, Stephenson JJ, Walsh JK. Insomnia and the performance of US workers: results from the America insomnia survey. Sleep. 2011 Sep 1;34(9):1161-71. Erratum in: Sleep. 2011;34(11):1608. Sleep. 2012 Jun;35(6):725.

8 Yaffe K, Tocco M, Petersen RC, Sigler C, Burns LC, Cornelius C, Khachaturian AS, Irizarry MC, Carrillo MC. The epidemiology of Alzheimer's disease: laying the foundation for drug design, conduct, and analysis of clinical trials. Alzheimers Dement. 2012 May;8(3):237-42.

9 Haas HS, Schauenstein K. Neuroimmunomodulation via limbic structures—the neuroanatomy of psychoimmunology. Prog Neurobiol. 1997 Feb;51(2):195-222.

10 Kiecolt-Glaser JK, McGuire L, Robles TF, Glaser R. Emotions, morbidity, and mortality: new perspectives from psychoneuroimmunology. Annu Rev Psychol. 2002;53:83-107.

11 Robson P. Elucidating the unexplained underperformance syndrome in endurance athletes: the interleukin-6 hypothesis. Sports Med. 2003;33(10):771-81.

[12] Rosa Neto JC, Lira FS, Venancio DP, Cunha CA, Oyama LM, Pimentel GD, Tufik S, Oller do Nascimento CM, Santos RV, de Mello MT. Sleep deprivation affects inflammatory marker expression in adipose tissue. Lipids Health Dis. 2010 Oct 30;9:125.

[13] O'Reilly S, Ciechomska M, Cant R, Hügle T, van Laar JM. Interleukin-6, its role in fibrosing conditions. Cytokine Growth Factor Rev. 2012 Jun;23(3):99-107. Epub 2012 May 5.

[14] Harrison NA, Brydon L, Walker C, Gray MA, Steptoe A, Critchley HD. Inflammation causes mood changes through alterations in subgenual cingulate activity and mesolimbic connectivity. Biol Psychiatry. 2009 Sep 1;66(5):407-14.

[15] Bob P, Raboch J, Maes M, Susta M, Pavlat J, Jasova D, Vevera J, Uhrova J, Benakova H, Zima T. Depression, traumatic stress and interleukin-6. J Affect Disord. 2010 Jan;120(1-3):231-4.

[16] Chiu IM, von Hehn CA, Woolf CJ. Neurogenic inflammation and the peripheral nervous system in host defense and immunopathology. Nat Neurosci. 2012 Jul 26;15(8):1063-7. doi: 10.1038/nn.3144.

[17] Levine JD, Moskowitz MA, Basbaum AI. The contribution of neurogenic inflammation in experimental arthritis. J Immunol. 1985 Aug;135(2 Suppl):843s-847s.

[18] Kelly GS. Nutritional and botanical interventions to assist with the adaptation to stress. Altern Med Rev. 1999 Aug;4(4):249-65.

[19] Singh B, Saxena AK, Chandan BK, Gupta DK, Bhutani KK, Anand KK. Adaptogenic activity of a novel, withanolide-free aqueous fraction from the roots of Withania somnifera Dun. Phytother Res. 2001 Jun;15(4):311-8.

[20] Rege NN, Thatte UM, Dahanukar SA. Adaptogenic properties of six rasayana herbs used in Ayurvedic medicine. Phytother Res. 1999 Jun;13(4):275-91.

[21] Azmathulla S, Hule A, Naik SR. Evaluation of adaptogenic activity profile of herbal preparation. Indian J Exp Biol. 2006 Jul;44(7):574-9.

[22] Nocerino E, Amato M, Izzo AA. The aphrodisiac and adaptogenic properties of ginseng. Fitoterapia. 2000 Aug;71 Suppl 1:S1-5.

CHAPTER SEVEN: BRAIN CIRCULATION AND OXYGEN

[1] Plassman BL, Langa KM, McCammon RJ, Fisher GG, Potter GG, Burke JR, Steffens DC, Foster NL, Giordani B, Unverzagt FW, Welsh-Bohmer KA, Heeringa SG, Weir DR, Wallace RB. Incidence of dementia and cognitive impairment, not dementia in the United States. Ann Neurol. 2011 Sep;70(3):418-26.

[2] Culotta E, Koshland DE Jr. NO news is good news. Science. 1992;258:1862-5.

[3] Southan GJ, Szabo C. Selective pharmacological inhibition of distinct nitric oxide synthase isoforms. Biochem Pharmacol. 1996;51(4):383-94.

[4] Song W, Kwak HB, Kim JH, Lawler JM. Exercise training modulates the nitric oxide synthase profile in skeletal muscle from old rats. Journal of Gerentology. Biological Sciences. 2009;64(5):540-549.

5   Nevzorova VA, Zakharchuk NV, Plotinokova IV. The state of cerebral blood flow in hypertensive crises and possibilities of its correction. Kardiologia. 2007;47(12):20-3.

6   Miyata n. Yamaura H. Tanaka M, Murmastsu M, Tsuchida K, Okuyma S, Otomo S. Effects of VA-045, a novel apovincaminic acid derivative, on isolated blood vessels: cerebroarterial selectivity. Life Sci.1993:51(18):PL181-6.

7   Szober A, Klein M. Examination of the relative fluidity in cerebrovascular disease patients. Ther Hung 1992:40(1):8-11.

8   Bagoly E, Fehr G, Szapary L. The role of vinpocetine in the treatment of cerebrovascular disease based in human studies. Orb Hetil. 2007;148(29):1353-8.

9   Evgenov OV, Busch CJ, Evgenov NV, et al. Inhibition of phosphodiesterase 1 augments the pulmonary vasodilator response to inhaled nitric oxide in awake labs with acute pulmonary hypertension. Am J Physiol Lung Cell Mol Physiol. 2006;290(4):L723-L729.

10 Mancina R, Filippi s, Marini M, et al. Expression and functional activity of phosphodiesterase type 5 in human and rabbit vas deferens. Mol Hum Reprod. 2005;11(2):107-115.

11 Oiu Y, Kraft P, Craig Ec, et al. Identification and functional study of phosphodiesterases in rat urinary bladder. Urol Res. 2001;29(6):388-92.

12 Kim D, Rybalkin SD, Pi X. Upregualtion of phosphodiesterase 1A1 expression is associated with development of nitrate tolerance. Circulation. 2001. 104(19):2263-5.

13 Peyter AC, Muehlethaler V, Liaudet L. Muscarinic receptor M1 phosphodiesterase 1 are key determinants in pulmonary vascular dysfunction following perinatal hypoxia in mice. Am J Physiol Lung Cell Mol Physiol. 2008;295(1):L201-213.

14 Kedia Gt, Ucker T S, Kedia M, Kuczyk MA. Effects of phosphodiesterase inhibitors on contraction induced by endothelin-1 of isolated human prostatic tissue. Urology.2009;73(6):1397-1401.

15 Souness Je, Brazdil R, Diocee BK, Jordan R. Role of selective cyclic GMP phosphodiesterase inhibition in the myorelaxant actions of M&B 22, 948, MY-5455, vinpocetine and 1-methyl-3-isobutyl-8-(methylamino)xanthine. Br J Pharmacol. 1989. 98(3):725-34.

16 Loew D. Value of Ginkgo biloba in treatment of Alzheimer's dementia. Wein Med Wochenschr. 2002;152(15-16):418-22.

17 Jezova D, Duncko R, Lassanova M, Kriska M, Moncek F. Reduction of rise in blood pressure and cortisol release during stress by Ginkgo biloba extract (EGb 761) in healthy volunteers. J Physiol Pharmacol. 2002;53(30:337-48.

18 Umegaki K, Shinozuka K, Wataarai K, Takenaka H, Yoshiura M, Daohua P, Esashi T. Ginkgo biloba extract attenuates the development of hypertension in deoxycorticosterone acetate-salt hypertensive rats. Clin Exp Pharmacol Physiol. 2000;27(4):277-82.

19 Oberpichler H, Beck T, Adel-Rahman MM, Bielenberg GW, Krieglstein J. Effects of Ginkgo biloba constituents related to protection against brain damage caused by hypoxia. Pharmacol Res Commun.1988:20(5):349-68.

20 Agretesch HJ, Dagnelie PC, et al. Adensoine triphosphate, established and potential clinical applications. Drugs. 1999;58:211-232.

21 Williams M, Bagwat SS. P2 purinoceptors: a family of novel therapeutic targets. Annual Reports in Medicinal Chemistry. 1996;31:21-30.

22 Haskell CM, Wong M, Williams A, and Leee LY. Phase 1 trial of extracellular adenosine 5'-triphosphate in patients with advanced cancer. Medicinal and Pediatric Oncology. 1996;27:165-173.

23 Mortensen DP, Gonzalez-Alonso J, Bune LT, et al. ATP-induced vasodilation and purinergic receptors in the human leg: roles of nitric oxide, prostaglandins and adenosine. Am J Physiol Regul Integr Comp Physiol. 2009;296:R1140-R1148.

24 Yegutkin GG, Henttiner T, Jalkanen S. Extracellular ATP formation on vascular endothelial cells is mediated by ectonucleotide kinase activities via phosphotransfer reactions. FASEB. 2001;15:251-260.

25 Persechini PM, Bisaggio RC, Alves Neto JL, Coutinho-Silva R. Extracellular ATP in the lymphohematopoiectic system: P2Z purinoceptors and membrane permeabilization. Braz J of Med and Bio Res.1998;31(1):25-34.

26 Silva G, Beierwaltes WH, Garvin JL. Extracellular ATP stimulates NO production in rat thick ascending limb. Hypertension.2006;47(3):563-7.

27 Tongguang W, Guangxiang H, Shuanke W, et al. Effects of extracellular ATP on survival of sensory neurons in the dorsal root ganglia of rats. J Tongi Med Univ. 2001;21(1):44-7.

28 McCullough WT, Collins DM, Ellsworth ML. Arteriolar responses to extracellular ATP in striated muscle. Am J Physiol Heart Cir Physiol. 1997;272:H1886-H1891.

29 Tonetti M, Sturia L, Bistolfi T, Benatti U, De Flora A. Extracellular ATP potentiates nitric oxide synthase expression induced by lipopolysaccharide in RAW 264.7 murine macrophages. Biochem Biophys Res Commun. 1994;203(1):430-5.

30 Li W, Mak M, Jian H, et al. Novel anti-Alzheimer's dimmer Bis(7)-cognition: cellular and molecular mechanisms of neuroprotection through multiple targets. Neurotherapeutics. 2009: 6(1):187-201.

31 Li J , Wu HM, Zhou RL, Liu GJ, Dong BR. Huperzine A for Alzheimer's disease. Cochrane Database Sys Rev. 2008:16(2):CD005592.

32 Wang ZF, Tang XC. Huperzine A protects C6 rat glioma cells against oxygen-glucose deprivation –induced injury. FEBS Lett. 2007;581(4):596-602.

33 Zhao HW, Li XY. Ginkgolide A, B, and huperzine A inhibit nitric oxide-induced neurotoxicity. Int Immunopharmacol. 2002;2(11):1551-6.

34 Wang ZF, Tang XC. Huperzine A protects C6 rat glioma cells against oxygen-glucose deprivation –induced injury. FEBS Lett. 2007;581(4):596-602.

35 Pavlov VA, Parrish WR, Rosas-Ballina M. Brain acetylcholinesterase activity controls systemic levels through the cholinergic anti-inflammatory pathway. Brain Behav Immun. 2009;23(1):41-5.

36 Wang ZF, Wang J, Zhang HY, Tang XC. Huperzine A exhibits anti-inflammatory and neuroprotective effects in a rat model of transient focal cerebral ischemia. J Neurochem. 2008;106(4):1594-603.

37 Seiwart H, Winterfeld HJ, Strangeld, et al. Effect of a 3-month interval running exercise in combination with vasodilative therapy on microcirculation of the lower leg in peripheral arterial circulation disorders (stage I and II). ZFA.1983;38(5):377-81.

38 Bieron K, Swies J, Kostka-Trabka E, Gryglewski RJ. Thrombolytic and anti-platelet action of xanithinol nicotinate (Sadmin):possible mechanisms. J Physiol Pharmacol. 1998:49(2):241-9.

39 Sharma PL. Comparative effects of placebo and plain and slow-slow release tablets of xanithinol nicotinate on exercise tolerance in normal subjects. Int J Clin Pharmacol Biopharm. 1978;16(1):19-21.

40 Starikov VI. The use of antioxidants and preparations improving the microcirculation in the surgical treatment of cancer of the lung in elderly patients. Klin Khir. 1991;10:4-6.

41 Gomez RD, Rojad HE. Therapeutic results with xanithine derivatives in the intermittent claudication syndrome in diabetic patients. Rev Clin Esp. 1988:182(1):3-6.

42 Janaki S. Pentoxifylline in strokes: a clinical study. J Int Med Res. 1980: 8(1):56-62.

43 Mensen H. Rehabilitation course in patients with peripheral and coronary angioorganopathies. Studies with special reference to serum uric acid and cholesterl under xanthinol nicotinate. Ther Ggw. 1977:116(10):1853-81.

44 Lopez Cm, Govoni S, Battaini F, et al. Effect of a new cognition enhancer alpha-glycerlphosphorylcholine, on scopolamine induced amnesia and brain acetylcholine. Pharmacol Biochem Behav 1991;39(4):835-40.

45 Sigala S, Imperato A , Rizzoneli P, et al. L-alpha glycerylphosphorylcholine antagonizes scopolamine-induced amnesia and enhances hippocampal cholinergic transmission in the rat. Eur J Pharmacol 1992;211(3):351-8.

46 Sterin-Borda L, Echague AV, Leiros CP,et al. Endogenous nitrix oxide signaling system and the cardiac muscarinic acetylcholine receptor-inotropic response. Br J of Pharm. 1995;115:1525-1531.

47 Graves AR, Lewin KA, Lindgren CA. Nitrix oxide, camp and the biphasic muscarinic modulation of Ach release at the lizard neuromuscular junction. J Physiol. 2004;559.2:423-432.

48 Lindgren CA, Younk KM. The inhibition of Ach release by muscarinic agonists at the neuromuscular junction required nitric oxide synthesis. Soc Neurosci Abstr. 2002;28:838.3.

49 Lindgren CA, Graves AR, Lake B. Nitric oxide is necessary but not sufficient for the biphasic muscarinic modulation of synaptic transmission at the lizard neuromuscular junction. Soc Neurosci Abstr. 2003:29:168.11

50 Zyad Rm, Qazi S, Morton DB, Trimmer, BA. Nicotinic-acetylcholine receptors are functionally coupled to the nitric oxide/cGMP-pathways in insect neruons. J neurochem. 2002;83(2):421-431.

51 Arvalho FA, Martine-Silva J, Mesquirea r, Salanha C. Acetylcholine and choline effects on erthrocyte nitrite and nitrate levels. J Appl Tox.2004:24(6): 419-427.

52 Redman DA. Ruscus aculeatus (Butcher's broom) as a potential treatment for orthostatic hypotension, with case report. J Altern Complement Med. 2000; 6(6):539-49.

53 Bouskela E, Cyrino FZ, Marcelon G. Possible mechanisms for the inhibitory effect of Ruscus extract on increased microvascular permeability induced by histamine in haster cheek pouch. J Cardivasc Pharmacol. 1994;24(2):281-5.

54 Bourkela E, Cyrino FZ, Marcelon G. Effects of Ruscus extract on the internal diameter of arterioles and venules of the hamster cheek pouch microcirculation. J Cardivasc Pharmacol. 1993:22(2):221-4.

55 Prusinski A, Durko A, Niczyporuk-Turek A. Feverfew as a prophylactic treatment of migraine. Neurol Neurochir Pol. 1999: 33(5):89-95.

56 Ernst E, Pittler MH. The efficacy and safety of Feverfew (tanacetum parthenium L.): an update of a systematic review. Public Health Nutr. 2000. 3(4A):509-14.

57 Evans RW, Taylor FR. "Natural" or alternative medication for migraine prevention. Headache. 2006:46(6):1012-8.

58 Henneicke-von-Zepelin HH. Feverfew for migraine prophylaxis. Headache. 2006:46(3):531.

59 Diener HC, Pfaffenrath VJ, Schnitker J, Friede M, Henneicke-von-Zepelin HH. Efficacy and safety of 6.25 mg t.i.d. feverfew CO2 extract (MIG-99) in migraine prevention—a randomized, double-blind, multicentre, placebo-controlled study. Cephalagia. 2005;25(11):1031-41.

60 Cady RK, Schreiber CP, Beach ME, hart CC. Gelstat Migraine (sublingual administered feverfew and ginger compound) for acute treatment of migraine when administered during the mild pain phase. Med Sci Monit. 2005.

61 Kwok BJ, Koh B, Ndubuisi MI, Elofsson M, Crews CW. The anti-inflammatory natural product parthenolide from the medicinal herb Feverfew directly binds to and inhibits IkappaB kinase. Chem Biol. 2001;8(8):759-66.

CHAPTER EIGHT: GLUTEN SENSITIVITY AND BEYOND

1 Rubio-Tapia A, Murray JA. Celiac disease. Curr Opin Gastroenterol. 2010 Mar;26(2):116-22.

2 Rubio-Tapia A, Kyle RA, Kaplan EL, Johnson DR, Page W, Erdtmann F, Brantner TL, Kim WR, Phelps TK, Lahr BD, Zinsmeister AR, Melton LJ 3rd, Murray JA. Increased prevalence and mortality in undiagnosed celiac disease. Gastroenterology. 2009 Jul;137(1):88-93.

3 Yuan Z, Liu D, Zhang L, Zhang L, Chen W, Yan Z, Zheng Y, Zhang H, Yen Y. Mitotic illegitimate recombination is a mechanism for novel changes in high-molecular-weight glutenin subunits in wheat-rye hybrids. PLoS One. 2011;6(8):e23511.

4 Molnár-Láng M, Kruppa K, Cseh A, Bucsi J, Linc G. Identification and phenotypic description of new wheat: six-rowed winter barley disomic additions. Genome. 2012 Apr;55(4):302-11.

[5] Szakács E, Molnár-Láng M. Identification of new winter wheat—winter barley addition lines (6HS and 7H) using fluorescence in situ hybridization and the stability of the whole 'Martonvásári 9 kr1' - 'Igri' addition set. Genome. 2010 Jan;53(1):35-44.

[6] Leduc V, Moneret-Vautrin DA, Guerin L, Morisset M, Kanny G. Anaphylaxis to wheat isolates: immunochemical study of a case proved by means of double-blind, placebo-controlled food challenge. J Allergy Clin Immunol. 2003 Apr;111(4):897-9.

[7] Vojdani A, O'Bryan T, Kellermann GH. The immunology of immediate and delayed hypersensitivity reaction to gluten. European J of Inflammation. 2008 ; 6(1): 1-10.

[8] Lakatos PL, Kiss LS, Miheller P. Nutritional influences in selected gastrointestinal diseases. Dig Dis. 2011;29(2):154-65.

[9] Admou B, Essaadouni L, Krati K, Zaher K, Sbihi M, Chabaa L, Belaabidia B, Alaoui-Yazidi A. Atypical celiac disease: from recognizing to managing. Gastroenterol Res Pract. 2012;2012:637187. Epub 2012 Jul 3.

[10] Grossman G. Neurological complications of coeliac disease: what is the evidence? Pract Neurol. 2008 Apr;8(2):77-89.

[11] Hadjivassiliou M, Grünewald RA, Davies-Jones GA. Gluten sensitivity as a neurological illness. J Neurol Neurosurg Psychiatry. 2002 May;72(5):560-3.

[12] Hadjivassiliou M, Grünewald RA, Lawden M, Davies-Jones GA, Powell T, Smith CM. Headache and CNS white matter abnormalities associated with gluten sensitivity. Neurology. 2001 Feb 13;56(3):385-8.

[13] Ford RP. The gluten syndrome: a neurological disease. Med Hypotheses. 2009 Sep;73(3):438-40. Epub 2009 Apr 29.

[14] Hadjivassiliou M, Sanders DS, Grünewald RA, Woodroofe N, Boscolo S, Aeschlimann D. Gluten sensitivity: from gut to brain. Lancet Neurol. 2010 Mar;9(3):318-30.

[15] Ruuskanen A, Kaukinen K, Collin P, Krekelä I, Patrikainen H, Tillonen J, Nyrke T, Laurila K, Haimila K, Partanen J, Valve R, Mäki M, Luostarinen L. Gliadin antibodies in older population and neurological and psychiatric disorders. Acta Neurol Scand. 2012 Apr 12.

[16] Baizabal-Carvallo JF, Jankovic J. Movement disorders in autoimmune diseases. Mov Disord. 2012 Jul;27(8):935-46.

[17] Savolainen H. Sensory ganglionopathy due to gluten sensitivity. Neurology. 2011 Jul 5;77(1):87; author reply 87.

[18] Rashtak S, Rashtak S, Snyder MR, Pittock SJ, Wu TT, Gandhi MJ, Murray JA. Serology of celiac disease in gluten-sensitive ataxia or neuropathy: role of deamidated gliadin antibody. J Neuroimmunol. 2011 Jan;230(1-2):130-4.

[19] Volta U, De Giorgio R. Gluten sensitivity: an emerging issue behind neurological impairment? Lancet Neurol. 2010 Mar;9(3):233-5.

[20] Jarius S, Jacob S, Waters P, Jacob A, Littleton E, Vincent A. Neuromyelitis optica in patients with gluten sensitivity associated with antibodies to aquaporin-4. J Neurol Neurosurg Psychiatry. 2008 Sep;79(9):1084.

21 Borhani Haghighi A, Ansari N, Mokhtari M, Geramizadeh B, Lankarani KB. Multiple sclerosis and gluten sensitivity. Clin Neurol Neurosurg. 2007 Oct;109(8):651-3. Epub 2007 May 29

22 Chin RL, Sander HW, Brannagan TH, Green PH, Hays AP, Alaedini A, Latov N. Celiac neuropathy. Neurology. 2003 May 27;60(10):1581-5.

23 Zhang Y, Menkes DL, Silvers DS. Propriospinal myoclonus associated with gluten sensitivity in a young woman. J Neurol Sci. 2012 Apr 15;315(1-2):141-2.

24 Morris CR, Agin MC. Syndrome of allergy, apraxia, and malabsorption: characterization of a neurodevelopmental phenotype that responds to omega 3 and vitamin E supplementation. Altern Ther Health Med. 2009 Jul-Aug;15(4):34-43.

25 Hadjivassiliou M, Chattopadhyay AK, Grünewald RA, Jarratt JA, Kandler RH, Rao DG, Sanders DS, Wharton SB, Davies-Jones GA. Myopathy associated with gluten sensitivity. Muscle Nerve. 2007 Apr;35(4):443-50.

26 Serratrice J, Attarian S, Disdier P, Weiller PJ, Serratrice G. Neuromuscular diseases associated with antigliadin antibodies. A contentious concept. Acta Myol. 2004 Dec;23(3):146-50.

27 Pellecchia MT, Ambrosio G, Salvatore E, Vitale C, De Michele G, Barone P. Possible gluten sensitivity in multiple system atrophy. Neurology. 2002 Oct 8;59(7):1114-5.

28 Bürk K, Bösch S, Müller CA, Melms A, Zühlke C, Stern M, Besenthal I, Skalej M, Ruck P, Ferber S, Klockgether T, Dichgans J. Sporadic cerebellar ataxia associated with gluten sensitivity. Brain. 2001 May;124(Pt 5):1013-9.

29 Schlesinger I, Hering R. Antigliadin antibodies in migraine patients. Cephalalgia. 1997 Oct;17(6):712.

30 Solmaz F, Unal F, Apuhan T. Celiac disease and sensorineural hearing loss in children. Acta Otolaryngol. 2012 Feb;132(2):146-51.

31 Hu WT, Murray JA, Greenaway MC, Parisi JE, Josephs KA. Cognitive impairment and celiac disease. Arch Neurol. 2006 Oct;63(10):1440-6.

32 Konishi T. [Dementia due to celiac disease]. Nihon Rinsho. 2004 Jan;62 Suppl:450-5.

33 Moccia M, Pellecchia MT, Erro R, Zingone F, Marelli S, Barone DG, Ciacci C, Strambi LF, Barone P. Restless legs syndrome is a common feature of adult celiac disease. Mov Disord. 2010 May 15;25(7):877-81.

34 Alaedini A, Okamoto H, Briani C, Wollenberg K, Shill HA, Bushara KO, Sander HW, Green PH, Hallett M, Latov N. Immune cross-reactivity in celiac disease: anti-gliadin antibodies bind to neuronal synapsin I. J Immunol. 2007 May 15;178(10):6590-5.

35 Hadjivassiliou M, Boscolo S, Davies-Jones GA, Grünewald RA, Not T, Sanders DS, Simpson JE, Tongiorgi E, Williamson CA, Woodroofe NM. The humoral response in the pathogenesis of gluten ataxia. Neurology. 2002 Apr 23;58(8):1221-6.

36 Hadjivassiliou M. Immune-mediated acquired ataxias. Handb Clin Neurol. 2012;103:189-99.

[37] Thomas H, Beck K, Adamczyk M, Aeschlimann P, Langley M, Oita RC, Thiebach L, Hils M, Aeschlimann D. Transglutaminase 6: a protein associated with central nervous system development and motor function. Amino Acids. 2011 Oct 8.

[38] Stamnaes J, Dorum S, Fleckenstein B, Aeschlimann D, Sollid LM. Gluten T cell epitope targeting by TG3 and TG6; implications for dermatitis herpetiformis and gluten ataxia. Amino Acids. 2010 Nov;39(5):1183-91.

[39] Hemmings WA. The entry into the brain of large molecules derived from dietary protein. Proc R Soc Lond B Biol Sci. 1978 Feb 23;200(1139): 175-92.

[40] Visser J, Rozing J, Sapone A, Lammers K, Fasano A. Tight junctions, intestinal permeability, and autoimmunity: celiac disease and type 1 diabetes paradigms. Ann N Y Acad Sci. 2009 May;1165:195-205.

[41] Pastore L, Campisi G, Compilato D, Lo Muzio L. Orally based diagnosis of celiac disease: current perspectives. J Dent Res. 2008 Dec;87(12):1100-7.

[42] Pastore L, Campisi G, Compilato D, Lo Muzio L. Orally based diagnosis of celiac disease: current perspectives. J Dent Res. 2008 Dec;87(12):1100-7.

[43] Pastore L, Campisi G, Compilato D, Lo Muzio L. Orally based diagnosis of celiac disease: current perspectives. J Dent Res. 2008 Dec;87(12):1100-7.

[44] Quarsten H, McAdam SN, Jensen T, Arentz-Hansen H, Molberg Ø, Lundin KE, Sollid LM. Staining of celiac disease-relevant T cells by peptide-DQ2 multimers. J Immunol. 2001 Nov 1;167(9):4861-8.

[45] Vader W, Kooy Y, Van Veelen P, De Ru A, Harris D, Benckhuijsen W, Peña S, Mearin L, Drijfhout JW, Koning F. The gluten response in children with celiac disease is directed toward multiple gliadin and glutenin peptides. Gastroenterology. 2002 Jun;122(7):1729-37.

[46] van de Wal Y, Kooy YM, van Veelen P, Vader W, August SA, Drijfhout JW, Peña SA, Koning F. Glutenin is involved in the gluten-driven mucosal T cell response. Eur J Immunol. 1999 Oct;29(10):3133-9.

[47] Leduc V, Moneret-Vautrin DA, Guerin L, Morisset M, Kanny G. Anaphylaxis to wheat isolates: immunochemical study of a case proved by means of double-blind, placebo-controlled food challenge. J Allergy Clin Immunol. 2003 Apr;111(4):897-9.

[48] Hashimoto S, Hagino A. Wheat germ agglutinin, concanavalin A, and lens culinalis agglutinin block the inhibitory effect of nerve growth factor on cell-free phosphorylation of Nsp100 in PC12h cells. Cell Struct Funct. 1989 Feb;14(1):87-93.

[49] Ross-Smith P, Jenner FA. Diet (gluten) and schizophrenia. J Hum Nutr. 1980 Apr;34(2):107-12.

[50] Dohan FC. Hypothesis: genes and neuroactive peptides from food as cause of schizophrenia. Adv Biochem Psychopharmacol. 1980;22:535-48.

[51] Alessio MG, Tonutti E, Brusca I, Radice A, Licini L, Sonzogni A, Florena A, Schiaffino E, Marus W, Sulfaro S, Villalta D; Study Group on Autoimmune Diseases of Italian Society of Laboratory Medicine. Correlation between IgA tissue transglutaminase antibody ratio and histological finding in celiac disease. J Pediatr Gastroenterol Nutr. 2012 Jul;55(1):44-9.

52 Stamnaes J, Dorum S, Fleckenstein B, Aeschlimann D, Sollid LM. Gluten T cell epitope targeting by TG3 and TG6; implications for dermatitis herpetiformis and gluten ataxia. Amino Acids. 2010 Nov;39(5):1183-91.

53 Thomas H, Beck K, Adamczyk M, Aeschlimann P, Langley M, Oita RC, Thiebach L, Hils M, Aeschlimann D. Transglutaminase 6: a protein associated with central nervous system development and motor function. Amino Acids. 2011 Oct 8.

54 Craig L, Sanschagrin PC, Rozek A, Lackie S, Kuhn LA, Scott JK. The role of structure in antibody cross-reactivity between peptides and folded proteins. J Mol Biol. 1998 Aug 7;281(1):183-201.

55 Kristjánsson G, Venge P, Hällgren R. Mucosal reactivity to cow's milk protein in coeliac disease. Clin Exp Immunol. 2007 Mar;147(3):449-55.

56 Tiruppathi C, Miyamoto Y, Ganapathy V, Leibach FH. Genetic evidence for role of DPP IV in intestinal hydrolysis and assimilation of prolyl peptides. Am J Physiol. 1993;265:G81-9.

57 Kozakova H, Stepankova R, Kolinska J, et al. Brush border enzyme activities in the small intestine after long-term gliadin feeding in animal models of human celiac disease. Folia Microbiol(Phraha). 1998;43(5):497-500.

58 Hausch F, Shan L, Nilda A, et al. Intestinal digestive resistance of immunodominant gliadin peptides. Am J Gastrointest Liver Physiol. 2002;283:G9996-G1003.

59 Detel D, Persic M, Varljen J. Serum and intestinal dipeptidyl peptidase IV (DPP IV/CD26) activity in children with celiac disease. J Pediatr Gastroenterol Nutr. 2007;45(1):65-70.

60 Smith MW, Phillips D. Abnormal expression of dipeptidylpeptidase IV activity enterocyte brush-border membranes of children suffering from celiac disease. Exp Phys. 1990;75:613-616.

61 Vojdani A, Bazaragan M, Vojdani E, et al. Heat shock protein and gliadin peptide promote development of peptidase antibodies in children with autism and patients with autoimmune disease. Clin Diagn Lab Immunol. 2004;11(3):515-24.

62 Vojdani A, Pangborn JB, Vojdani E, Cooper EL. Infections, toxic chemicals and dietary peptides binding to lymphocyte receptors and tissue enzymes are major instigators of autoimmunity in autism. Int J Immunopathol Pharmacol. 2003;16(3):189-99.

63 Maiuri MC, De Stefano D, Mele G, et al. Nuclear factor kappa B is activated in small intestinal mucosa of celiac patients. J Mol Med. 2003;81(6):373-9.

64 Ruiz PA, Haller D. Functional diversity of flavonoids in the inhibition of the proinflammatory NF-kappa B, IRF, and Akt signaling pathways in murine and epithelial cells. J Nutr. 2006;136(3):664-71.

65 Peng IW, Kuo SM. Flavonoid structure affects the inhibition of lipid peroxidation in Caco-2 intestinal cells at physiological concentrations. J Nutr. 2003;133(7):2184-7.

66 De Stafano D, Maiuri MC, Simeon V, et al. Lycopene, Quercetin and tyrosol prevent macrophage activation induced by gliadin and IFN-gamma. Eur J Pharmacol. 2007;566(1-3):192-9.

67 Simons Al, Renouf M, Hendrich S, Murphy PA. Human gut microbial degradation of flavonoids: structure-function relationships. J Agric Food Chem. 2005;53(10):4258-63.

68 Panes J, Gerritsen Me, Anderson DC, et al. Apigenin inhibits tumor necrosis factor-induced intercellular adhesion molecule-1 upregulation in vivo. Microcirculation. 1996;3(3):279-86.

69 Pearce Fl, Befus AD, Bienenstock J. Mucosal mast cells. III. Effect of quercetin and other flavonoids on antigen-induced histamine secretion from rat intestinal mast cells. J Allergy Clin Immunol. 1984:73(60:819-23.

70 Kim JS, Jobin C. The flavonoid luteolin prevents lipopolysaccharide-induced NF-kappa B signalling and gene expression by blocking IkappaB kinase activity in intestinal epithelial cells and bone-marrow derived dendritic cells. Immunology. 2005;115(3):375-87.

71 Ashokkumar P, Sudhandiran G. Protective role of luteolin on the status of lipid peroxidation and antioxidant defense against azoxymethane-induced experimental colon carcinogenesis. Biomed Pharmacother. 2008;62 (9):590-7.

72 Manju V, Nalini N. Protective role of luteolin in 1,2-dimethylhydrazine induced experimental colon carcinogenesis. Cell Biochem Funct. 2007;25(2):189-94.

73 Kim JA, Kim DK, Kang OH, et al. Inhibitory effect of luteolin on TNF-alpha-induced IL-8 production in human colon epithelial cells. Int Immunopharmacol. 2005;5(1):209-17.

CHAPTER NINE: THE GUT-BRAIN AXIS

1 Chang L. Brain responses to visceral and somatic stimuli in irritable bowel syndrome: a central nervous system disorder? Gastroenterol Clin North Am. 2005 Jun;34(2):271-9.

2 Harris LA, Chang L. Irritable bowel syndrome: new and emerging therapies. Curr Opin Gastroenterol. 2006 Mar;22(2):128-35.

3 Cuomo R, D'Alessandro A, Andreozzi P, Vozzella L, Sarnelli G. Gastrointestinal regulation of food intake: do gut motility, enteric nerves and entero-hormones play together? Minerva Endocrinol. 2011 Dec;36(4):281-93.

4 Ohman L, Simrén M. Pathogenesis of IBS: role of inflammation, immunity and neuroimmune interactions. Nat Rev Gastroenterol Hepatol. 2010 Mar;7(3):163-73.

5 Wang Y, Kondo T, Suzukamo Y, Oouchida Y, Izumi S. Vagal nerve regulation is essential for the increase in gastric motility in response to mild exercise. Tohoku J Exp Med. 2010;222(2):155-63.

6 Arai E, Arai M, Uchiyama T, Higuchi Y, Aoyagi K, Yamanaka Y, Yamamoto T, Nagano O, Shiina A, Maruoka D, Matsumura T, Nakagawa T, Katsuno T, Imazeki F, Saeki N, Kuwabara S, Yokosuka O. Subthalamic deep brain stimulation can improve gastric emptying in Parkinson's disease. Brain. 2012 May;135(Pt 5):1478-85.

7 Taché Y, Vale W, Rivier J, Brown M. Brain regulation of gastric acid secretion in rats by neurogastrointestinal peptides. Peptides. 1981;2 Suppl 2:51-5.

8 Catalioto RM, Maggi CA, Giuliani S. Intestinal epithelial barrier dysfunction in disease and possible therapeutical interventions. Curr Med Chem. 2011;18(3):398-426.

9 Bansal V, Costantini T, Kroll L, Peterson C, Loomis W, Eliceiri B, Baird A, Wolf P, Coimbra R. Traumatic brain injury and intestinal dysfunction: uncovering the neuro-enteric axis. J Neurotrauma. 2009 Aug;26(8):1353-9.

10 1: Bansal V, Costantini T, Ryu SY, Peterson C, Loomis W, Putnam J, Elicieri B, Baird A, Coimbra R. Stimulating the central nervous system to prevent intestinal dysfunction after traumatic brain injury. J Trauma. 2010 May;68(5):1059-64.

11 Hollander D. Intestinal permeability, leaky gut, and intestinal disorders. Curr Gastroenterol Rep. 1999 Oct;1(5):410-6.

12 Wade PR, Cowen T. Neurodegeneration: a key factor in the ageing gut. Neurogastroenterol Motil. 2004 Apr;16 Suppl 1:19-23.

13 Lebouvier T, Neunlist M, Bruley des Varannes S, Coron E, Drouard A, N'Guyen JM, Chaumette T, Tasselli M, Paillusson S, Flamand M, Galmiche JP, Damier P, Derkinderen P. Colonic biopsies to assess the neuropathology of Parkinson's disease and its relationship with symptoms. PLoS One. 2010 Sep 14;5(9):e12728.

14 Pothoulakis C. The role of neuroenteric hormones in intestinal infectious diseases. Curr Opin Gastroenterol. 2000 Nov;16(6):536-40.

15 Yang J, Wang BJ, Ding M, Pang H, Sun XF, Li ZJ. [The relationship between SNP of cholecystokinin gene and certain mental status and its forensic significance]. Fa Yi Xue Za Zhi. 2008 Aug;24(4):284-7.

16 Diano S, Farr SA, Benoit SC, McNay EC, da Silva I, Horvath B, Gaskin FS, Nonaka N, Jaeger LB, Banks WA, Morley JE, Pinto S, Sherwin RS, Xu L, Yamada KA, Sleeman MW, Tschöp MH, Horvath TL. Ghrelin controls hippocampal spine synapse density and memory performance. Nat Neurosci. 2006 Mar;9(3):381-8.

17 Diano S, Farr SA, Benoit SC, McNay EC, da Silva I, Horvath B, Gaskin FS, Nonaka N, Jaeger LB, Banks WA, Morley JE, Pinto S, Sherwin RS, Xu L, Yamada KA, Sleeman MW, Tschöp MH, Horvath TL. Ghrelin controls hippocampal spine synapse density and memory performance. Nat Neurosci. 2006 Mar;9(3):381-8.

18 Yang J, Wang BJ, Ding M, Pang H, Sun XF, Li ZJ. [The relationship between SNP of cholecystokinin gene and certain mental status and its forensic significance]. Fa Yi Xue Za Zhi. 2008 Aug;24(4):284-7.

19 Whitcomb DC, Taylor IL. A new twist in the brain-gut axis. Am J Med Sci. 1992 Nov;304(5):334-8.

20 Fetissov SO, Déchelotte P. The new link between gut-brain axis and neuropsychiatric disorders. Curr Opin Clin Nutr Metab Care. 2011 Sep;14(5):477-82.

21 Desbonnet L, Garrett L, Clarke G, Bienenstock J, Dinan TG. The probiotic Bifidobacteria infantis: An assessment of potential antidepressant properties in the rat. J Psychiatr Res. 2008 Dec;43(2):164-74.

22   Maes M, Kubera M, Leunis JC. The gut-brain barrier in major depression: intestinal mucosal dysfunction with an increased translocation of LPS from gram negative enterobacteria (leaky gut) plays a role in the inflammatory pathophysiology of depression. Neuro Endocrinol Lett. 2008 Feb; 29(1):117-24.

23   Geissler A, Andus T, Roth M, Kullmann F, Caesar I, Held P, Gross V, Feuerbach S, Schölmerich J. Focal white-matter lesions in brain of patients with inflammatory bowel disease. Lancet. 1995 Apr 8;345(8954):897-8.

24   Dejaco C, Fertl E, Prayer D, Oberhuber G, Wyatt J, Gasché C, Gangl A. Symptomatic cerebral microangiopathy preceding initial manifestation of ulcerative colitis. Dig Dis Sci. 1996 Sep;41(9):1807-10.

25   Levine JB, Lukawski-Trubish D. Extraintestinal considerations in inflammatory bowel disease. Gastroenterol Clin North Am. 1995 Sep;24(3):633-46.

26   Agranoff D, Schon F. Are focal white matter lesions in patients with inflammatory bowel disease linked to multiple sclerosis? Lancet. 1995 Jul 15;346(8968):190-1.

27   Fasano A. Zonulin and its regulation of intestinal barrier function: the biological door to inflammation, autoimmunity, and cancer. Physiol Rev. 2011 Jan;91(1):151-75.

28   Turner JR. Molecular basis of epithelial barrier regulation: from basic mechanisms to clinical application. Am J Pathol. 2006 Dec;169(6):1901-9.

29   Cuvelier C, Barbatis C, Mielants H, De Vos M, Roels H, Veys E. Histopathology of intestinal inflammation related to reactive arthritis. Gut. 1987 Apr;28(4):394-401.

30   Rakoff-Nahoum S, Paglino J, Eslami-Varzaneh F, Edberg S, Medzhitov R. Recognition of commensal microflora by toll-like receptors is required for intestinal homeostasis. Cell. 2004 Jul 23;118(2):229-41

31   Cario E, Gerken G, Podolsky DK. Toll-like receptor 2 enhances ZO-1-associated intestinal epithelial barrier integrity via protein kinase C. Gastroenterology. 2004 Jul;127(1):224-38.

32   Lee J, Mo JH, Katakura K, Alkalay I, Rucker AN, Liu YT, Lee HK, Shen C, Cojocaru G, Shenouda S, Kagnoff M, Eckmann L, Ben-Neriah Y, Raz E. Maintenance of colonic homeostasis by distinctive apical TLR9 signalling in intestinal epithelial cells. Nat Cell Biol. 2006 Dec;8(12):1327-36.

33   Karper WB. Intestinal permeability, moderate exercise, and older adult health. Holist Nurs Pract. 2011 Jan-Feb;25(1):45-8.

34   Maes M, Kubera M, Leunis JC. The gut-brain barrier in major depression: intestinal mucosal dysfunction with an increased translocation of LPS from gram negative enterobacteria (leaky gut) plays a role in the inflammatory pathophysiology of depression. Neuro Endocrinol Lett. 2008 Feb; 29(1):117-24.

35   Lammers KM, Lu R, Brownley J, Lu B, Gerard C, Thomas K, Rallabhandi P, Shea-Donohue T, Tamiz A, Alkan S, Netzel-Arnett S, Antalis T, Vogel SN, Fasano A. Gliadin induces an increase in intestinal permeability and zonulin release by binding to the chemokine receptor CXCR3. Gastroenterology. 2008 Jul;135(1):194-204.e3.

36 Purohit V, Bode JC, Bode C, Brenner DA, Choudhry MA, Hamilton F, Kang YJ, Keshavarzian A, Rao R, Sartor RB, Swanson C, Turner JR. Alcohol, intestinal bacterial growth, intestinal permeability to endotoxin, and medical consequences: summary of a symposium. Alcohol. 2008 Aug;42(5):349-61.

37 Gareau MG, Silva MA, Perdue MH. Pathophysiological mechanisms of stress-induced intestinal damage. Curr Mol Med. 2008 Jun;8(4):274-81.

38 van Ampting MT, Schonewille AJ, Vink C, Brummer RJ, van der Meer R, Bovee-Oudenhoven IM. Intestinal barrier function in response to abundant or depleted mucosal glutathione in Salmonella-infected rats. BMC Physiol. 2009 Apr 17;9:6.

39 Machowska A, Brzozowski T, Sliwowski Z, Pawlik M, Konturek PC, Pajdo R, Szlachcic A, Drozdowicz D, Schwarz M, Stachura J, Konturek SJ, Pawlik WW. Gastric secretion, proinflammatory cytokines and epidermal growth factor (EGF) in the delayed healing of lingual and gastric ulcerations by testosterone. Inflammopharmacology. 2008 Feb;16(1):40-7.

40 Money SR, Cheron RG, Jaffe BM, Zinner MJ. The effects of thyroid hormones on the formation of stress ulcers in the rat. J Surg Res. 1986 Feb;40(2): 176-80.

41 Braniste V, Leveque M, Buisson-Brenac C, Bueno L, Fioramonti J, Houdeau E. Oestradiol decreases colonic permeability through oestrogen receptor beta-mediated up-regulation of occludin and junctional adhesion molecule-A in epithelial cells. J Physiol. 2009 Jul 1;587(Pt 13):3317-28

42 Drago F, Montoneri C, Varga C, Làszlò F. Dual effect of female sex steroids on drug-induced gastroduodenal ulcers in the rat. Life Sci. 1999;64(25):2341-50.

43 Zen K, Chen CX, Chen YT, Wilton R, Liu Y. Receptor for advanced glycation endproducts mediates neutrophil migration across intestinal epithelium. J Immunol. 2007 Feb 15;178(4):2483-90.

44 Korenaga K, Micci MA, Taglialatela G, Pasricha PJ. Suppression of nNOS expression in rat enteric neurones by the receptor for advanced glycation end-products. Neurogastroenterol Motil. 2006 May;18(5):392-400.

45 1: Dijkstra G, van Goor H, Jansen PL, Moshage H. Targeting nitric oxide in the gastrointestinal tract. Curr Opin Investig Drugs. 2004 May;5(5):529-36.

46 Keklikoglu N, Koray M, Kocaelli H, Akinci S. iNOS expression in oral and gastrointestinal tract mucosa. Dig Dis Sci. 2008 Jun;53(6):1437-42.

47 Braniste V, Leveque M, Buisson-Brenac C, Bueno L, Fioramonti J, Houdeau E. Oestradiol decreases colonic permeability through oestrogen receptor beta-mediated up-regulation of occludin and junctional adhesion molecule-A in epithelial cells. J Physiol. 2009 Jul 1;587(Pt 13):3317-28. Epub 2009 May 11.

48 Fasano A. Zonulin and its regulation of intestinal barrier function: the biological door to inflammation, autoimmunity, and cancer. Physiological Reviews. 2011; 91 (1):151-75.

49 Marchiando AM, L Shen, WV Graham, KL Edelblum, CA Duckworth, Y Guan, MH Montrose, JR Turner, and AJ Watson. The epithelial barrier is maintained by in vivo tight junction expansion during pathologic intestinal epithelial shedding. Gastroenterology. 2011;140 (4):1208-1218.e1-2.

50 Clayburgh, D.R., et al. "A porous defense: the leaky epithelial barrier in intestinal disease." Lab Invest, 2004; 84:282-291.

51 El Asmar, R., et al. „Host-dependent zonulin secretion causes the impairment of the small intestine barrier function after bacterial exposure." Gastroenterol, 2002; 123:1607-1615.

52 Wang, W., et al. "Human zonulin, a potential modulator of intestinal tight junctions." J Cell Sci, 2000; 113:4435-4440.

53 El Asmar, R., et al. „Host-dependent zonulin secretion causes the impairment of the small intestine barrier function after bacterial exposure." Gastroenterol, 2002; 123:1607-1615.

54 Wang, W., et al. "Human zonulin, a potential modulator of intestinal tight junctions." J Cell Sci, 2000; 113:4435-4440.

55 Wang, W., et al. "Human zonulin, a potential modulator of intestinal tight junctions." J Cell Sci, 2000; 113:4435-4440.

56 Yasuoka T, M Sasaki, T Fukunaga, T Tsujikawa, Y Fujiyama, R Kushima, and RA Goodlad. The effects of lectins on indomethacin-induced small intestinal ulceration. International Journal of Experimental Pathology. 2003; 84 (5):231-7.

57 Bajaj M, A Hinge, LS Limaye, RK Gupta, A Surolia, and VP Kale. 2011. Mannose-binding dietary lectins induce adipogenic differentiation of the marrow-derived mesenchymal cells via an active insulin-like signaling mechanism. Glycobiology. 2011; 21 (4):521-9.

58 Noyer CM, Simon D, Borczuk A, Brandt LJ, Lee MJ, Nehra V. A double-blind placebo-controlled pilot study of glutamine therapy for abnormal intestinal permeability in patients with AIDS. Am J Gastroenterol. 1998 Jun;93(6):972-5.

59 Klimberg VS, Souba WW, Dolson DJ, Salloum RM, Hautamaki RD, Plumley DA, Mendenhall WM, Bova FJ, Khan SR, Hackett RL, et al. Prophylactic glutamine protects the intestinal mucosa from radiation injury. Cancer. 1990 Jul 1;66(1):62-8.

60 Chamorro S, de Blas C, Grant G, Badiola I, Menoyo D, Carabaño R. Effect of dietary supplementation with glutamine and a combination of glutamine-arginine on intestinal health in twenty-five-day-old weaned rabbits. J Anim Sci. 2010 Jan;88(1):170-80.

61 Amasheh M, Andres S, Amasheh S, Fromm M, Schulzke JD. Barrier effects of nutritional factors. Ann N Y Acad Sci. 2009 May;1165:267-73

62 Kul M, Vurucu S, Demirkaya E, Tunc T, Aydinoz S, Meral C, Kesik V, Alpay F. Enteral glutamine and/or arginine supplementation have favorable effects on oxidative stress parameters in neonatal rat intestine. J Pediatr Gastroenterol Nutr. 2009 Jul;49(1):85-9.

63 Azuma H, Mishima S, Oda J, Homma H, Sasaki H, Hisamura M, Ohta S, Yukioka T. Enteral supplementation enriched with glutamine, fiber, and oligosaccharide prevents gut translocation in a bacterial overgrowth model. J Trauma. 2009 Jan;66(1):110-4.

64 Maes M, Leunis JC. Normalization of leaky gut in chronic fatigue syndrome (CFS) is accompanied by a clinical improvement: effects of age, duration of illness and the translocation of LPS from gram-negative bacteria. Neuro Endocrinol Lett. 2008 Dec;29(6):902-10.

65 Tian J, Hao L, Chandra P, Jones DP, Willams IR, Gewirtz AT, Ziegler TR. Dietary glutamine and oral antibiotics each improve indexes of gut barrier function in rat short bowel syndrome. Am J Physiol Gastrointest Liver Physiol. 2009 Feb;296(2):G348-55.

66 Coëffier M, Claeyssens S, Lecleire S, Leblond J, Coquard A, Bôle-Feysot C, Lavoinne A, Ducrotté P, Déchelotte P. Combined enteral infusion of glutamine, carbohydrates, and antioxidants modulates gut protein metabolism in humans. Am J Clin Nutr. 2008 Nov;88(5):1284-90.

67 Wang WW, Qiao SY, Li DF. Amino acids and gut function. Amino Acids. 2009 May;37(1):105-10. Epub 2008 Aug 1. Review. PubMed PMID: 18670730.

68 Xue H, Sawyer MB, Field CJ, Dieleman LA, Murray D, Baracos VE. Bolus oral glutamine protects rats against CPT-11-induced diarrhea and differentially activates cytoprotective mechanisms in host intestine but not tumor. J Nutr. 2008 Apr;138(4):740-6.

69 Vicario M, Amat C, Rivero M, Moretó M, Pelegrí C. Dietary glutamine affects mucosal functions in rats with mild DSS-induced colitis. J Nutr. 2007 Aug;137(8):1931-7.

70 Harsha WT, Kalandarova E, McNutt P, Irwin R, Noel J. Nutritional supplementation with transforming growth factor-beta, glutamine, and short chain fatty acids minimizes methotrexate-induced injury. J Pediatr Gastroenterol Nutr. 2006 Jan;42(1):53-8.

71 Yeh CL, Hsu CS, Yeh SL, Chen WJ. Dietary glutamine supplementation modulates Th1/Th2 cytokine and interleukin-6 expressions in septic mice. Cytokine. 2005 Sep 7;31(5):329-34.

72 Basivireddy J, Jacob M, Balasubramanian KA. Oral glutamine attenuates indomethacin-induced small intestinal damage. Clin Sci (Lond). 2004 Sep;107(3):281-9.

73 Li N, Liboni K, Fang MZ, Samuelson D, Lewis P, Patel R, Neu J. Glutamine decreases lipopolysaccharide-induced intestinal inflammation in infant rats. Am J Physiol Gastrointest Liver Physiol. 2004 Jun;286(6):G914-21.

74 Zhou X, Li YX, Li N, Li JS. Glutamine enhances the gut-trophic effect of growth hormone in rat after massive small bowel resection. J Surg Res. 2001 Jul;99(1):47-52.

75 Li N, Li J, Li Y. [Nutritional rehabilitation for patients with extreme short bowel]. Zhonghua Wai Ke Za Zhi. 1997 Dec;35(12):707-9.

76 Gismondo MR, Drago L, Fassina MC, Vaghi I, Abbiati R, Grossi E. Immunostimulating effect of oral glutamine. Dig Dis Sci. 1998 Aug;43(8):1752-4.

77 Ameho CK, Adjei AA, Harrison EK, Takeshita K, Morioka T, Arakaki Y, Ito E, Suzuki I, Kulkarni AD, Kawajiri A, Yamamoto S. Prophylactic effect of dietary glutamine supplementation on interleukin 8 and tumour necrosis factor alpha production in trinitrobenzene sulphonic acid induced colitis. Gut. 1997 Oct;41(4):487-93.

[78] Elia M, Lunn PG. The use of glutamine in the treatment of gastrointestinal disorders in man. Nutrition. 1997 Jul-Aug;13(7-8):743-7.

[79] Wu G, Meier SA, Knabe DA. Dietary glutamine supplementation prevents jejunal atrophy in weaned pigs. J Nutr. 1996 Oct;126(10):2578-84.

[80] Marks IN. Site-protective agents. Baillieres Clin Gastroenterol. 1988 Jul;2(3):609-20. Review. 81 Marks IN, Boyd E. Mucosal protective agents in the long-term management of gastric ulcer. Med J Aust. 1985 Feb 4;142(3):S23-5.

[82] Russell RI, Morgan RJ, Nelson LM. Studies on the protective effect of deglycyrrhinised liquorice against aspirin (ASA) and ASA plus bile acid-induced gastric mucosal damage, and ASA absorption in rats. Scand J Gastroenterol Suppl. 1984;92:97-100.

[83] Bennett A. Gastric mucosal formation of prostanoids and the effects of drugs. Acta Physiol Hung. 1984;64(3-4):215-7.

[84] Morgan RJ, Nelson LM, Russell RI, Docherty C. The protective effect of deglycyrrhinized liquorice against aspirin and aspirin plus bile acid-induced gastric mucosal damage, and its influence on aspirin absorption in rats. J Pharm Pharmacol. 1983 Sep;35(9):605-7.

[85] Glick L. Deglycyrrhizinated liquorice for peptic ulcer. Lancet. 1982 Oct 9;2(8302):817.

[86] van Marle J, Aarsen PN, Lind A, van Weeren-Kramer J. Deglycyrrhizinised liquorice (DGL) and the renewal of rat stomach epithelium. Eur J Pharmacol. 1981 Jun 19;72(2-3):219-25.

[87] Datla R, Rao SR, Murthy KJ. Excretion studies of nitrofurantoin and nitrofurantoin with deglycyrrhizinated liquorice. Indian J Physiol Pharmacol. 1981 Jan-Mar;25(1):59-63.

[88] Rees WD, Rhodes J, Wright JE, Stamford LF, Bennett A. Effect of deglycyrrhizinated liquorice on gastric mucosal damage by aspirin. Scand J Gastroenterol. 1979;14(5):605-7.

[89] Balakrishnan V, Pillai MV, Raveendran PM, Nair CS. Deglycyrrhizinated liquorice in the treatment of chronic duodenal ulcer. J Assoc Physicians India. 1978 Sep;26(9):811-4.

[90] D'Imperio N, Giuliani Piccari G, Sarti F, Soffritti M, Spongano P, Benvenuti C, Dal Monte PR. Double-blind trial in duodenal and gastric ulcers. Cimetidine and deglycyrrhizinized liquorice. Acta Gastroenterol Belg. 1978 Jul-Aug;41(7-8):427-34.

[91] Bardhan KD, Cumberland DC, Dixon RA, Holdsworth CD. Proceedings: Deglycyrrhizinated liquorice in gastric ulcer: a double blind controlled study. Gut. 1976 May;17(5):397.

[92] Larkworthy W, Holgate PF. Deglycyrrhizinized liquorice in the treatment of chronic duodenal ulcer. A retrospective endoscopic survey of 32 patients. Practitioner. 1975 Dec;215(1290):787-92.

[93] Aarsen PN. Standardization method of deglycyrrhizinized liquorice on experimental gastric ulcers in rats. Arzneimittelforschung. 1973 Sep;23(9):1346-8.

[94] Engqvist A, von Feilitzen F, Pyk E, Reichard H. Double-blind trial of deglycyrrhizinated liquorice in gastric ulcer. Gut. 1973 Sep;14(9):711-5.

[95] Håkanson R, Liedberg G, Oscarson J, Rehfeld JF, Stadil F. Effect of deglycyrrhizinized liquorice on gastric acid secretion, histidine decarboxylase activity and serum gastrin level in the rat. Experientia. 1973 May 15;29(5):570-1.

[96] Whiting B, Thomson TJ. Deglycyrrhizinized liquorice in duodenal ulcer. Br Med J. 1971 Oct 2;4(5778):48.

[97] Whiting B, Thomson TJ. Deglycyrrhizinized liquorice in duodenal ulcer. Br Med J. 1971 Oct 2;4(5778):48.

[98] Feldman H, Gilat T. A trial of deglycyrrhizinated liquorice in the treatment of duodenal ulcer. Gut. 1971 Jun;12(6):449-51.

[99] Andersson S, Bárány F, Caboclo JL, Mizuno T. Protective action of deglycyrrhizinized liquorice on the occurrence of stomach ulcers in pylorus-ligated rats. Scand J Gastroenterol. 1971;6(8):683-6.

[100] Khan A, Ahmad A, Manzoor N, Khan LA. Antifungal activities of Ocimum sanctum essential oil and its lead molecules. Nat Prod Commun. 2010 Feb;5(2):345-9.

[101] Fawole OA, Amoo SO, Ndhlala AR, Light ME, Finnie JF, Van Staden J. Anti-inflammatory, anticholinesterase, antioxidant and phytochemical properties of medicinal plants used for pain-related ailments in South Africa. J Ethnopharmacol. 2010 Feb 3;127(2):235-41.

[102] Ozsoy N, Candoken E, Akev N. Implications for degenerative disorders: Antioxidative activity, total phenols, flavonoids, ascorbic acid, beta-carotene and beta-tocopherol in Aloe vera. Oxid Med Cell Longev. 2009 Apr;2 (2):99-106.

[103] Kigondu EV, Rukunga GM, Keriko JM, Tonui WK, Gathirwa JW, Kirira PG, Irungu B, Ingonga JM, Ndiege IO. Anti-parasitic activity and cytotoxicity of selected medicinal plants from Kenya. J Ethnopharmacol. 2009 Jun 25;123(3):504-9.

[104] Chen W, Lu Z, Viljoen A, Hamman J. Intestinal drug transport enhancement by Aloe vera. Planta Med. 2009 May;75(6):587-95.

[105] Pogribna M, Freeman JP, Paine D, Boudreau MD. Effect of Aloe vera whole leaf extract on short chain fatty acids production by Bacteroides fragilis, Bifidobacterium infantis and Eubacterium limosum. Lett Appl Microbiol. 2008 May;46(5):575-80.

[106] Rosca-Casian O, Parvu M, Vlase L, Tamas M. Antifungal activity of Aloe vera leaves. Fitoterapia. 2007 Apr;78(3):219-22.

[107] Iena IaM. [The therapeutic properties of aloe]. Lik Sprava. 1993 Feb-Mar;(2-3):142-5.

[108] t'Hart LA, van den Berg AJ, Kuis L, van Dijk H, Labadie RP. An anti-complementary polysaccharide with immunological adjuvant activity from the leaf parenchyma gel of Aloe vera. Planta Med. 1989 Dec;55(6):509-12.

[109] Brossat JY, Ledeaut JY, Ralamboranto L, Rakotovao LH, Solar S, Gueguen A, Coulanges P. [Immunostimulating properties of an extract isolated from Aloe vahombe. 2. Protection in mice by fraction F1 against infections by Listeria monocytogenes, Yersinia pestis, Candida albicans and Plasmodium berghei]. Arch Inst Pasteur Madagascar. 1981;48(1):11-34.

[110] Delaporte RH, Sarragiotto MH, Takemura OS, Sánchez GM, Filho BP, Nakamura CV. Evaluation of the antioedematogenic, free radical scavenging and antimicrobial activities of aerial parts of Tillandsiastreptocarpa Baker-Bromeliaceae. J Ethnopharmacol. 2004 Dec;95(2-3):229-33.

[111] de Queiroga MA, de Andrade LM, Florêncio KC, de Fátima Agra M, da Silva MS, Barbosa-Filho JM, da-Cunha EV. Chemical constituents from Tillandsia recurvata. Fitoterapia. 2004 Jun;75(3-4):423-5.

[112] Arslanian RL, Stermitz FR, Castedo L. 3-Methoxy-5-hydroxyflavonols from Tillandsia purpurea. J Nat Prod. 1986 Nov-Dec;49(6):1177-8.

[113] FEURT SD, FOX LE. Effects of oral administration of Spanish moss, Tillandsia usneoides L. Science. 1953 Nov 20;118(3073):626-7.

[114] FEURT SD, FOX LE. The pharmacological activity of substances extracted from Spanish moss, Tillandsia usneoides L. J Am Pharm Assoc Am Pharm Assoc (Baltim). 1952 Aug;41(8):453-4.

[115] WEBBER MG, LAUTER WM, FOOTE PA. A preliminary phytochemical study of Tillandsia usneoides L. (Spanish moss). J Am Pharm Assoc Am Pharm Assoc. 1952 May;41(5):230-5.

[116] Wang DF, Shang JY, Yu QH. [Analgesic and anti-inflammatory effects of the flower of Althaea rosea (L.) Cav.]. Zhongguo Zhong Yao Za Zhi. 1989 Jan;14(1):46-8, 64.

[117] Deters A, Zippel J, Hellenbrand N, Pappai D, Possemeyer C, Hensel A. Aqueous extracts and polysaccharides from Marshmallow roots (Althea officinalis L.): cellular internalisation and stimulation of cell physiology of human epithelial cells in vitro. J Ethnopharmacol. 2010 Jan 8;127(1):62-9.

[118] Iauk L, Lo Bue AM, Milazzo I, Rapisarda A, Blandino G. Antibacterial activity of medicinal plant extracts against periodontopathic bacteria. Phytother Res. 2003 Jun;17(6):599-604.

[119] Satia JA, Littman A, Slatore CG, Galanko JA, White E. Associations of herbal and specialty supplements with lung and colorectal cancer risk in the VITamins and Lifestyle study. Cancer Epidemiol Biomarkers Prev. 2009 May;18(5):1419-28.

[120] Marañón G, Muñoz-Escassi B, Manley W, García C, Cayado P, de la Muela MS, Olábarri B, León R, Vara E. The effect of methyl sulphonyl methane supplementation on biomarkers of oxidative stress in sport horses following jumping exercise. Acta Vet Scand. 2008 Nov 7;50:45.

[121] Brien S, Prescott P, Bashir N, Lewith H, Lewith G. Systematic review of the nutritional supplements dimethyl sulfoxide (DMSO) and methylsulfonylmethane (MSM)in the treatment of osteoarthritis. Osteoarthritis Cartilage. 2008 Nov;16(11):1277-88.

[122] Parcell S. Sulfur in human nutrition and applications in medicine. Altern Med Rev. 2002 Feb;7(1):22-44.

[123] Maoka T, Tanimoto F, Sano M, Tsurukawa K, Tsuno T, Tsujiwaki S, Ishimaru K, Takii K. Effects of dietary supplementation of ferulic acid and gamma-oryzanol on integument color and suppression of oxidative stress in cultured red sea bream, Pagrus major. J Oleo Sci. 2008;57(2):133-7.

[124] Accinni R, Rosina M, Bamonti F, Della Noce C, Tonini A, Bernacchi F, Campolo J, Caruso R, Novembrino C, Ghersi L, Lonati S, Grossi S, Ippolito S, Lorenzano E, Ciani A, Gorini M. Effects of combined dietary supplementation on oxidative and inflammatory status in dyslipidemic subjects. Nutr Metab Cardiovasc Dis. 2006 Mar;16(2):121-7.

[125] Sierra S, Lara-Villoslada F, Olivares M, Jiménez J, Boza J, Xaus J. Increased immune response in mice consuming rice bran oil. Eur J Nutr. 2005 Dec;44(8):509-16.

[126] Jariwalla RJ. Rice-bran products: phytonutrients with potential applications in preventive and clinical medicine. Drugs Exp Clin Res. 2001;27(1):17-26.

[127] Sugano M, Tsuji E. Rice bran oil and human health. Biomed Environ Sci. 1996 Sep;9(2-3):242-6.

[128] Hirose M, Ozaki K, Takaba K, Fukushima S, Shirai T, Ito N. Modifying effects of the naturally occurring antioxidants gamma-oryzanol, phytic acid, tannic acid and n-tritriacontane-16, 18-dione in a rat wide-spectrum organ carcinogenesis model. Carcinogenesis. 1991 Oct;12(10):1917-21.

[129] Wheeler KB, Garleb KA. Gamma oryzanol-plant sterol supplementation: metabolic,endocrine, and physiologic effects. Int J Sport Nutr. 1991 Jun;1(2):170-7.

[130] Itaya K, Kitonaga J, Ishikawa M. [Studies of gamma-oryzanol. (2) The antiulcerogenic action]. Nippon Yakurigaku Zasshi. 1976 Nov;72(8): 1001-11.

[131] Brown AC, Hairfield M, Richards DG, McMillin DL, Mein EA, Nelson CD. Medical nutrition therapy as a potential complementary treatment for psoriasis—five case reports. Altern Med Rev. 2004 Sep;9(3):297-307.

[132] Choi HR, Choi JS, Han YN, Bae SJ, Chung HY. Peroxynitrite scavenging activity of herb extracts. Phytother Res. 2002 Jun;16(4):364-7.

[133] Majchrowicz MA. Essiac. Notes Undergr. 1995 Winter;(no 29):6-7.

[134] GILL RE, HIRST EL, JONES JK. Constitution of the mucilage from the bark of Ulmus fulva (slippery elm mucilage); the sugars formed in the hydrolysis of the methylated mucilage. J Chem Soc. 1946 Nov:1025-9.

[135] Jarrahi M, Vafaei AA, Taherian AA, Miladi H, Rashidi Pour A. Evaluation of topical Matricaria chamomilla extract activity on linear incisional wound healing in albino rats. Nat Prod Res. 2010 May;24(8):697-702.

[136] Bezerra SB, Leal LK, Pinto NA, Campos AR. Bisabolol-induced gastroprotection against acute gastric lesions: role of prostaglandins, nitric oxide, and KATP+ channels. J Med Food. 2009 Dec;12(6):1403-6.

[137] Moura Rocha NF, Venâncio ET, Moura BA, Gomes Silva MI, Aquino Neto MR, Vasconcelos Rios ER, de Sousa DP, Mendes Vasconcelos SM, de França Fonteles MM, de Sousa FC. Gastroprotection of (-)-alpha-bisabolol on acute gastric mucosal lesions in mice: the possible involved pharmacological mechanisms. Fundam Clin Pharmacol. 2009 Aug 3.

[138] Pereira RP, Fachinetto R, de Souza Prestes A, Puntel RL, Santos da Silva GN, Heinzmann BM, Boschetti TK, Athayde ML, Bürger ME, Morel AF, Morsch VM, Rocha JB.Antioxidant effects of different extracts from Melissa officinalis, Matricaria recutita and Cymbopogon citratus. Neurochem Res. 2009 May;34(5):973-83.

139 Nogueira JC, Diniz Mde F, Lima EO. In vitro antimicrobial activity of plants in Acute Otitis Externa. Braz J Otorhinolaryngol. 2008 Jan-Feb;74(1):118-24.

140 Shikov AN, Pozharitskaya ON, Makarov VG, Kvetnaya AS. Antibacterial activity of Chamomilla recutita oil extract against Helicobacter pylori. Phytother Res. 2008 Feb;22(2):252-3.

141 Capasso R, Savino F, Capasso F. Effects of the herbal formulation ColiMil on upper gastrointestinal transit in mice in vivo. Phytother Res. 2007 Oct;21(10):999-1101.

142 Mahady GB, Pendland SL, Stoia A, Hamill FA, Fabricant D, Dietz BM, Chadwick LR. In vitro susceptibility of Helicobacter pylori to botanical extracts used traditionally for the treatment of gastrointestinal disorders. Phytother Res. 2005 Nov;19(11):988-91.

143 Madisch A, Holtmann G, Mayr G, Vinson B, Hotz J. Treatment of functional dyspepsia with a herbal preparation. A double-blind, randomized, placebo-controlled, multicenter trial. Digestion. 2004;69(1):45-52.

144 Elango G, Rahuman AA, Kamaraj C, Zahir AA, Bagavan A. Studies on effects of indigenous plant extracts on filarial vector Culex tritaeniorhynchus Giles. Parasitol Res. 2010 Apr 7.

145 Aguilar HH, de Gives PM, Sánchez DO, Arellano ME, Hernández EL, Aroche UL, Valladares-Cisneros G. In vitro nematocidal activity of plant extracts of Mexican flora against Haemonchus contortus fourth larval stage. Ann N Y Acad Sci. 2008 Dec;1149:158-60.

146 Bashir S, Gilani AH. Studies on the antioxidant and analgesic activities of Aztec marigold (Tagetes erecta) flowers. Phytother Res. 2008 Dec;22(12):1692-4.

147 Wang M, Tsao R, Zhang S, Dong Z, Yang R, Gong J, Pei Y. Antioxidant activity, mutagenicity/anti-mutagenicity, and clastogenicity/anti-clastogenicity of lutein from marigold flowers. Food Chem Toxicol. 2006 Sep;44(9):1522-9.

148 Wang M, Tsao R, Zhang S, Dong Z, Yang R, Gong J, Pei Y. Antioxidant activity, mutagenicity/anti-mutagenicity, and clastogenicity/anti-clastogenicity of lutein from marigold flowers. Food Chem Toxicol. 2006 Sep;44(9):1522-9.

149 Breithaupt DE, Bamedi A, Wirt U. Carotenol fatty acid esters: easy substrates for digestive enzymes? Comp Biochem Physiol B Biochem Mol Biol. 2002 Aug;132(4):721-8.

150 Garg SC, Dengre SL. Antibacterial activity of essential oil of Tagetes erecta Linn. Hindustan Antibiot Bull. 1986 Feb-Nov;28(1-4):27-9.

151 Jones K. Probiotics: preventing antibiotic-associated diarrhea. J Spec Pediatr Nurs. 2010 Apr;15(2):160-2.

152 Girard P, Coppé MC, Pansart Y, Gillardin JM. Gastroprotective effect of Saccharomyces boulardii in a rat model of ibuprofen-induced gastric ulcer. Pharmacology. 2010;85(3):188-93.

153 Whelan K, Myers CE. Safety of probiotics in patients receiving nutritional support: a systematic review of case reports, randomized controlled trials, and nonrandomized trials. Am J Clin Nutr. 2010 Mar;91(3):687-703.

[154] Krasowska A, Murzyn A, Dyjankiewicz A, Łukaszewicz M, Dziadkowiec D. The antagonistic effect of Saccharomyces boulardii on Candida albicans filamentation, adhesion and biofilm formation. FEMS Yeast Res. 2009 Dec;9(8):1312-21.

[155] Krasowska A, Murzyn A, Dyjankiewicz A, Łukaszewicz M, Dziadkowiec D. The antagonistic effect of Saccharomyces boulardii on Candida albicans filamentation, adhesion and biofilm formation. FEMS Yeast Res. 2009 Dec;9(8):1312-21.

[156] Pothoulakis C. Review article: anti-inflammatory mechanisms of action of Saccharomyces boulardii. Aliment Pharmacol Ther. 2009 Oct 15;30(8):826-33. Epub 2008 Jul 23. Review.

[157] Buts JP. The probiotic Saccharomyces boulardii upgrades intestinal digestive functions by several mechanisms. Acta Gastroenterol Belg. 2009 Apr-Jun;72(2):274-6.

[158] Thomas S, Przesdzing I, Metzke D, Schmitz J, Radbruch A, Baumgart DC. Saccharomyces boulardii inhibits lipopolysaccharide-induced activation of human dendritic cells and T cell proliferation. Clin Exp Immunol. 2009 Apr;156(1):78-87. Epub 2009 Jan 21.

[159] Zanello G, Meurens F, Berri M, Salmon H. Saccharomyces boulardii effects on gastrointestinal diseases. Curr Issues Mol Biol. 2009;11(1):47-58.

[160] Fidan I, Kalkanci A, Yesilyurt E, Yalcin B, Erdal B, Kustimur S, Imir T. Effects of Saccharomyces boulardii on cytokine secretion from intraepithelial lymphocytes infected by Escherichia coli and Candida albicans. Mycoses. 2009 Jan;52(1):29-34.

[161] Czerucka D, Piche T, Rampal P. Review article: yeast as probiotics—Saccharomyces boulardii. Aliment Pharmacol Ther. 2007 Sep 15;26(6): 767-78.

[162] Dalmasso G, Cottrez F, Imbert V, Lagadec P, Peyron JF, Rampal P, Czerucka D, Groux H, Foussat A, Brun V. Saccharomyces boulardii inhibits inflammatory bowel disease by trapping T cells in mesenteric lymph nodes. Gastroenterology. 2006 Dec;131(6):1812-25.

[163] Buts JP, De Keyser N. Effects of Saccharomyces boulardii on intestinal mucosa. Dig Dis Sci. 2006 Aug;51(8):1485-92. Epub 2006 Jul 13. Review.

[164] Sougioultzis S, Simeonidis S, Bhaskar KR, Chen X, Anton PM, Keates S, Pothoulakis C, Kelly CP. Saccharomyces boulardii produces a soluble anti-inflammatory factor that inhibits NF-kappaB-mediated IL-8 gene expression. Biochem Biophys Res Commun. 2006 Apr 28;343(1):69-76.

[165] Singhi SC, Baranwal A. Probiotic use in the critically ill. Indian J Pediatr. 2008 Jun;75(6):621-7. Epub 2008 Aug 31

[166] Astegiano M, Pellicano R, Terzi E, Simondi D, Rizzetto M. Treatment of irritable bowel syndrome. A case control experience. Minerva Gastroenterol Dietol. 2006 Dec;52(4):359-63.

[167] Hernández D, Cardell E, Zárate V. Antimicrobial activity of lactic acid bacteria isolated from Tenerife cheese: initial characterization of plantaricin TF711, a bacteriocin-like substance produced by Lactobacillus plantarum TF711. J Appl Microbiol. 2005;99(1):77-84

[168] Lactobacillus sporogenes. Altern Med Rev. 2002 Aug;7(4):340-2. Review.

[169] La Rosa M, Bottaro G, Gulino N, Gambuzza F, Di Forti F, Inì G, Tornambè E. [Prevention of antibiotic-associated diarrhea with Lactobacillus sporogens and fructo-oligosaccharides in children. A multicentric double-blind vs placebo study]. Minerva Pediatr. 2003 Oct;55(5):447-52.

[170] ten Brink B, Minekus M, van der Vossen JM, Leer RJ, Huis in't Veld JH. Antimicrobial activity of lactobacilli: preliminary characterization and optimization of production of acidocin B, a novel bacteriocin produced by Lactobacillus acidophilus M46. J Appl Bacteriol. 1994 Aug;77(2):140-8

[171] used for colonization of the vagina. Obstet Gynecol. 1990 Feb;75(2):244-8.

[172] [Probiotic properties of industrial strains of lactobacilli and bifidobacteria]. Mikrobiol Z. 2010 Jan-Feb;72(1):9-17. Ukrainian.

[173] de Roock S, van Elk M, van Dijk ME, Timmerman HM, Rijkers GT, Prakken BJ, Hoekstra MO, de Kleer IM. Lactic acid bacteria differ in their ability to induce functional regulatory T cells in humans. Clin Exp Allergy. 2010 Jan;40(1):103-10.

[174] Ostad SN, Salarian AA, Ghahramani MH, Fazeli MR, Samadi N, Jamalifar H. Live and heat-inactivated lactobacilli from feces inhibit Salmonella typhi and Escherichia coli adherence to Caco-2 cells. Folia Microbiol (Praha). 2009;54(2):157-60.

[175] Jain S, Yadav H, Sinha PR, Naito Y, Marotta F. Dahi containing probiotic Lactobacillus acidophilus and Lactobacillus casei has a protective effect against Salmonella enteritidis infection in mice. Int J Immunopathol Pharmacol. 2008 Oct-Dec;21(4):1021-9.

[176] Nanda Kumar NS, Balamurugan R, Jayakanthan K, Pulimood A, Pugazhendhi S, Ramakrishna BS. Probiotic administration alters the gut flora and attenuates colitis in mice administered dextran sodium sulfate. J Gastroenterol Hepatol. 2008 Dec;23(12):1834-9

[177] Moorthy G, Murali MR, Devaraj SN. Lactobacilli facilitate maintenance of intestinal membrane integrity during Shigella dysenteriae 1 infection in rats. Nutrition. 2009 Mar;25(3):350-8.

[178] Kanzato H, Fujiwara S, Ise W, Kaminogawa S, Sato R, Hachimura S. Lactobacillus acidophilus strain L-92 induces apoptosis of antigen-stimulated T cells by modulating dendritic cell function. Immunobiology. 2008;213(5):399-408.

[179] Eremina EIu, Bondarenko VM, Zvereva SI, Nikitina OI, Shaposhnikova LI. [Dysbiotic manifestations during eradication therapy of Helicobacter pylori and their corrections]. Zh Mikrobiol Epidemiol Immunobiol. 2008 May-Jun;(3):62-6.

[180] Pascher M, Hellweg P, Khol-Parisini A, Zentek J. Effects of a probiotic Lactobacillus acidophilus strain on feed tolerance in dogs with non-specific dietary sensitivity. Arch Anim Nutr. 2008 Apr;62(2):107-16.

[181] Ma FZ, Ma HS, Yu Q, Han SX. [Effects of Lactobacilli on regulating NF-kappaB activation and IL-8 secretion in SGC7901 cell impacted by Helicobacter pylori]. Sichuan Da Xue Xue Bao Yi Xue Ban. 2007 Sep;38(5):795-8

[182] Su P, Henriksson A, Mitchell H. Selected prebiotics support the growth of probiotic mono-cultures in vitro. Anaerobe. 2007 Jun-Aug;13(3-4):134-9.

[183] Daniel C, Poiret S, Goudercourt D, Dennin V, Leyer G, Pot B. Selecting lactic acid bacteria for their safety and functionality by use of a mouse colitis model. Appl Environ Microbiol. 2006 Sep;72(9):5799-805.

[184] Saide JA, Gilliland SE. Antioxidative activity of lactobacilli measured by oxygen radical absorbance capacity. J Dairy Sci. 2005 Apr;88(4):1352-7. 185 Klein G. [Use of molecular methods in food microbiology with the example of probiotic use of lactobacilli]. Berl Munch Tierarztl Wochenschr. 2003 Nov-Dec;116(11-12):510-6.

[186] Juárez Tomás MS, Ocaña VS, Wiese B, Nader-Macías ME. Growth and lactic acid production by vaginal Lactobacillus acidophilus CRL 1259, and inhibition of uropathogenic Escherichia coli. J Med Microbiol. 2003 Dec;52(Pt 12):1117-24.

[187] Hamilton-Miller JM. The role of probiotics in the treatment and prevention of Helicobacter pylori infection. Int J Antimicrob Agents. 2003 Oct;22(4): 360-6.

[188] Sullivan A, Barkholt L, Nord CE. Lactobacillus acidophilus, Bifidobacterium lactis and Lactobacillus F19 prevent antibiotic-associated ecological disturbances of Bacteroides fragilis in the intestine. J Antimicrob Chemother. 2003 Aug;52(2):308-11.

[189] Alonso L, Cuesta EP, Gilliland SE. Production of free conjugated linoleic acid by Lactobacillus acidophilus and Lactobacillus casei of human intestinal origin. J Dairy Sci. 2003 Jun;86(6):1941-6.

[190] Fernández MF, Boris S, Barbés C. Probiotic properties of human lactobacilli strains to be used in the gastrointestinal tract. J Appl Microbiol. 2003;94(3):449-55.

[191] Gukasian GB, Akopian LG, Charian LM, Aleksanian IuT. [Antibiotic properties of Lactobacillus acidophilus, "Narine" strain, and the ways for their improvement]. Zh Mikrobio

[192] Ellis M, Egelund J, Schultz CJ, Bacic A. Arabinogalactan-proteins (AGPs): Key regulators at the cell surface? Plant Physiol. 2010 Apr 13.

[193] Bodera P. Influence of prebiotics on the human immune system (GALT). Recent Pat Inflamm Allergy Drug Discov. 2008;2(2):149-53. Review.

[194] Wolucka BA. Biosynthesis of D-arabinose in mycobacteria—a novel bacterial pathway with implications for antimycobacterial therapy. FEBS J. 2008 Jun;275(11):2691-711. Epub 2008 Apr 15.

[195] Choi EM, Kim AJ, Kim YO, Hwang JK. Immunomodulating activity of arabinogalactan and fucoidan in vitro. J Med Food. 2005 Winter;8(4):446-53.

[196] Inngjerdingen KT, Kiyohara H, Matsumoto T, Petersen D, Michaelsen TE, Diallo D, Inngjerdingen M, Yamada H, Paulsen BS. An immunomodulating pectic polymer fromGlinus oppositifolius. Phytochemistry. 2007 Apr;68(7):1046-58.

[197] Schepetkin IA, Faulkner CL, Nelson-Overton LK, Wiley JA, Quinn MT. Macrophage immunomodulatory activity of polysaccharides isolated from Juniperus scopolorum. Int Immunopharmacol. 2005 Dec;5(13-14): 1783-99.

[198] Brecker L, Wicklein D, Moll H, Fuchs EC, Becker WM, Petersen A. Structural and immunological properties of arabinogalactan polysaccharides from pollen of timothy grass (Phleum pratense L.). Carbohydr Res. 2005 Mar 21;340(4):657-63.

[199] Kiyohara H, Matsumoto T, Yamada H. Intestinal immune system modulating polysaccharides in a Japanese herbal (Kampo) medicine, Juzen-Taiho-To. Phytomedicine. 2002 Oct;9(7):614-24.

[200] Qiao H, Duffy LC, Griffiths E, Dryja D, Leavens A, Rossman J, Rich G, Riepenhoff-Talty M, Locniskar M. Immune responses in rhesus rotavirus-challenged BALB/c mice treated with bifidobacteria and prebiotic supplements. Pediatr Res. 2002 Jun;51(6):750-5.

[201] Grieshop CM, Flickinger EA, Fahey GC Jr. Oral administration of arabinogalactan affects immune status and fecal microbial populations in dogs. J Nutr. 2002 Mar;132(3):478-82.

[202] Larch arabinogalactan. Altern Med Rev. 2000 Oct;5(5):463-6.

[203] Robinson RR, Feirtag J, Slavin JL. Effects of dietary arabinogalactan on gastrointestinal and blood parameters in healthy human subjects. J Am Coll Nutr. 2001 Aug;20(4):279-85.

[204] Van Laere KM, Hartemink R, Bosveld M, Schols HA, Voragen AG. Fermentation of plant cell wall derived polysaccharides and their corresponding oligosaccharides by intestinal bacteria. J Agric Food Chem. 2000 May;48(5):1644-52.

[205] Salyers AA, Arthur R, Kuritza A. Digestion of larch arabinogalactan by a strain of human colonic Bacteroides growing in continuous culture. J Agric Food Chem. 1981 May-Jun;29(3):475-80.

[206] Salyers AA, Vercellotti JR, West SE, Wilkins TD. Fermentation of mucin and plant polysaccharides by strains of Bacteroides from the human colon. Appl Environ Microbiol. 1977 Feb;33(2):319-22.

[207] Li XC, Jacob MR, Khan SI, Ashfaq MK, Babu KS, Agarwal AK, Elsohly HN, Manly SP, Clark AM. Potent in vitro antifungal activities of naturally occurring acetylenic acids. Antimicrob Agents Chemother. 2008 Jul;52(7):2442-8.

[208] McDonough V, Stukey J, Cavanagh T. Mutations in erg4 affect the sensitivity of Saccharomyces cerevisiae to medium-chain fatty acids. Biochim Biophys Acta. 2002 Apr 15;1581(3):109-18.

[209] McLain N, Ascanio R, Baker C, Strohaver RA, Dolan JW. Undecylenic acid inhibits morphogenesis of Candida albicans. Antimicrob Agents Chemother. 2000 Oct;44(10):2873-5.

[210] Watson W. Fungal infections of the skin in children. Pediatr Ann. 1976 Dec;5(12):800-11.

[211] Tabernero E, Guaithero E, Ercoli N. Therapeutic action of antimicrobial agents in localized infections of mice. Chemotherapy. 1974;20(1):52-60.

[212] Ishidate K, Mizugaki M, Uchiyama M. Biohydrogenation accompanying the beta-oxidation of unsaturated fatty acids by Candida. J Biochem. 1973 Aug;74(2):279-83.

[213] Knüsel F, Weirich EG. [Microbiological evaluation of salicyclic acid and other broad spectrum antimicrobials]. Dermatologica. 1972;145(4):233-44.

214 Capek A, Simek A. [Antimicrobial effective substances. X. Comparative study of the fungicidal effect of Hexadecyl, Irgasan and 2-aminotridekan and their salts on yeast microorganisms]. Cesk Epidemiol Mikrobiol Imunol. 1971 Jul;20(4):209-11.

215 Morgan LW, Cronk DH, Knott RP. Synthesis and in vitro fungistatic evaluation of some N-substituted amides and amine salts of sorbic acid. J Pharm Sci. 1969 Aug;58(8):942-5.

216 ZULIANI F, MASONI S. [Ultimate potentiation in the antibacterial and fungicidal action of chemotherapeutic agents combined with vitamin K5 (2-methyl-4-amino-1-naphthol HC1).]. Arch Sci Biol (Bologna). 1956 Jan-Feb;40(1):58-65.

217 Scherrer M, Knüsel F, Weirich EG. [Antimicrobial activity of broad-spectrum antimicrobial agents, with special reference to salicylic acid]. Mykosen. 1971 Jul 1;7(6):323-34.

218 McLain N, Ascanio R, Baker C, Strohaver RA, Dolan JW. Undecylenic acid inhibits morphogenesis of Candida albicans. Antimicrob Agents Chemother. 2000 Oct;44(10):2873-5.

219 Loebenberg D, Parmegiani R, Hanks M, Waitz JA. Comparative in vitro and in vivo antifungal activity of tolnaftate and various undecylenates. J Pharm Sci. 1980 Jun;69(6):739-41.

220 Morgan LW, Cronk DH, Knott RP. Synthesis and in vitro fungistatic evaluation of some N-substituted amides and amine salts of sorbic acid. J Pharm Sci. 1969 Aug;58(8):942-5.

221 ZULIANI F, MASONI S. [Ultimate potentiation in the antibacterial and fungicidal action of chemotherapeutic agents combined with vitamin K5 (2-methyl-4-amino-1-naphthol HC1).]. Arch Sci Biol (Bologna). 1956 Jan-Feb;40(1):58-65

222 imenes EC, Sant'Ana AE. Antimicrobial activities of components of the glandular secretions of leaf cutting ants of the genus Atta. Antonie Van Leeuwenhoek. 2009 May;95(4):295-303.

223 Skrivanová E, Molatová Z, Marounek M. Effects of caprylic acid and triacylglycerols of both caprylic and capric acid in rabbits experimentally infected with enteropathogenic Escherichia coli O103. Vet Microbiol. 2008 Jan 25;126(4):372-6.

224 Rayan P, Stenzel D, McDonnell PA. The effects of saturated fatty acids on Giardia duodenalis trophozoites in vitro. Parasitol Res. 2005 Oct;97(3): 191-200.

225 Hoshimoto A, Suzuki Y, Katsuno T, Nakajima H, Saito Y. Caprylic acid and medium-chain triglycerides inhibit IL-8 gene transcription in Caco-2 cells: comparison with the potent histone deacetylase inhibitor trichostatin A. Br J Pharmacol. 2002 May;136(2):280-6.

226 Mu H, Høy CE. Effects of different medium-chain fatty acids on intestinal absorption of structured triacylglycerols. Lipids. 2000 Jan;35(1):83-9.

227 Petschow BW, Batema RP, Ford LL. Susceptibility of Helicobacter pylori to bactericidal properties of medium-chain monoglycerides and free fatty acids. Antimicrob Agents Chemother. 1996 Feb;40(2):302-6.

228 Nair MK, Abouelezz H, Hoagland T, Venkitanarayanan K. Antibacterial effect of monocaprylin on Escherichia coli O157:H7 in apple juice. J Food Prot. 2005Sep;68(9):1895-9.

229 Head KA. Natural approaches to prevention and treatment of infections of the lower urinary tract. Altern Med Rev. 2008 Sep;13(3):227-44.

230 Kruszewska H, Zareba T, Tyski S. Examination of antimicrobial activity of selected non-antibiotic drugs. Acta Pol Pharm. 2004 Dec;61 Suppl:18-21.

231 Bousová I, Martin J, Jahodár L, Dusek J, Palicka V, Drsata J. Evaluation of in vitro effects of natural substances of plant origin using a model of protein glycoxidation. J Pharm Biomed Anal. 2005 Apr 29;37(5):957-62.

232 Hu JF, Yoo HD, Williams CT, Garo E, Cremin PA, Zeng L, Vervoort HC, Lee CM, Hart SM, Goering MG, O'Neil-Johnson M, Eldridge GR. Miniaturization of the structure elucidation of novel natural products—two trace antibacterial acylated caprylic alcohol glycosides from Arctostaphylos pumila. Planta Med. 2005 Feb;71(2):176-80.

233 Edozien JC, Udo UU, Young VR, Scrimshaw NS. Effects of high levels of yeast feeding on uric acid metabolism of young man. Nature. 1970 Oct 10;228(5267):180. PubMed PMID: 5460023.

234 Shiota S, Shimizu M, Sugiyama J, Morita Y, Mizushima T, Tsuchiya T. Mechanisms of action of corilagin and tellimagrandin I that remarkably potentiate the activity of beta-lactams against methicillin-resistant Staphylococcus aureus. Microbiol Immunol. 2004;48(1):67-73.

235 Joksić G, Stanković M, Novak A. Antibacterial medicinal plants Equiseti herba and Ononidis radix modulate micronucleus formation in human lymphocytes in vitro.J Environ Pathol Toxicol Oncol. 2003;22(1):41-8.

236 Yarnell E. Botanical medicines for the urinary tract. World J Urol. 2002 Nov;20(5):285-93. Epub 2002 Oct 17.

237 Newton M, Combest W, Kosier JH. Select herbal remedies used to treat common urologic conditions. Urol Nurs. 2001 Jun;21(3):232-4.

238 Bol'shakova IV, Lozovskaia EL, Sapezhinski II. [Antioxidant properties of plant extracts]. Biofizika. 1998 Mar-Apr;43(2):186-8.

239 Ritch-Krc EM, Thomas S, Turner NJ, Towers GH. Carrier herbal medicine: traditional and contemporary plant use. J Ethnopharmacol. 1996 Jun;52(2):85-94.

240 Jahodár L, Jílek P, Páktová M, Dvoráková V. [Antimicrobial effect of arbutin and an extract of the leaves of Arctostaphylos uva-ursi in vitro]. Cesk Farm. 1985 Jun;34(5):174-8.

241 Schaufelberger D, Hostettmann K. On the molluscicidal activity of tannin containing plants. Planta Med. 1983 Jun;48(6):105-7

242 Groom SN, Johns T, Oldfield PR. The potency of immunomodulatory herbs may be primarily dependent upon macrophage activation. J Med Food. 2007 Mar;10(1):73-9.

243 Allen-Hall L, Cano P, Arnason JT, Rojas R, Lock O, Lafrenie RM. Treatment of THP-1 cells with Uncaria tomentosa extracts differentially regulates the expression if IL-1beta and TNF-alpha. J Ethnopharmacol. 2007 Jan 19;109(2):312-7.

244 Spelman K, Burns J, Nichols D, Winters N, Ottersberg S, Tenborg M. Modulation of cytokine expression by traditional medicines: a review of herbal immunomodulators. Altern Med Rev. 2006 Jun;11(2):128-50.

245 Setty AR, Sigal LH. Herbal medications commonly used in the practice of rheumatology: mechanisms of action, efficacy, and side effects. Semin Arthritis Rheum. 2005 Jun;34(6):773-84.

246 Sheng Y, Akesson C, Holmgren K, Bryngelsson C, Giamapa V, Pero RW. An active ingredient of Cat's Claw water extracts identification and efficacy of quinic acid. J Ethnopharmacol. 2005 Jan 15;96(3):577-84.

247 Sheng Y, Li L, Holmgren K, Pero RW. DNA repair enhancement of aqueous extracts of Uncaria tomentosa in a human volunteer study. Phytomedicine. 2001 Jul;8(4):275-82.

248 Cat's claw scratching away at the immune system? TreatmentUpdate. 1999 Nov 1;11(8):1-2.

249 Steinberg PN. [Cat's Claw: an herb from the Peruvian Amazon]. Sidahora. 1995 Apr-May:35-6.

250 Reinhard KH. Uncaria tomentosa (Willd.) D.C.: cat's claw, uña de gato, or savéntaro. J Altern Complement Med. 1999 Apr;5(2):143-51.

251 Coelho JM, Antoniolli AB, Nunes e Silva D, Carvalho TM, Pontes ER, Odashiro AN. [Effects of silver sulfadiazine, ipê roxo (tabebuia avellanedae) extract and barbatimão (stryphnodendron adstringens) extract on cutaneous wound healing in rats]. Rev Col Bras Cir. 2010 Feb;37(1):45-51.

252 Melo e Silva F, de Paula JE, Espindola LS. Evaluation of the antifungal potential of Brazilian Cerrado medicinal plants. Mycoses. 2009 Nov;52(6):511-7.

253 Kung HN, Yang MJ, Chang CF, Chau YP, Lu KS. In vitro and in vivo wound healing-promoting activities of beta-lapachone. Am J Physiol Cell Physiol. 2008 Oct;295(4):C931-43.

254 Byeon SE, Chung JY, Lee YG, Kim BH, Kim KH, Cho JY. In vitro and in vivo anti-inflammatory effects of taheebo, a water extract from the inner bark of Tabebuia avellanedae. J Ethnopharmacol. 2008 Sep 2;119(1):145-52.

255 Twardowschy A, Freitas CS, Baggio CH, Mayer B, dos Santos AC, Pizzolatti MG, Zacarias AA, dos Santos EP, Otuki MF, Marques MC. Antiulcerogenic activity of bark extract of Tabebuia avellanedae, Lorentz ex Griseb. J Ethnopharmacol. 2008 Aug 13;118(3):455-9.

256 Ekanem AP, Brisibe EA. Effects of ethanol extract of Artemisia annua L. against monogenean parasites of Heterobranchus longifilis. Parasitol Res. 2010 Apr;106(5):1135-9. Epub 2010 Feb 18.

257 Adams M, Zimmermann S, Kaiser M, Brun R, Hamburger M. A protocol for HPLC-based activity profiling for natural products with activities against tropical parasites. Nat Prod Commun. 2009 Oct;4(10):1377-81.

258 de Oliveira TC, Silva DA, Rostkowska C, Béla SR, Ferro EA, Magalhães PM, Mineo JR. Toxoplasma gondii: effects of Artemisia annua L. on susceptibility to infection in experimental models in vitro and in vivo. Exp Parasitol. 2009 Jul;122(3):233-41. Epub 2009 Apr 21.

259 Abdel-Shafy S, El-Khateeb RM, Soliman MM, Abdel-Aziz MM. The efficacy of some wild medicinal plant extracts on the survival and development of third instar larvae of Chrysomyia albiceps (Wied) (Diptera: Calliphoridae). Trop Anim Health Prod. 2009 Dec;41(8):1741-53.

260 Tariq KA, Chishti MZ, Ahmad F, Shawl AS. Anthelmintic activity of extracts of Artemisia absinthium against ovine nematodes. Vet Parasitol. 2009 Mar 9;160(1-2):83-8.

261 Caner A, Döşkaya M, Değirmenci A, Can H, Baykan S, Uner A, Başdemir G, Zeybek U, Gürüz Y. Comparison of the effects of Artemisia vulgaris and Artemisia absinthium growing in western Anatolia against trichinellosis (Trichinella spiralis) in rats. Exp Parasitol. 2008 May;119(1):173-9.

262 Caner A, Döşkaya M, Değirmenci A, Can H, Baykan S, Uner A, Başdemir G, Zeybek U, Gürüz Y. Comparison of the effects of Artemisia vulgaris and Artemisia absinthium growing in western Anatolia against trichinellosis (Trichinella spiralis) in rats. Exp Parasitol. 2008 May;119(1):173-9.

263 Iqbal Z, Lateef M, Ashraf M, Jabbar A. Anthelmintic activity of Artemisia brevifolia in sheep. J Ethnopharmacol. 2004 Aug;93(2-3):265-8.

264 Tagboto S, Townson S. Antiparasitic properties of medicinal plants and other naturally occurring products. Adv Parasitol. 2001;50:199-295. Review.

265 Kim JT, Park JY, Seo HS, Oh HG, Noh JW, Kim JH, Kim DY, Youn HJ. In vitro antiprotozoal effects of artemisinin on Neospora caninum. Vet Parasitol. 2002 Jan3;103(1-2):53-63.

266 Darwish RM, Aburjai TA. Effect of ethnomedicinal plants used in folklore medicine in Jordan as antibiotic resistant inhibitors on Escherichia coli. BMC Complement Altern Med. 2010 Feb 28;10:9.

267 Ahameethunisa AR, Hopper W. Antibacterial activity of Artemisia nilagirica leaf extracts against clinical and phytopathogenic bacteria. BMC Complement Altern Med. 2010 Jan 29;10:6.

268 Vega AE, Wendel GH, Maria AO, Pelzer L. Antimicrobial activity of Artemisia douglasiana and dehydroleucodine against Helicobacter pylori. J Ethnopharmacol. 2009 Jul 30;124(3):653-5.

269 Cha JD, Jeong MR, Jeong SI, Moon SE, Kim JY, Kil BS, Song YH. Chemical composition and antimicrobial activity of the essential oils of Artemisia scoparia and A. capillaris. Planta Med. 2005 Feb;71(2):186-90.

270 Lee OH, Lee BY. Antioxidant and antimicrobial activities of individual and combined phenolics in Olea europaea leaf extract. Bioresour Technol. 2010 May;101(10):3751-4. Epub 2010 Jan 27.

271 Dell'Agli M, Fagnani R, Galli GV, Maschi O, Gilardi F, Bellosta S, Crestani M, Bosisio E, De Fabiani E, Caruso D. Olive oil phenols modulate the expression of metalloproteinase 9 in THP-1 cells by acting on nuclear factor-kappaB signaling. J Agric Food Chem. 2010 Feb 24;58(4):2246-52.

272 Medina E, Brenes M, García A, Romero C, de Castro A. Bactericidal activity of glutaraldehyde-like compounds from olive products. J Food Prot. 2009 Dec;72(12):2611-4.

273 El SN, Karakaya S. Olive tree (Olea europaea) leaves: potential beneficial effects on human health. Nutr Rev. 2009 Nov;67(11):632-8. Review.

274 Zhao G, Yin Z, Dong J. Antiviral efficacy against hepatitis B virus replication of oleuropein isolated from Jasminum officinale L. var. grandiflorum. J Ethnopharmacol. 2009 Sep 7;125(2):265-8.

275 Jiang JH, Jin CM, Kim YC, Kim HS, Park WC, Park H. Anti-toxoplasmosis effects of oleuropein isolated from Fraxinus rhychophylla. Biol Pharm Bull. 2008 Dec;31(12):2273-6.

276 Waterman E, Lockwood B. Active components and clinical applications of olive oil. Altern Med Rev. 2007 Dec;12(4):331-42. Review.

277 Medina E, Brenes M, Romero C, García A, de Castro A. Main antimicrobial compounds in table olives. J Agric Food Chem. 2007 Nov 28;55(24):9817-23. Epub 2007 Oct 31.

278 Pereira AP, Ferreira IC, Marcelino F, Valentão P, Andrade PB, Seabra R, Estevinho L, Bento A, Pereira JA. Phenolic compounds and antimicrobial activity of olive (Olea europaea L. Cv. Cobrançosa) leaves. Molecules. 2007 May 26;12(5):1153-62.

279 Medina E, de Castro A, Romero C, Brenes M. Comparison of the concentrations of phenolic compounds in olive oils and other plant oils: correlation with antimicrobial activity. J Agric Food Chem. 2006 Jul 12;54(14):4954-61.

280 Corona G, Tzounis X, Assunta Dessì M, Deiana M, Debnam ES, Visioli F, Spencer JP. The fate of olive oil polyphenols in the gastrointestinal tract: implications of gastric and colonic microflora-dependent biotransformation. Free Radic Res. 2006 Jun;40(6):647-58.

281 Hamdi HK, Castellon R. Oleuropein, a non-toxic olive iridoid, is an anti-tumor agent and cytoskeleton disruptor. Biochem Biophys Res Commun. 2005 Sep2;334(3):769-78.

282 Zanichelli D, Baker TA, Clifford MN, Adams MR. Inhibition of Staphylococcus aureus by oleuropein is mediated by hydrogen peroxide. J Food Prot. 2005 Jul;68(7):1492-6.

283 Miles EA, Zoubouli P, Calder PC. Effects of polyphenols on human Th1 and Th2 cytokine production. Clin Nutr. 2005 Oct;24(5):780-4.

284 Micol V, Caturla N, Pérez-Fons L, Más V, Pérez L, Estepa A. The olive leaf extract exhibits antiviral activity against viral haemorrhagic septicaemia rhabdovirus (VHSV). Antiviral Res. 2005 Jun;66(2-3):129-36.

285 Furneri PM, Marino A, Saija A, Uccella N, Bisignano G. In vitro antimycoplasmal activity of oleuropein. Int J Antimicrob Agents. 2002 Oct;20(4):293-6.

286 Sadjjadi SM, Zoharizadeh MR, Panjeshahin MR. In vitro screening of different Allium sativum extracts on hydatid cysts protoscoleces. J Invest Surg. 2008 Nov-Dec;21(6):318-22.

287 Peyghan R, Powell MD, Zadkarami MR. In vitro effect of garlic extract and metronidazole against Neoparamoeba pemaquidensis, page 1987 and isolated amoebae from Atlantic salmon. Pak J Biol Sci. 2008 Jan 1;11(1): 41-7.

288 Toulah FH, Al-Rawi MM. Efficacy of garlic extract on hepatic coccidiosis in infected rabbits (Oryctolagus cuniculus): histological and biochemical studies. J Egypt Soc Parasitol. 2007 Dec;37(3):957-68.

[289] Ghazanfari T, Hassan ZM, Khamesipour A. Enhancement of peritoneal macrophage phagocytic activity against Leishmania major by garlic (Allium sativum)treatment. J Ethnopharmacol. 2006 Feb 20;103(3):333-7.

[290] Sréter T, Széll Z, Varga I. Attempted chemoprophylaxis of cryptosporidiosis in chickens, using diclazuril, toltrazuril, or garlic extract. J Parasitol. 1999 Oct;85(5):989-91.

[291] Nok AJ, Williams S, Onyenekwe PC. Allium sativum-induced death of African trypanosomes. Parasitol Res. 1996;82(7):634-7.

[292] Soffar SA, Mokhtar GM. Evaluation of the antiparasitic effect of aqueous garlic (Allium sativum) extract in hymenolepiasis nana and giardiasis. J Egypt Soc Parasitol. 1991 Aug;21(2):497-502.

[293] Harjai K, Kumar R, Singh S. Garlic blocks quorum sensing and attenuates the virulence of Pseudomonas aeruginosa. FEMS Immunol Med Microbiol. 2009 Sep 18.

[294] Ivanova A, Mikhova B, Najdenski H, Tsvetkova I, Kostova I. Chemical composition and antimicrobial activity of wild garlic Allium ursinum of Bulgarian origin. Nat Prod Commun. 2009 Aug;4(8):1059-62.

[295] Fani MM, Kohanteb J, Dayaghi M. Inhibitory activity of garlic (Allium sativum) extract on multidrug-resistant Streptococcus mutans. J Indian Soc Pedod Prev Dent. 2007 Oct-Dec;25(4):164-8.

[296] Lal M, Kaur H, Gupta LK. Anticryptococcal activity of garlic extract—A preliminary report. Indian J Med Microbiol. 2003 Jul-Sep;21(3):214.

[297] Gomaa NF, Hashish MH. The inhibitory effect of garlic (Allium sativum) on growth of some microorganisms. J Egypt Public Health Assoc. 2003;78(5-6):361-72.

[298] Bjarnsholt T, Jensen PØ, Rasmussen TB, Christophersen L, Calum H, Hentzer M, Hougen HP, Rygaard J, Moser C, Eberl L, Høiby N, Givskov M. Garlic blocks quorum sensing and promotes rapid clearing of pulmonary Pseudomonas aeruginosa infections. Microbiology. 2005 Dec;151(Pt 12):3873-80.

[299] Amin M, Kapadnis BP. Heat stable antimicrobial activity of Allium ascalonicum against bacteria and fungi. Indian J Exp Biol. 2005 Aug;43(8):751-4.

[300] Shuford JA, Steckelberg JM, Patel R. Effects of fresh garlic extract on Candida albicans biofilms. Antimicrob Agents Chemother. 2005 Jan;49(1):473.

[301] Dikasso D, Lemma H, Urga K, Debella A, Addis G, Tadele A, Yirsaw K. Investigation on the antibacterial properties of garlic (Allium sativum) on pneumonia causing bacteria. Ethiop Med J. 2002 Jul;40(3):241-9.

[302] Belknap JK. Black walnut extract: an inflammatory model. Vet Clin North Am Equine Pract. 2010 Apr;26(1):95-101.

[303] McConnico RS, Stokes AM, Eades SC, Moore RM. Investigation of the effect of black walnut extract on in vitro ion transport and structure of equine colonic mucosa. Am J Vet Res. 2005 Mar;66(3):443-9.

[304] Quave CL, Plano LR, Pantuso T, Bennett BC. Effects of extracts from Italian medicinal plants on planktonic growth, biofilm formation and adherence of methicillin-resistant Staphylococcus aureus. J Ethnopharmacol. 2008 Aug 13;118(3):418-28.

305 Amarowicz R, Dykes GA, Pegg RB. Antibacterial activity of tannin constituents from Phaseolus vulgaris, Fagoypyrum esculentum, Corylus avellana and Juglans nigra. Fitoterapia. 2008 Apr;79(3):217-9.

306 Lans C, Turner N, Khan T, Brauer G. Ethnoveterinary medicines used to treat endoparasites and stomach problems in pigs and pets in British Columbia, Canada. Vet Parasitol. 2007 Sep 30;148(3-4):325-40.

307 Maes M, Kubera M, Leunis JC. The gut-brain barrier in major depression: intestinal mucosal dysfunction with an increased translocation of LPS from gram negative enterobacteria (leaky gut) plays a role in the inflammatory pathophysiology of depression. Neuro Endocrinol Lett. 2008 Feb; 29(1):117-24.

308 Purohit V, Bode JC, Bode C, Brenner DA, et al. Alcohol, intestinal bacterial growth, intestinal permeability to endotoxin, and medical consequences: summary of a symposium. Alcohol. 2008 Aug;42(5):349-61. Epub 2008 May 27.

309 Amin AH, Subbaiah TV, Abbasi KM. Berberine sulfate: antimicrobial activity, bioassay, and mode of action. Can J Microbiol 1969; 15:1067-1076.

310 Rabbani GH, Butler T, Knight J, et al. Randomized controlled trial of berberine sulfate therapy for diarrhea due to enterotoxigenic Escherichia coli and Vibrio cholerae. J Inf Dis 1987;155:979-984.

311 Sack RB, Froehlich JL. Berberine inhibits intestinal secretory response of Vibrio cholerae and Escherichia coli enterotoxins. Infect Immun 1982;35:471-475.

312 Sun D, Courtney HS, Beachey EH. Berberine sulfate blocks adherence of Streptococcus pyogenes to epithelial cells, fibronectin, and hexadecane. Antimicrob Agents Chemother 1988;32:1370-1374.

313 Mahajan VM, Sharma A, Rattan A. Antimycotic activity of berberine sulphate: An alkaloid from an Indian medicinal herb. Sabouraudia 1982;20:79-81.

314 Nakamoto K, Sadamori S, Hamada T. Effects of crude drugs and berberine hydrochloride on the activities of fungi. J Prosthet Dent 1990;64:691-694.

315 Subbaiah TV, Amin AH. Effect of berberine sulphate on Entamoeba histolytica. Nature 1967;215:527-528

316 Kaneda Y, Tanaka T, Saw T. Effects of berberine, a plant alkaloid, on the growth of anaerobic protozoa in axenic culture. Tokai J Exp Clin Med 1990;15: 417-423.

317 Ghosh AK, Bhattacharyya FK, Ghosh DK. Leishmania donovani: Amastigote inhibition and mode of action of berberine. Exp Parasitol 1985;60:404-413.

318 Singhal KC. Anthelmintic activity of berberine hydrochloride against Syphacia obvelata in mice. Indian J Exp Biol 1976;14:345-347.

319 Mohan M, Pant CR, Angra SK, Mahajan VM. Berberine in trachoma. Indian J Ophthalmol 1982;30:69-75.

320 Sabir M, Mahajan VM, Mohapatra LN, Bhide NK. Experimental study of the antitrachoma action of berberine. Indian J Med Res 1976;64:1160-1167.

321 Gudima SO, Memelova LV, Borodulin VB, et al. Kinetic analysis of interaction of human immunodeficiency virus reverse transcriptase with alkaloids. Mol Biol (Mosk) 1994;28:1308-1314.

[322] Kaneda Y, Torii M, Tanaka T, Aikawa M. In vitro effects of berberine sulphate on the growth and structure of Entamoeba histolytica, Giardia lamblia and Trichomonas vaginalis. Ann Trop Med Parasitol 1991;85:417-425.

[323] Kumazawa Y, Itagaki A, Fukumoto M, et al. Activation of peritoneal macrophages by berberine alkaloids in terms of induction of cytostatic activity. Int J Immunopharmacol 1984;6:587-592.

[324] Huang CG, Chu ZL, Yang ZM. Effects of berberine on synthesis of platelet TXA2 and plasma PGI2 in rabbits. Chung Kuo Yao Li Hsueh Pao 1991;12:526-528.

[325] Fleming, Thomas ed. PDR for Herbal Medicines 1st ed. Medical Economics Company, Montvale, NJ, 1998.

[326] Moore, Michael. Medicinal Plants of the Desert and Canyon West. Museum of New Mexico Press, Santa Fe, NM, 1989.

[327] Kay, M.A. Healing with Plants in the American and Mexican West. University of Arizona Press, Tucson, AZ, 1996.

[328] Arcila-Lozano CC, Loarca-Pina G, Lecona-Uribe S, Gonzalez de Mejia E. Oregano: properties, composition and biological activity. Arch Latinoam Nutr. 2004 Mar;54(1):100-11.

[329] Force M, Sparks WS, Ronzio RA. Inhibition of enteric parasites by emulsified oil of oregano in vivo. Phytother Res. 2000 May;14(3):213-4.

[330] Walter BM, Bilkei G. Immunostimulatory effect of dieatary oregano etheric oils on lymphocytes from growth-retarded, low-weight growing-finishing pigs and productivity. Tijdschr Diergeneeskd. 2004 Mar 15;129(6):178-81.

[331] Park BS, Lee HK, Lee SE, Piao XL, Takeoka GR, Wong RY, Ahn YJ, Kim JH. Antibacterial activity of Tabebuia impetiginosa Martius ex DC (Taheebo) against Helicobacter pylori. J Ethnopharmacol. 2006 Apr 21;105(1-2): 255-62

[332] Park BS, Kim JR, Lee SE, Kim KS, Takeoka GR, Ahn YJ, Kim JH. Selective growth-inhibiting effects of compounds identified in Tabebuia impetiginosa inner bark on human intestinal bacteria. J Agric Food Chem. 2005 Feb 23;53(4):1152-7.

[333] Warashina T, Nagatani Y, Noro T. Constituents from the bark of Tabebuia impetiginosa. Phytochemistry. 2004 Jul;65(13):2003-11.

CHAPTER TEN: BRAIN INFLAMMATION

[1] Perry VH. The influence of systemic inflammation on inflammation in the brain: implications for chronic neurodegenerative disease. Brain Behav Immun. 2004 Sep;18(5):407-13.

[2] Perry VH. Contribution of systemic inflammation to chronic neurodegeneration. Acta Neuropathol. 2010 Sep;120(3):277-86.

[3] Vichaya EG, Young EE, Frazier MA, Cook JL, Welsh CJ, Meagher MW. Social disruption induced priming of CNS inflammatory response to Theiler's virus is dependent upon stress induced IL-6 release. J Neuroimmunol. 2011 Oct 28;239(1-2):44-52.

4   Pascoe MC, Crewther SG, Carey LM, Crewther DP. What you eat is what you are—a role for polyunsaturated fatty acids in neuroinflammation induced depression? Clin Nutr. 2011 Aug;30(4):407-15.

5   Burton MD, Sparkman NL, Johnson RW. Inhibition of interleukin-6 trans-signaling in the brain facilitates recovery from lipopolysaccharide-induced sickness behavior. J Neuroinflammation. 2011 May 19;8:54.

6   Miyake S, Yamamura T. Ghrelin: friend or foe for neuroinflammation. Discov Med. 2009 Aug;8(41):64-7.

7   Dénes A, Ferenczi S, Kovács KJ. Systemic inflammatory challenges compromise survival after experimental stroke via augmenting brain inflammation, blood-brain barrier damage and brain oedema independently of infarct size. J Neuroinflammation. 2011 Nov 24;8:164.

8   Meerman EE, Verkuil B, Brosschot JF. Decreasing pain tolerance outside of awareness. J Psychosom Res. 2011 Mar;70(3):250-7.

9   McDougall JJ. Arthritis and pain. Neurogenic origin of joint pain. Arthritis Res Ther. 2006;8(6):220.

10 McDougall JJ. Arthritis and pain. Neurogenic origin of joint pain. Arthritis Res Ther. 2006;8(6):220.

11 Walton KD, Dubois M, Llinás RR. Abnormal thalamocortical activity in patients with Complex Regional Pain Syndrome (CRPS) type I. Pain. 2010 Jul;150(1):41-51.

12 Schulze J, Troeger C. [Increased sympathetic activity assessed by spectral analysis of heart rate variability in patients with CRPS I]. Handchir Mikrochir Plast Chir. 2010 Feb;42(1):44-8.

13 Kwan CL, Diamant NE, Pope G, Mikula K, Mikulis DJ, Davis KD. Abnormal forebrain activity in functional bowel disorder patients with chronic pain. Neurology. 2005 Oct 25;65(8):1268-77.

14 Brian L, Michael M. Mechanistic explanations how cell-mediated immune activation, inflammation and oxidative and nitrosative stress pathways and their sequels and concomitants play a role in the pathophysiology of unipolar depression. Neurosci Biobehav Rev. 2011 Dec 19.

15 Ekmekcioglu C. Are proinflammatory cytokines involved in an increased risk for depression by unhealthy diets? Med Hypotheses. 2012 Feb;78(2):337-40.

16 Van Zuiden M, Heijnen CJ, van de Schoot R, Amarouchi K, Maas M, Vermetten E, Geuze E, Kavelaars A. Cytokine production by leukocytes of military personnel with depressive symptoms after deployment to a combat-zone: a prospective, longitudinal study. PLoS One. 2011;6(12):e29142.

17 Bansal V, Costantini T, Kroll L, Peterson C, Loomis W, Eliceiri B, Baird A, Wolf P, Coimbra R. Traumatic brain injury and intestinal dysfunction: uncovering the neuro-enteric axis. J Neurotrauma. 2009 Aug;26(8):1353-9.

18 Peng YP, Qiu YH, Qiu J, Wang JJ. Cerebellar interposed nucleus lesions suppress lymphocyte function in rats. Brain Res Bull. 2006 Dec 11;71(1-3):10-7.

19 Ghoshal D, Sinha S, Sinha A, Bhattacharyya P. Immunosuppressive effect of vestibulo-cerebellar lesion in rats. Neurosci Lett. 1998 Nov 27;257(2):89-92.

20 Ni SJ, Qiu YH, Lu JH, Cao BB, Peng YP. Effect of cerebellar fastigial nuclear lesions on differentiation and function of thymocytes. J Neuroimmunol. 2010 May;222(1-2):40-7.

21 Barneoud P, Neveu PJ, Vitiello S, Le Moal M. Functional heterogeneity of the right and left cerebral neocortex in the modulation of the immune system. Physiol Behav. 1987;41(6):525-30.

22 Neveu PJ. [Cerebral lateralization and immune response]. Encephale. 1989 Jul-Aug;15(4):405-8.

23 Gao HM, Hong JS. Why neurodegenerative diseases are progressive: uncontrolled inflammation drives disease progression. Trends Immunol. 2008 Aug;29(8):357-65.

24 Block ML, Hong JS. Microglia and inflammation-mediated neurodegeneration: multiple triggers with a common mechanism. Prog Neurobiol. 2005 Jun;76(2):77-98.

25 Drake C, Boutin H, Jones MS, et al. Brain inflammation is induced by co-morbidities and risk factors for stroke. Brain Behav Immun. 2011 Aug;25(6):1113-22.

26 Streit WJ. Microglial response to brain injury: a brief synopsis. Toxicol Pathol. 2000 Jan-Feb;28(1):28-30.

27 Block ML, Hong JS. Microglia and inflammation-mediated neurodegeneration: multiple triggers with a common mechanism. Prog Neurobiol. 2005 Jun;76(2):77-98.

28 Lull ME, Block ML. Microglial activation and chronic neurodegeneration. Neurotherapeutics. 2010 Oct;7(4):354-65.

29 Carty ML, Wixey JA, Reinebrant HE, Gobe G, Colditz PB, Buller KM. Ibuprofen inhibits neuroinflammation and attenuates white matter damage following hypoxia-ischemia in the immature rodent brain. Brain Res. 2011 Jul 21;1402:9-19.

30 Friese MA, Fugger L. T cells and microglia as drivers of multiple sclerosis pathology. Brain. 2007 Nov;130(Pt 11):2755-7.

31 Kraft AD, Harry GJ. Features of microglia and neuroinflammation relevant to environmental exposure and neurotoxicity. Int J Environ Res Public Health. 2011 Jul;8(7):2980-3018. Epub 2011 Jul 20.

32 Harry GJ, Kraft AD. Neuroinflammation and microglia: considerations and approaches for neurotoxicity assessment. Expert Opin Drug Metab Toxicol. 2008 Oct;4(10):1265-77.

33 Jovanović Z, Jovanović S. [Resistance of nerve cells to oxidative injury]. Med Pregl. 2011 Jul-Aug;64(7-8):386-91.

34 Mittelbronn M, Schittenhelm J, Bakos G, de Vos RA, Wehrmann M, Meyermann R, Bürk K. CD8(+)/perforin/granzyme B(+) effector cells infiltrating cerebellum and inferior olives in gluten ataxia. Neuropathology. 2010 Feb 1;30(1):92-6.

35 Smith, Quentin, Transport of glutamate and other amino acids at the blood-brain barrier. Journal of Nutrition. 2000;130:1016S-1022S.

36 Lockman PR, et al. Nanoparticle technology for drug delivery across the blood-brain barrier. Drug Dev Ind Pharm. 2002 Jan;28 (1):1-13

[37] Lefauconnier JM. Transport processes through the blood-brain barrier. Reprod Nutr Dev. 1989;29(6):689-702.

[38] Haorah J, et al. Alcohol-induced oxidative stress in brain endothelial cells causes blood-brain-barrier dysfunction. Journal of Leukocyte Biology. 2005.;78:1223-1232.

[39] Espositie, P, et al. Acute stress increases permeability of the blood-brain-barrier through activation of brain mast cells. Brain Research. 2001;888(1): 117-127.

[40] Atul F, et al. Elevated levels of homocysteine compromise blood-brain-barrier integrity in mice. Blood. 2005.

[41] Homocysteine attenuates blood brain barrier function by inducing oxidative stress and the junctional proteins. FASEB.2008;22:734-7.

[42] Kamada H, et al. Influence of hyperglycemia on oxidative stress and matrix metalloproteinase-9 activation after focal cerebral ischemia/reperfusion in rats. Stroke. 2007;38:1044-1049.

[43] Jali C, et al. Cyclooxygenase inhibition limits blood-brain-barrier disruption following intracerebral injection of tumor necrosis factor-alpha in the rat. JPET. 2007;323(2):488-498.

[44] Haroh J, et al. Oxidative stress activates protein tyrosine kinase and matrix metalloproteinases leading to blood-brain barrier dysfunction. J Neurochem. 2007;22(1).

[45] Hedley-Whyte ET & Hsu DW. Efect of dexamethasone on blood-brain-barrier in normal mouse. Ann Neurol. 1986;19:373-377.

[46] Long JB & Holaday JW. Blood-brain barrier:endogenous modulation by adrenal-cortical function. Science. 1985;227:15801583.

[47] Neuwelt EA, Barnett PA, Bigner DD, and Frenkel EP. Effects of adrenal cortical steroids and osmotic blood-brain-barrier opening on methotrexate delivery to gliomos in the rodentL the factor of the blood-brain-barrier. Proc Natl Acad Sci. 1982:79:4420-4423.

[48] Reid AC, Teasdale GM, McCulloch J. The effects of dexamethasone administration and withdrawal on water permeability across the blood-brain-barrier. Ann Neurool. 1983;13:28-31.

[49] Ziylan YZ, et al. Efect of dexamethasone on transport of alpha-aminoisobutyric acid and sucrose across the blood-brain-barrier. J Neurochem. 1988;51:1338-1342

[50] Rezai-Zaldeh K, Ehrhart J, Bai Y, Sansberg PR, Bickfored P, Tan J, Shytel D. Apigenin and luteolin modulate microglial activation via inhibition of STAT-1 induced CD40 expression. J Neuroinflammation. 2008;25(5):41.

[51] Elsisi NS, Darling-Reed S, Lee EY, Oriaku ET, Soiman KF. Ibuprofen and apigenin induce apoptosis and cell cycle arrest in activated microglia. Neurosci Lett. 2005;375(2):91-6.

[52] Ha SK, Lee P, Park JA, Oh HR, Lee SY, Park JH, Lee EH, Ryu JH, Lee KR, Kim SY. Apigenin inhibits the production of NO and PGE2 in microglia and inhibits neuronal cell death in a middle cerebral artery occlusion-induced focal ischemia mice model. Neurochem Int. 2008;52(4-5):878-886.

53 Shanmugam K, Holmquist L, Steele M, Stuchbury G, Berbaum K, Schulz O, Benavente GO, Castillo J, Burnell J, Garcia Rivas V, Munch G. Plant-derived polypheonls attenuate lipopolysaccharide-induced nitric oxide and tumour necrosis factor production in murine microglia and macrophages. Mol Nutr Food Res. 2008;52(4):427-38.

54 Chen HO, Jin ZY, Wang XJ, Xu XM, Deng L, Zhao JW. Luteolin protects dopaminergic neurons from inflammation-induced injury through inhibition of microglial activation. Neurosci Lett. 2008;448(2):175-179.

55 Rezai-Zaldeh K, Ehrhart J, Bai Y, Sansberg PR, Bickfored P, Tan J, Shytel D. Apigenin and luteolin modulate microglial activation via inhibition of STAT-1 induced CD40 expression. J Neuroinflammation. 2008;25(5):41.

56 Jang S, Kelly KW, Johnson RW. Luteolin reduces IL-6 produciton in microglia by inhibiting JNK phosphorylation and activation of AP-1. Proc Natl Acad Sci USA. 2008;105(21):7534-7539.

57 Kim JS, Lee HJ, Lee MH, Kim J, Jin C, Ryu JH. Luteolin inhibits LPS-stimulated inducible nitric oxide synthase expression in BV-2 microglial cells. Planta Med. 2006;72(1):65-8.

58 Suk K, Lee H, Kang SS, CHO GJ, Choi WS. Flavonoid baicalein attenuates activation-induced cell death of brain microglia. J Pharmacol Exp Ther. 2003;305(2):638-45.

59 Tarrago T, Kickik N, Claasen B, Prades R, Teixido M, Giralt E. Baicalin, a prodrug able to reach the CNS, is a prolyl olgiopeptidase inhibitor. Bioorg Med Chem. 2008:16(15):7516-24.

60 Cheng Y, He G, Mu X, Zhang T, Li X, Hu J, Xu B, Du G. Neuroprotective effect of baicelein against MPTP neurotoxicity: behavioral, biochemical and immunohistochemical profile. Neurosci Lett. 2008;441(1):16-20.

61 Wu PH, Shen YC, Wang YH, Chi CW, Yen JC. Baicalein attenuates methamphetamine-induced loss of dopamine transporter in mouse striatum. Toxicology. 2006;226(2-3):238-45.

62 Im HI, Joo WS, Nam E, Lee ES, Hwang YJ, Kim YS. Baicalein prevents 6-hydroxydopamine dysfunction and lipid peroxidation in mice. J Pharmacol Sci. 2005;98(2):185-9.

63 Lee HJ, Noh YH, Lee DY, Kim YS, Kim KY, Chung YH, Lee WB, Kim SS. Baicalein attenuates 6-hydroxydopamine-induced neurotoxicityin SH-SY5Y cells. Eur J Cell Biol. 2005;84(11):897-905.

64 Labeau A, Esclaire F, Rostene W, Pelaprat D. Baicalein protects cortical neurons from beta-amyloid (25-350 induced toxicity. Neuroreport. 2001;12(10):2199-202.

65 Yang L, Sun HL, Wu LM, Guo XJ, Dou H, Tso MO, Zhao L, Li SM. Baicalein Reduces Inflammatory process in a Rodent Model of Diabetic Retinopathy. Invest Opthalmol Vis Sci. 2008; Nov 14. [Epub ahead of print].

66 He XL, Wang YH, Gao M, Li XX, Zhang TT, Du GH. Baicalein protects rat brain mitochondria against chronic cerebral hypoperfusion-induced oxidative damage. Brain Res. 2008; Oct 18 [Epub ahead of print]

67 Baicalein improves cognitive deficits induced by chronic cerebral hypoperfusion in rats. Pharmacol Biochem Behav. 2007. 86(3):423-30.

[68] Chen SF, Hsu CW, Huan WH, Wang JY. Post-injury baicalein improves histological and functional outcomes and reduces inflammatory cytokines after experimental traumatic brain injury. Br J Pharmacol. 2008 [Epub ahead of print].

[69] Meng XL, Chen GL, Yank JY, Wang S, Wu CF, Wang JM. Inhibitory effect of a novel resveratrol derivative on nitric oxide production in lipopolysaccharide-activated microglia. Pharmazie. 2008;63(9):671-5.

[70] Bi XL, Yang JY, Dong YX, Wang JM, Cui YH, Ikeshima T, Zhao YO, Wu CF. Resveratrol inhibits nitric oxide and TNF-alpha production by lipopolysaccharide-activated microglia. Int Immunopharmacol. 2005;5(1)185-93.

[71] Lorenz P, Roychowdhury S, Engelmann M, Wolf G, Thomas H. Oxyresveratrol and resveratrol are potent antioxidants and free radical scavengers: effect on nitrosative and oxidative stress derived from microglia cells. J of Nitric Oxide Society. 2003;9(2):64-76.

[72] Meng XL, Yang JY, Chen GL, Zhang LJ, Wang LH, Li J, Wang JM, Wu CF. RV09, a novel resveratrol analogue, inhibits NO and TNF-alpha production by LPS-activated microglia. Int Immunopharmacol. 2008; 8(8): 1074-82.

[73] Candelario-Jalil E, de Oliveira AC, Graf S, Bhatia HS, Hull M, Munoz E, Fiebich BL. Resveratrol potently reduces prostaglandin E2 production and free radical formation in lipopolysaccharide-activated primary rat microglia. J Neuroinflammation. 2007;4:25.

[74] Kim YA, Kim GY, Park KY, Choi YH. Resveratrol inhibits nitric oxide and prostaglandin E2 production by lipopolysaccharide-activated C6 microglia. J Med Food. 2007;10(2):218-24.

[75] Chen J, Zhou Y, Mueller-Steiner S, Chen Lf, Kwon H, Yi S, Mucke L, Gan L. SIRT1 protects against microglia-dependent amyloid-beta toxicity through inhibiting NF-kappaB signaling. J Bio Chem. 2005;280(48):40364-74.

[76] Meng XL, Yang JY, Chen GI, Wang LH, Zhang LJ, Wang S, Wu CE. Effects of resveratrol and its derivatives on lipopolysaccharide-induced microglia activation and their structure-activity relationships. Chem Biol Interact. 2008;174(1):51-9.

[77] Bureau G, Longpre F, Martinoli MG. Resveratrol and quercetin, two natural polyphenols, reduce apoptotic neuronal cell death induced by neuroinflammation. J Neurosci Res. 2008;86(2):403-10.

[78] Milde J, Eistner EF, Grassmann J. Synergistic inhibition of low-density lipoprotein oxidation by rutin, gamma-terpineine, and ascorbic acid. Phytomedicine. 2004;11(2-3):105-13.

[79] Silva AR, Pinheiro Am, Souza CS, Freitas Sr, Vasconcellos V, Freire SM, Velozo ES, Tardy M, El Bacha RS, Costa MF, Costa SL. The flavonoid rutin induces astrocyte and microglia activation and regulates TNF-alpha and NO release in primary glia cell cultures. Cell Biol Toxicol. 2008;24(1):75-86.

[80] Koda T, Kuroda Y, Imai H. Rutin supplementation in the diet has protective effects against toxicant induced hippocampal injury by suppression of microglia activation and pro-inflammatory cytokines: protective effect of rutin against toxicant-induced hippcampal injury. Cell Mol Neurobiol. 2009 Jan 21 [Epub ahead of print].

81 Huang O, Wu LJ, Tashiro S, Onedera S, Ikejima T. Elevated levels of DNA repair enzymes and antioxidative enzymes by (+)-catechin in murine microglia cells after oxidative stress. J Asian Nat Prod Res. 8(1-2):61-71.

82 Huang O, Wu LJ, Tashiro S, Gao HY, Onodera S, Ikejima T. (=)- Catechin, an ingredient of green tea, protects murine microglia from oxidative stress-induced DNA damage and cell cycle arrest. J Pharmacol Sci. 98(1):Epub 2005 May.

83 Mandel S, Amit T, Reznichenko L, Weinreb O, Youdim MB. Green tea catechins as brain-permeable, matural iron chelators-antioxidants for the treatment of neurodegenerative disorders. Mol Nutr Food Res. 50(2): 229-34.

84 Mandel S, Maor G, Youdim MB. Iron and alpha-synuclein in the substantia nigra of MPTP-treated mice: effect of neuroprotective drugs R-ampomorpine and green tea polyphenol (-)- epigallocatechin-3-gallate. J Mol Neurosci. 2004;24(3):401-6.

85 Li R, Huang YG, Fang D, Le WD. (-)-Epigallocatechin gallate inhibits lipopolysaccharide-induced microglial actiation and protects against inflammation-mediated dopaminergic neuron injury. J Neurosci Res. 2004;78(5):723-31.

86 Yang S, Zhang D, Yang Z, Hu X, Liu J, Wilson B, Block M, Hong JS. Curcumin protects dopaminergic neuron against LPS induced neurotoxicity in primary rat neuron/gllia culture. Neurochem Res. 2008;33(10):2044-53.

87 Jin CY, Lee JD, Park C, Choi YH, Kim GY. Curcumin attenuates the release of pro-inflammatory cytokines in lipoplysaccharide-stimulated BV2 microglia. Acta Pharmacol Sin. 2007;28(10):1645-51.

88 Jung KK, Lee HS, Cho JY, Shin WC, Rhee MH, Kim TG, Kang JH, Hong S. Kang SY. Inhibitory effect of curcumin on nitric oxide production from lipopolysaccharide-activated primary microglia. Life Sci. 79(21):2022-31.

89 Wang O, Sun AY, Simonyi Jensen MD, Shelat PB, Rottinghaus GE, MacDonald RS, Miller DK, Lubahn DE, Weisman GA, Sun GY. Neuroprotectivemechanisms of / curcumin against cerebral ischemia-induced neuronal apoptosis and behavioral deficits. J Neurosci Res. 2005;82(1):138-48.

90 Kang G, Kong PJ, Yuh YJ, Lim SY, Yim SV, Chun W, Kim SS. Curcumin suppresses liopolysaccharide-induced cyclooxygenase-2 expresiion by inhibiting activator protein 1 and nuclear factor kappaB binding in BV2 microglia cells. J Pharmacol Sci. 2004;94(3):325-8.

91 Natarajan C & Bright JJ. Curcumin inhibits experimental allergic encephalomyelitis by blocking IL-2 signaling through Jana Kinase-STAT pathway in T lymphocytes. J Immunol. 2002;168(12):6506-13.

92 Giri Rk, Rajagopal V, Kalra VK. Curcumin, the active constituent of tumeric, inhibits amyloid peptide-induced cythchemokine gene expression and CCR5-mediated chemotaxis of THP-1 monocytes by modulating early growth response-1 transcription factor. J Neurochem. 2004 91(5):1199-210.

CHAPTER ELEVEN: WHAT IS NEUROLOGICAL AUTOIMMUNITY?

[1] http://www.niaid.nih.gov/topics/autoimmune/Documents/adccreport.pdf

[2] http://www.aarda.org/

[3] http://www.aarda.org/

[4] Braunschweig D, Van de Water J. Maternal autoantibodies in autism. Arch Neurol. 2012 Jun;69(6):693-9.

[5] Cohly HH, Panja A. Immunological findings in autism. Int Rev Neurobiol. 2005;71:317-41.

[6] Gruden MA, Sewell RD, Yanamandra K, Davidova TV, Kucheryanu VG, Bocharov EV, Bocharova OR, Polyschuk VV, Sherstnev VV, Morozova-Roche LA. Immunoprotection against toxic biomarkers is retained during Parkinson's disease progression. J Neuroimmunol. 2011 Apr;233(1-2):221-7.

[7] Papachroni KK, Ninkina N, Papapanagiotou A, Hadjigeorgiou GM, Xiromerisiou G, Papadimitriou A, Kalofoutis A, Buchman VL. Autoantibodies to alpha-synuclein in inherited Parkinson's disease. J Neurochem. 2007 May;101(3):749-56.

[8] Murinson BB, Vincent A. Stiff-person syndrome: autoimmunity and the central nervous system. CNS Spectr. 2001 May;6(5):427-33.

[9] Honnorat J, Saiz A, Giometto B, Vincent A, Brieva L, de Andres C, Maestre J, Fabien N, Vighetto A, Casamitjana R, Thivolet C, Tavolato B, Antoine J, Trouillas P, Graus F. Cerebellar ataxia with anti-glutamic acid decarboxylase antibodies: study of 14 patients. Arch Neurol. 2001 Feb;58(2):225-30.

[10] Takagi M, Yamasaki H, Endo K, Yamada T, Kaneko K, Oka Y, Mori E. Cognitive decline in a patient with anti-glutamic acid decarboxylase autoimmunity; case report. BMC Neurol. 2011 Dec 21;11:156.

[11] Peltola J, Kulmala P, Isojärvi J, Saiz A, Latvala K, Palmio J, Savola K, Knip M, Keränen T, Graus F. Autoantibodies to glutamic acid decarboxylase in patients with therapy-resistant epilepsy. Neurology. 2000 Jul 12;55(1):46-50.

[12] Pearce DA, Atkinson M, Tagle DA. Glutamic acid decarboxylase autoimmunity in Batten disease and other disorders. Neurology. 2004 Dec 14;63(11):2001-5.

[13] Singh A, Kamen DL. Potential benefits of vitamin D for patients with systemic lupus erythematosus. Dermatoendocrinol. 2012 Apr 1;4(2):146-51.

[14] Antico A, Tampoia M, Tozzoli R, Bizzaro N. Can supplementation with vitamin D reduce the risk or modify the course of autoimmune diseases? A systematic review of the literature. Autoimmun Rev. 2012 Jul 7.

[15] Muñoz-Ortego J, Torrente-Segarra V, Prieto-Alhambra D, Salman-Monte T, Carbonell-Abello J. Prevalence and predictors of vitamin D deficiency in non-supplemented women with systemic lupus erythematosus in the Mediterranean region: a cohort study. Scand J Rheumatol. 2012 Jul 26.

[16] Tewthanom K, Janwityanuchit S, Totemchockchyakarn K, Panomvana D. Correlation of lipid peroxidation and glutathione levels with severity of systemic lupus erythematosus: a pilot study from single center. J Pharm Pharm Sci. 2008;11(3):30-4.

[17] Yan Z, Banerjee R. Redox remodeling as an immunoregulatory strategy. Biochemistry. 2010 Feb 16;49(6):1059-66.

18 Yan Z, Banerjee R. Redox remodeling as an immunoregulatory strategy. Biochemistry. 2010 Feb 16;49(6):1059-66.

19 Hushmendy S, Jayakumar L, Hahn AB, Bhoiwala D, Bhoiwala DL, Crawford DR. Select phytochemicals suppress human T-lymphocytes and mouse splenocytes suggesting their use in autoimmunity and transplantation. Nutr Res. 2009 Aug;29(8):568-78.

20 Shindler KS, Ventura E, Dutt M, Elliott P, Fitzgerald DC, Rostami A. Oral resveratrol reduces neuronal damage in a model of multiple sclerosis. J Neuroophthalmol. 2010 Dec;30(4):328-39.

21 Petro TM. Regulatory role of resveratrol on Th17 in autoimmune disease. Int Immunopharmacol. 2011 Mar;11(3):310-8. Epub 2010 Aug 12.

22 Anekonda TS, Adamus G. Resveratrol prevents antibody-induced apoptotic death of retinal cells through upregulation of Sirt1 and Ku70. BMC Res Notes. 2008 Dec 1;1:122.

23 Yoshida Y, Shioi T, Izumi T. Resveratrol ameliorates experimental autoimmune myocarditis. Circ J. 2007 Mar;71(3):397-404.

24 Mito S, Watanabe K, Harima M, Thandavarayan RA, Veeraveedu PT, Sukumaran V, Suzuki K, Kodama M, Aizawa Y. Curcumin ameliorates cardiac inflammation in rats with autoimmune myocarditis. Biol Pharm Bull. 2011;34(7):974-9.

25 Xie L, Li XK, Takahara S. Curcumin has bright prospects for the treatment of multiple sclerosis. Int Immunopharmacol. 2011 Mar;11(3):323-30. Epub 2010 Sep 8.

26 Kurien BT, D'Souza A, Scofield RH. Heat-solubilized curry spice curcumin inhibits antibody-antigen interaction in in vitro studies: a possible therapy to alleviate autoimmune disorders. Mol Nutr Food Res. 2010 Aug;54(8): 1202-9.

27 Xie L, Li XK, Funeshima-Fuji N, Kimura H, Matsumoto Y, Isaka Y, Takahara S. Amelioration of experimental autoimmune encephalomyelitis by curcumin treatment through inhibition of IL-17 production. Int Immunopharmacol. 2009 May;9(5):575-81.

CHAPTER TWELVE: INTRODUCTION TO NEUROTRANSMITTERS

1 Kandel ER, Schwartz JH, and Jessel TM. Principles of Neural Science, 4th edition, New York:McGraw-Hill, 2000.

2 Bear M, Bear MF, Connors BW, Paradiso MA. Neuroscience: Exploring the Brain, Hagerstown, MD: Lippinocottt Williams and Wilkens, 2001.

3 Vöhringer PA, Ghaemi SN. Solving the antidepressant efficacy question: effect sizes in major depressive disorder. Clin Ther. 2011 Dec;33(12):B49-61.

CHAPTER THIRTEEN: ACETYLCHOLINE

[1] Easton A, Douchamps V, Eacott M, Lever C. A specific role for septohippocampal acetylcholine in memory? Neuropsychologia. 2012 Aug 3.

[2] Devanand DP, Pradhaban G, Liu X, Khandji A, De Santi S, Segal S, Rusinek H, Pelton GH, Honig LS, Mayeux R, Stern Y, Tabert MH, de Leon MJ. Hippocampal and entorhinal atrophy in mild cognitive impairment: prediction of Alzheimer disease. Neurology. 2007 Mar 13;68(11):828-36.

[3] Raves ML, Harel M, Pang YP, et al. Structure of acetylcholinesterase complexed with the nootropic alkaloid, (-)-huperzine A. Nat Struct Biol. 1997;4:57–63.

[4] Ashani Y, Peggins JO III, Doctor BP. Mechanism of inhibition of cholinesterases by huperzine A. Biochem Biophys Res Commun. 1992;184:719–726.

[5] Pang YP, Kozikowski AP. Prediction of the binding sites of huperzine A in acetylcholinesterase by docking studies. J Comput Aided Mol Des. 1994;8:669–681.

[6] Laganiere S, Corey J, Tang XC, et al. Acute and chronic studies with the anticholinesterase Huperzine A: effect on central nervous system cholinergic parameters. Neuropharmacology. 1991;30:763–768.

[7] Xu SS, Goa ZX, Weng Z, et al. Efficacy of tablet huperzine-A on memory, cognition, and behavior in Alzheimer's disease. Zhongguo Yao Li Xue Bao. 1995;16:391–395.

[8] Sun QQ, Xu SS, Pan JL, et al. Huperzine-A capsules enhance memory and learning performance in 34 pairs of matched adolescent students [abstract]. Zhongguo Yao Li Xue Bao. 1999;20:601–603.

[9] Zhou J, Zhang HY, Tang XC. Huperzine A attenuates cognitive deficits and hippocampal neuronal damage after transient global ischemia in gerbils. Neurosci Lett. 2001;313:137-140.

[10] Ved HS, Koenig ML, Dave JR, et al. Huperzine A, a potential therapeutic agent for dementia, reduces neuronal cell death caused by glutamate. Neuroreport. 1997;8:963–968.

[11] Lopez Cm, Govoni S, Battaini F, et al. Effect of a new cognition enhancer alpha-glycerlphosphorylcholine, on scopolamine induced amnesia and brain acetylcholine. Pharmacol Biochem Behav 1991;39(4):835-40.

[12] Sigala S, Imperato A , Rizzoneli P, et al. L-alpha glycerylphosphorylcholine antagonizes scopolamine-induced amnesia and enhances hippocampal cholinergic transmission in the rat. Eur J Pharmacol 1992;211(3):351-8.

[13] Moreno DJ and Moreno M. Cognitive improvement in mild to moderate Alzheimer's dementia after treatment with the acetylcholine precursor choline alfoscerete: a multicenter, double-blind, randomized, placebo-controlled trial. Clin Ther 2003;25(1):178-93.

[14] Sbbati C, et al. Nootropic therapy of cerebral aging. Adv Therapy 1991;8:268.

[15] Vezzetti V, Bettini R. Clinical and instrument evaluation of the effect of choline alfoscerate on cerebral decline. Presse Medicale 1992;5:141.

[16] Ban TA, et al. Choline alfoscerate in elderly patients with cognitive decline due to dementing illness. New Trends Clin Neuropharmacol 1991;5:87.

[17] Palleschi M, et al. Evaluation of effectiveness and tolerability of alpha-GFC (choline alfoscerate) in patients suffering from slight/moderate cognitive decline. Preliminary results. Geriatria 1992;4:13.

[18] Parnetti L, et al. Multicentre study of l-a-glyceryl-phosphorycholine vs ST200 among patients with probable senile dementia of Alzheimer's type. Drugs & Aging 1993;3:159.

[19] Aguglia E, et al. Choline alphoscerate in the treatment of mental pathology following acute cerebrovascular accident. Funct Neurol 1993;8 (Suppl):5.

[20] Barbagallo Sangiorgi G, et al. alpha-glycerophosphocholine in the mental recovery of cerebral ischemic attacks. Ann N Y Acad Sci 1994;717:253.

[21] Parnetti L, Amenta F, Gallai V. Choline alfoscerate in cognitive decline and in acute cerebrovascular disease: an analysis of published clinical data. Mechs Ageing Dev 2001;22:2041.

[22] Spagnolie A, et al. Long-term acetyl-L-carnitine treatment in Alzheimer's disease. Neurology 1991;41:1726-1732.

[23] Bowman B. Acetylcholine and Alzheimer's disease. Nutr Rev 1992; 50: 142-144.

[24] Careta A, et al. Acetyl-L-Carntine and Alzheimer's disease. Pharmacological considerations beyond cholinergic sphere. Ann NY Acad Sci 1993;695: 324-326.

[25] Pettegrew JW, et al. Clinical and neurochemical effects of acetyl-Lcarnitine in Alzheimer's disease. Neurobiol Aging 1995;16:1-4.

[26] Kimura S, Furukawa Y, Wakasugi J, Ishihara Y, Nakayama A. Antagonism of L (-) pantothenic acid on lipid metabolism in animals. J Nutr Sci Vitaminol (Tokyo). 1980;26(2):113-7.

[27] Rivera Calimlim L, Hartley D, Osterhout D. Effects of ethanol and pantothenic acid on brain acetylcholine synthesis. Br J Pharmacol 1988;95(1):77-82.

CHAPTER FOURTEEN: SEROTONIN

[1] Goodman N. The serotonergic system and mysticism: could LSD and the nondrug-induced mystical experience share common neural mechanisms? J Psychoactive Drugs. 2002 Jul-Sep;34(3):263-72.

[2] Mohr P, Bitter I, Svestka J, Seifritz E, Karamustafalioglu O, Koponen H, Sartorius N. Management of depression in the presence of pain symptoms. Psychiatr Danub. 2010 Mar;22(1):4-13. Erratum in: Psychiatr Danub. 2010 Sep;22(3):476.

[3] Lambru G, Matharu M. Serotonergic agents in the management of cluster headache. Curr Pain Headache Rep. 2011 Apr;15(2):108-17.

[4] Marazziti D, Carlini M, Dell'Osso L. Treatment strategies of obsessive-compulsive disorder and panic disorder/agoraphobia. Curr Top Med Chem. 2012;12(4):238-53.

[5] Camilleri M, Katzka DA. Irritable bowel syndrome: methods, mechanisms, and pathophysiology. Genetic epidemiology and pharmacogenetics in irritable bowel syndrome. Am J Physiol Gastrointest Liver Physiol. 2012 May 15;302(10):G1075-84.

6   Lewis CE. Neurochemical mechanisms of chronic antisocial behavior
     (psychopathy). A literature review. J Nerv Ment Dis. 1991 Dec;179(12):
     720-7.

7   Osterlund MK. Underlying mechanisms mediating the antidepressant effects of
     estrogens. Biochim Biophys Acta. 2010 Oct;1800(10):1136-44.

8   Sarzi Puttini P, Caruso I. Primary fibromylagia syndrome and 5-hydrox-L-
     tryptophan: a 90-day open study. J Int Med Res1992;20(2):182-9.

9   De Benedittis G, Massei R. Serotonin precursors in chronic primary headache.
     A double-blind cross-over study with L-5-hydroxytryptophan vs. placebo.
     Journal of Neurosurgical Sciences 1985;29(3):239-48.

10   Birdsall TC."5-Hydroxytryptophan: a clinically-effective serotonin precursor
     Alternative medicine review : a journal of clinical therapeutic 1998;3(4):
     271-80.

11   Meryer S. Use of neurotransmitter precursors for treatment of depression. Alter
     Med Rev 2000;5(1):64-71.

12   Turner EH, Loftis JM, Blackwell AD. Serotonin a la carte: supplementation
     with the serotonin precursor 5-hydroxytryptophan. Pharmacol.
     Ther2006;109 (3):325-38.

13   Randløv C, J. Mehlsen, CF, Thomsen, C. Hedman, H, von Fircks and K.
     Winther. The efficacy of St. John's Wort in patients with minor depressive
     symptoms or dysthymia—a double-blind placebo-controlled study"
     Phytomedicine. 2006; 13(4): 215–221.

14   Woelk H, et al. Comparison of St John's wort and imipramine for treating
     depression: randomised controlled trial. Br Med J 2000; 321:536-9.

15   Schrader E, et al. Equivalence of St John's wort extract (Ze 117) and fluoxetine:
     a randomised, controlled study in mild-moderate depression. Int Clin
     Psychopharmacology 2000;15:61-68.

16   Laakmann G, Schule C, Baghai T, Kieser M. St. John's wort in mild to
     moderate depression: the relevance of hyperforin for the clinical efficacy.
     Pharmacopsychiatry 1998;31 (Suppl 1):54-9.

17   Harrer G, Schmidt U, Kuhn U, Biller A. Comparison of equivalence between
     the St. John's wort extract LoHyp-57 and fluoxetine. Arzneimittelforschung
     1999;49 (4):289-96.

18   Philipp M, Kohnen R, Hiller KO. Hypericum extract versus imipramine or
     placebo in patients with moderate depression: randomised multicentre study
     of treatment for eight weeks. Br Med J 1999;319 (7224):1534-8.

19   Lecrubier et al. "Efficacy of St. John's wort extract WS 5570 in major
     depression: a double-blind, placebo-controlled trial." Am J Psychiatry.
     2002;159(8):1361-6.

20   Bressa GM. S-Adenosyl-L-methionine (SAMe) as antidepressant: meta-analysis
     of clinical studies. Acta Neurol Scand 1994;89:7-14.

21   Curcio M, Catto E, Stramentinoli G, Algeri S. Effect of S-adenosyl-
     L-methionine on serotonin metabolism in rat brain. Prog
     Neuropsychopharmacol Biol Psychiatry 1978;2:65-71.

[22] Fonlupt P, Barailler J, Roche M, Cronenberger L, Pacheco H. Effets de la S-adénosylméthionine et de la S-adénosylhomocystéine sur la synthèse, in vivo, de la noradrénaline et de la sérotonine dans différentes parties du cerveau de rat. C R Seances Acad Sci D 1979; 288: 283-6.

[23] Bottiglieri T, Laundy M, Martin R, Carney MWP, Nissenbaum H, Toone BK, et al. S-Adenosylmethionine influences monoamine metabolism. Lancet 1984;ii:224.

[24] B. Kagan et al,"Oral [SAMe] in depression: a... double-blind, placebo controlled trial. Am J Psychiat 1990;147:591-95.

[25] E. Reynolds et al.Methylation and mood" Lancet II, 1984:196-98.

CHAPTER FIFTEEN: GABA

[1] Remler MP, Marcussen WH. A GABA-EEG test of the blood-brain barrier near epileptic foci. Appl Neurophysiol. 1983;46(5-6):276-85.

[2] Bhaskar S, Tian F, Stoeger T, Kreyling W, de la Fuente JM, Grazú V, Borm P, Estrada G, Ntziachristos V, Razansky D. Multifunctional Nanocarriers for diagnostics, drug delivery and targeted treatment across blood-brain barrier: perspectives on tracking and neuroimaging. Part Fibre Toxicol. 2010 Mar 3;7:3.

[3] Holzl J, & Godau P. Receptor binding studies with Valeriana officinalis on the benzodiazepine receptor. Planta Medica 1989; 55.

[4] Mennini T, Bernasconi P, et al.In vitro study in the interaction of extracts and pure compounds from Valerian officinalis roots with GABA, benzodiazepine and barbiturate receptors. Fitoterapia 1993;64:291-300.

[5] Hendriks H, Bos R, Allersma DP, Malingre TM, Koster AS. Pharmacological screening of valerenal and some other components of essential oil of Valeriana officinalis. Planta Med 1981;42:62-8.

[6] Ortiz JG, Nieves-Natal J, Chavez P. Effects of Valeriana officinalis extracts on [3H] flunitrazepam binding, synaptosomal [3H] GABA uptake, and hippocampal [3H] GABA release. Neurochem Res 1999;24:1373-8.

[7] Houghton PJ. The scientific basis for the reputed activity of Valerian. J Pharm Pharmacol 1999;51(5):505-12.

[8] Houghton PJ. The scientific basis for the reputed activity of Valerian. J Pharm Pharmacol 1999;51(5):505-12.

[9] Ferreira F, Santos M, Faro, et al. Effect of extracts of Valeriana officinalis on [3H] GABA. Revista Portuguesa de Farmacia 1996; 46:74-77.

[10] Santos MS, Ferreira F, et al. Synatposmal GABA releases as influenced by valerian root extract – involvement of the GABA carrier. Arch Int Pharmacodyn Ther 1994; 327:220-31.

[11] Sevenja L Mayer R. et al. Interaction of valerian extracts of different polarity with adenosine receptors: Identification of isovaltrate as an inverse agonist at A1 receptors. Biochemical Pharmacology 2007;73:248-258.

[12] Reidel E, Hansel R, Ehrke G. Inhibition of gamma-aminobutyric acid catabolism by valerenic acid derivatives. Planta Medica 1982;48:219-220.

13   Dean W. and English J. Lithium Orotate: The Unique, Safe Mineral with Multiple Uses, Vitamin Research News, July, 1999.

14   Cade JKJ. Lithium salts in the treatment of psychotic excitement. Med J Aust 1949;349-352.

15   Schrauzer GN. Effects of nutritional lithium supplementation on mood. Biol Trace El Res 1994;40:89-101.

16   Schrauzer GN. and Shrestha KP. Lithium in Drinking Water and the Incidences of Crimes, Suicides, and Arrests Related to Drug Addictions, Biol. Trace Element Res.1990; 25:105-113.

17   Schrauzer G. Lithium Occurances, dietary intakes, nutritional essentiality. JACN 2002; 21(1):14-21.

18   Vanyo L, Vu T, et al. Lithium induced perturbations of vitamin B12, folic acid and DNA metabolism. In Schrauzer Gn, Klippel, KF(eds): Lithium in Biology and Medicine. Weinheim:VCH Verlag, pp 17-30, 1991.

19   Akhondzadeh S, Kashani L, Mobaseri M, Hosseini SH, Nikzad S, Khani M. Passionflower in the treatment of opiates withdrawl [sic]: a double-blind randomized controlled trial. Journal of Clinical Pharmacy and Therapeutics. 2001;25(5):369-373.

20   Dhawan K, Kumar S, Sharma A. Anti-anxiety studies on extracts of Passiflora incarnata Linneaus. Journal of Ethnopharmacology. 2001;78:165-170.

21   Dhawan K, Kumar S, Sharma A. Anxiolytic activity of aerial and underground parts of Passiflora incarnata. Fitoterapia. 2001;72(8):922-926.

22   Krenn L. Passion Flower (Passiflora incarnata L.)—a reliable herbal sedative. Wiener Medizinische Wochenschrift. 2002;152(15-16):404-406.

23   Wolfman C, Viola H, Paladini A, Dajas F, Medina JH. Possible anxiolytic effects of chrysin, a central benzodiazepine receptor ligand isolated from Passiflora coerulea. Pharmacology, Biochemistry, and Behavior. 1994;47(1):1-4.

24   Reginatto FH, De-Paris F, Petry RD, et al. Evaluation of anxiolytic activity of spray dried powders of two South Brazilian Passiflora species. Phytotherapy Research. 2006;20(5):348-351.

25   Speroni E, Minghetti A. Neuropharmacological activity of extracts from Passiflora incarnata. Planta Medica. 1988;54(6):488-491.

26   Yokogoshi H, Kobayashi M, Mochizuki M, Terashima T (1998). "Effect of theanine, r-glutamylethylamide, on brain monoamines and striatal dopamine release in conscious rats". Neurochem Res 1998;23(5):667-73.

27   Gomez-Ramirez M. "The Deployment of Intersensory Selective Attention: A High-density Electrical Mapping Study of the Effects of Theanine". Clin Neuropharmacol 30 (1): 25-38.

28   Kimura K, Ozeki M, Juneja L, Ohira H (2007). "L-Theanine reduces psychological and physiological stress responses. Biol Psychol 2007;74(1): 39-45.

29   Lu K, Gray M, Oliver C, Liley D, Harrison B, Bartholomeusz C, Phan K, Nathan P.The acute effects of L-theanine in comparison with alprazolam on anticipatory anxiety in humans. Hum Psychopharmacol 2004;19(7): 457-65.

30 Nathan P, Lu K, Gray M, Oliver C. The neuropharmacology of L-theanine(N-ethyl-L-glutamine): a possible neuroprotective and cognitive enhancing agent. J Herb Pharmacother 2006;6(2): 21-30.

31 McCown TJ, Givens BS, Breese GR. "Amino acid influences on seizures elicited within the inferior colliculus." J Pharmacol Exp Ther. 1987 Nov; 243(2): 603-8.

32 Batuev AS, Bragina TA, Aleksandrov AS, Riabinskaia EA. "Audiogenic epilepsy: a morphofunctional analysis." Zh Vyssh Nerv Deiat Im I P Pavlova 1997 Mar-Apr; 47(2) 431-8.

33 Saransaari P, Oja SS. "Release of endogenous glutamate, aspartate, GABA, and taurine from hippocampal slices from adult and developing mice under cell-damaging conditions." Neurochem Res 1998 Apr; 23(4): 563-70.

34 Dawson R Jr, Pelleymounter MA, Cullen NJ, Gollub M, Liu S. "An age-related decline in striatal taurine is correlated with a loss of dopaminergic markers." Brain Res Bull 1999 Feb; 48(3); 319-24.

35 Mizushima S, Nara Y, Sawamura M, Yamori Y. "Effects of oral taurine supplementation on lipids and sympathetic nerve tone." Adv Exp Med Biol 1996; 403:615-22.

36 Kuroda K, "Effects of excitatory sulfur amino acids on glutamate transport in synaptosomes isolated from the rat cerebral cortex." Rinsho Shinkeigaku 1998 Dec; 38(12): 1019-23.

37 Principles of Medicinal Chemistry. by Foye, W.O., T.L. Lemke and D.A. Williams. Williams & Wilkins. Fourth Edition, 1995.

38 Caglar E, Ugurlu S, Ozenoglu A, Can G, Kadioglu P, Dobrucali A. Autoantibody frequency in celiac disease. Clinics (Sao Paulo). 2009;64(12):1195-200.

39 Kakleas K, Paschali E, Kefalas N, Fotinou A, Kanariou M, Karayianni C, Karavanaki K. Factors for thyroid autoimmunity in children and adolescents with type 1 diabetes mellitus. Ups J Med Sci. 2009;114(4):214-20.

40 Lock RJ, Tengah DP, Williams AJ, Ward JJ, Bingley PJ, Wills AJ, Unsworth DJ. Cerebellar ataxia, peripheral neuropathy, "gluten sensitivity" and anti-neuronal autoantibodies. Clin Lab. 2006;52(11-12):589-92.

41 Rout UK, Dhossche DM. A pathogenetic model of autism involving Purkinje cell loss through anti-GAD antibodies. Med Hypotheses. 2008 Aug;71(2):218-21.

42 Bhaskar S, Tian F, Stoeger T, Kreyling W, de la Fuente JM, Grazú V, Borm P, Estrada G, Ntziachristos V, Razansky D. Multifunctional Nanocarriers for diagnostics, drug delivery and targeted treatment across blood-brain barrier: perspectives on tracking and neuroimaging. Part Fibre Toxicol. 2010 Mar 3;7:3.

43 Remler MP, Marcussen WH. A GABA-EEG test of the blood-brain barrier near epileptic foci. Appl Neurophysiol. 1983;46(5-6):276-85.

CHAPTER SIXTEEN: DOPAMINE

[1] Lim BK, Huang KW, Grueter BA, Rothwell PE, Malenka RC. Anhedonia requires MC4R-mediated synaptic adaptations in nucleus accumbens. Nature. 2012 Jul 11;487(7406):183-9.

[2] Nocjar C, Zhang J, Feng P, Panksepp J. The social defeat animal model of depression shows diminished levels of orexin in mesocortical regions of the dopamine system, and of dynorphin and orexin in the hypothalamus. Neuroscience. 2012 Aug 30;218:138-53.

[3] Howland RH. The use of dopaminergic and stimulant drugs for the treatment of depression. J Psychosoc Nurs Ment Health Serv. 2012 Feb;50(2):11-4.

[4] Forbes EE, Dahl RE. Research Review: altered reward function in adolescent depression: what, when and how? J Child Psychol Psychiatry. 2012 Jan;53(1):3-15.

[5] Beeler JA. Thorndike's Law 2.0: Dopamine and the Regulation of Thrift. Front Neurosci. 2012;6:116. Epub 2012 Aug 10.

[6] Buchheim A, Viviani R, Kessler H, Kächele H, Cierpka M, Roth G, George C, Kernberg OF, Bruns G, Taubner S. Changes in prefrontal-limbic function in major depression after 15 months of long-term psychotherapy. PLoS One. 2012;7(3):e33745. Epub 2012 Mar 28.

[7] Luciana M, Wahlstrom D, Porter JN, Collins PF. Dopaminergic modulation of incentive motivation in adolescence: age-related changes in signaling, individual differences, and implications for the development of self-regulation. Dev Psychol. 2012 May;48(3):844-61.

[8] Depue RA, Collins PF. Neurobiology of the structure of personality: dopamine, facilitation of incentive motivation, and extraversion. Behav Brain Sci. 1999 Jun;22(3):491-517; discussion 518-69.

[9] Salamone JD, Correa M. Motivational views of reinforcement: implications for understanding the behavioral functions of nucleus accumbens dopamine. Behav Brain Res. 2002 Dec 2;137(1-2):3-25.

[10] Fusar-Poli P, Meyer-Lindenberg A. Striatal Presynaptic Dopamine in Schizophrenia, Part II: Meta-Analysis of [18F/11C]-DOPA PET Studies. Schizophr Bull. 2012 Jan 26.

[11] Fusar-Poli P, Rubia K, Rossi G, Sartori G, Balottin U. Striatal dopamine transporter alterations in ADHD: pathophysiology or adaptation to psychostimulants? A meta-analysis. Am J Psychiatry. 2012 Mar;169(3):264-72.

[12] Henderson HL, Townsend J, Tortonese DJ. Direct effects of prolactin and dopamine on the gonadotroph response to GnRH. J Endocrinol. 2008 May;197(2):343-50.

[13] Tharakan B, Dhanasekaran M, Mize-Berge J, Manyam BV. Anti-parkinson botanical Mucuna pruriens prevents levodopa induced plasmid and genomic DNA damage. Phytother Res 2007;11

[14] Mizra L and Wagner H. Extraction of bioactive principles from Mucuna pruriens seeds. Indian J Biochem Biophys 2007;44(1):56-60.

[15] Katzenschlager R, Evans A, Manson A, et al. Mucuna pruriens in Parkinson's disease: a double blind clinical and pharmacological study. J Neurol Neurosrug Psychiatry 2004; 75(12);1672-7.

[16] Manyam BV, Dhanasekaran M, Hare TA. Neuroprotective effects of the antiparkinson drug Mucuna pruriens. Phytother Res 2004;18(9):706-12.

[17] Singhal B, Lalkaka J, Sankhia C. Epidemiology and treatment of Parkinson's disease in India. Parkinsonism Relat Disord 2003;9 Suppl 2:S105-9.

[18] Mayam BV & Sanchez-Ramos JR. Traditional and complimentary therapies for Parkinson's disease. Adv Neurol 1999;80:565-74.

[19] Sebelli H, Fink P, Fawcett J. Tom C. Sustained antidepressant effect of PEA replacement. J Neuropsychiatry Clin Neurosci 1996;8(2): 168-71.

[20] Guang-Xi Z, Hiroshi S, et al. Decreased B-phenylethylamine in CSF in Parkinson's Disease. J Neurol Neurosurg Psychiatry 1997;63:754-758.

[21] Karoum F, Wolf M, Mosniam AD. Effects of the administration of amphetmaine eithier alone or in combination with resperine or cocaine, or regional brain beta-phenetylamine and dopamine release. Am J Ther 1997;4(9/10):333-342.

[22] Kausage A. Decrease beta-phenletyamine in urin of children with attention deficit hyperactivity disorder and autistic disorder. No To Hattatsu 2002; 34(3):243-8.

[23] Michell S, Lewis G, et al. Biomarkers of Parkinso's disease 2004;127(8): 1693-1705.

[24] McGuire S, Sortwell C, et al. Dietary supplementation with blueberry extract improves survival of transplanted dopamine neurons. Nutritional Neuroscience 2006;9:251-258.

[25] Crews F, Nixon K, et al. BHT blocks NF-kappa B activation and ethanol-induced brain damage. Alcohol Clin Exp Res 2006;30(11):1938-49.

[26] Ahukitt-Hale B, Carey AN, et al. Beneficial effects of fruit extracts on neuronal function and behavior in a rodent model of accelerated aging. Neurobiol Aging 2006:10:1187-94.

[27] Lau FC, Shukitt Hale B, Joseph JA. The beneficial effects of fruit polyphenols on brain aging. Neurobiol Aging 2005;26(1):128-32.

[28] Russell AL, McCarty MF. DL-phenylalanine markedly potentiates opiate analgesia—an example of nutrient/pharmaceutical up-regulation of the endogenous analgesia system. Med Hypotheses. 2000;55(4):283-8.

[29] Beckmann H, Athen D, Olteanu M, Zimmer R. DL-phenylalanine versus imipramine: a double-blind controlled study. Arch Psychiatr Nervenkr. 1979;227(1):49-58.

[30] Wood DR, Reimherr FW, Wender PH. Treatment of attention deficit disorder with DL-phenylalanine. Psychiatry Res. 1985;16(1):21-6.

[31] Borison RL, Maple PJ, Havdala HS, Diamond BI. Metabolism of an amino acid with antidepressant properties. Res Commun Chem Pathol Pharmacol. 1978;21(2):363-6.

[32] Ehrenpreis S. Analgesic properties of enkephalinase inhibitors: animal and human studies. Prog Clin Biol Res;192:363-70.

[33] Harmer CJ, McTavish SF, Clark L, Goodwin GM, Cowen PJ. Tyrosine depletion attenuates dopamine function in healthy volunteers. Psychopharmacology (Berl). 2001;154(1):105-11.

34 Rasmussen DD, Ishizuka B, Quigley ME, Yen SS. Effects of tyrosine and tryptophan ingestion on plasma catecholamine and 3,4-dihydroxyphenylacetic acid concentrations. J Clin Endocrinol Metab. 1983;57(4):760-3.

35 Meyers S. Use of neurotransmitter precursors for treatment of depression. Altern Med Rev. 2000 5(1):64-71.

36 Young SN. Behavioral effects of dietary neurotransmitter precursors: basic and clinical aspects. Neurosci Biobehav Rev. 1996;20(2):313-23.

37 Montgomery AJ, McTavish SF, Cowen PJ, Grasby PM. Reduction of brain dopamine concentration with dietary tyrosine plus phenylalanine depletion: an [11C]raclopride PET study. Am J Psychiatry. 2003;160(10):1887-9.

38 Guilarate TR. Effects of vitamin B-6 nutrition on the levels of dopamine, dopamine metabolites, dopa decarboxylase activity, tyrosine, and GABA in the developing rat corpus striatum. Neurochemical Research 1989;14: 571-578.

39 Tang F, Wei LL. Vitamin B-6 deficiency prolongs the time course of evoked dopamine release from rat striatum. 2004; 134:3350-3354.

40 Guilarte, T. R., Wagner, H. N., Jr & Frost, J. J. Effects of perinatal vitamin B6 deficiency on dopaminergic neurochemistry. J. Neurochem 1987;48: 432-439.

41 Guilarte, T. R.Effect of vitamin B-6 nutrition on the levels of dopamine, dopamine metabolites, dopa decarboxylase activity, tyrosine, and GABA in the developing rat corpus striatum. Neurochem. Res 1989;14:571-578.

CHAPTER SEVENTEEN: THE HORMONE-BRAIN CONNECTION

1 Okoroh EM, Hooper WC, Atrash HK, Yusuf HR, Boulet SL. Prevalence of polycystic ovary syndrome among the privately insured, United States, 2003-2008. Am J Obstet Gynecol. 2012 Jul 20.

2 Golden SH, Robinson KA, Saldanha I, Anton B, Ladenson PW. Clinical review: Prevalence and incidence of endocrine and metabolic disorders in the United States: a comprehensive review. J Clin Endocrinol Metab. 2009 Jun;94(6):1853-78.

3 De Nicola AF, Brocca ME, Pietranera L, Garcia-Segura LM. Neuroprotection and Sex Steroid Hormones: Evidence of Estradiol-Mediated Protection in Hypertensive Encephalopathy. Mini Rev Med Chem. 2012 Jul 18.

4 Singh M, Su C. Progesterone and neuroprotection. Horm Behav. 2012 Jun 23.

5 Scott E, Zhang QG, Wang R, Vadlamudi R, Brann D. Estrogen neuroprotection and the critical period hypothesis. Front Neuroendocrinol. 2012 Jan;33(1):85-104.

6 Vest RS, Pike CJ. Gender, sex steroid hormones, and Alzheimer's disease. Horm Behav. 2012 Apr 19.

7 Ooishi Y, Kawato S, Hojo Y, Hatanaka Y, Higo S, Murakami G, Komatsuzaki Y, Ogiue-Ikeda M, Kimoto T, Mukai H. Modulation of synaptic plasticity in the hippocampus by hippocampus-derived estrogen and androgen. J Steroid Biochem Mol Biol. 2012 Aug;131(1-2):37-51.

8   Hulshoff Pol HE Changing your sex changes your brain: influences of testosterone and estrogen on adult human brain structure. European Journal of Endocrinology. 2006;155:S107-S114.

9   Ishii H, Tsurugizawa T, Ogiue-Ikeda M, Asashima M, Mukai H, Murakami G, Hojo Y, Kimoto T, Kawato S. Local production of sex hormones and their modulation of hippocampal synaptic plasticity. Neuroscientist. 2007 Aug;13(4):323-34.

10 Garcia-Segura LM. Aromatase in the brain: not just for reproduction anymore. J Neuroendocrinol. 2008;20(6):705-712.

11 Gottfried-Blackmore A, Sierra A, Jellinck PH, McEwen BS, Bulloch K. Brain microglia express steroid-converting enzymes in the mouse. J Steroid Biochem Mol Biol. 2008 Mar;109(1-2):96-107.

12 Fernández G, Weis S, Stoffel-Wagner B, Tendolkar I, Reuber M, Beyenburg S, Klaver P, Fell J, de Greiff A, Ruhlmann J, Reul J, Elger CE. Menstrual cycle-dependent neural plasticity in the adult human brain is hormone, task, and region specific. J Neurosci. 2003 May 1;23(9):3790-5.

13 Mc Ewens BS, Alves SE. Estrogen actions in the central nervous system. Endocr Rev. 1999.20:279-307.

14 Lesek A, Rybacyxk MJ, et al. Effect of estrogen-serotonin interaction on mood and cognition. Behavioral and Cognitive Neuroscience Reviews. 2205;4:43-58.

15 Henderson V. Estrogen, cognition, and a women's risk of Alzheimer's disease. Am J Med. 1997;103:11S-18S.

16 Paganini-Hill A. Estrogen replacement therapy and stroke. Prog Cardiovasc Dis. 1995;38:223-242.

17 Segal M, Murdphy D. Oestradiol induces formation of dendritic spines in hippocampal neurons: functional correlates. Horm Behav;40:156-159.

18 Santagati S, et al. Estrogen receptor is expressed in different types of glials cells in culture. J Neurochem. 1994;63:2058-2064.

19 Mor G, et al. Estrogen and microglia: a regulatory system that affects the brain. J Neurobiol. 1999. J Neurobiol;40:484-496.

20 Goodman Y, Bruce AJ, et al. Estrogens attenuate and corticosterone exasperates excitotoxicity, oxidative injury, and amyloid B-peptide toxicity in hippocampal neurons. J Neurochem. 1996;66:1836-1844.

21 Singer CA, et al. The mitogen-activated protein kinase pathway mediated estrogen neuroprotection after glutamate toxicity in primary cortical neurons. J Neurosci. 1999;19:2455-2463.

22 Pfeilschifter J, Köditz R, Pfohl M, Schatz H. Changes in proinflammatory cytokine activity after menopause. Endocr Rev. 2002 Feb;23(1):90-119.

23 Pacifici R, Rifas L, McCracken R, Vered I, McMurtry C, Avioli LV, Peck WA. Ovarian steroid treatment blocks a postmenopausal increase in blood monocyte interleukin 1 release. Proc Natl Acad Sci U S A. 1989 Apr;86(7):2398-402.

24 Iliev A, Traykov V, Stoykov I, Yakimova K. Estradiol inhibits astrocytic GFAP expression in an animal model of neuroinflammation. Methods Find Exp Clin Pharmacol. 2001 Jan-Feb;23(1):29-35.

[25] Henderson V. Estrogen, cognition, and a women's risk of Alzheimer's disease. Am J Med. 1997;103:11S-18S.

[26] Baulieu E, et al. Progesterone as a neuroactive neurosteroid, with special reference to the effect of progesterone on myelination. Steroids.2000;65(10-11):605-612.

[27] Arafat ES, et al. Sedative an hypnotic effects of oral administration of micronized progesterone may be mediated through its metabolites. Am J Obstet Gynecol.1988;159(5):1203-9.

[28] Steiner TH, et al. Brain metabolism of progesterone, coping behavior and emotional reactivity in male rats from tow psychogentically selected lines. J of Neuroendocrinology. 2002;9:169-175.

[29] Bishnoi M, Chopra K, Kulkarni SK. Progesterone attenuates neuroleptic-induced orofacial dyskinesia via the activity of its metabolite, allopregnanolone, a positive GABA(A) modulating neurosteroid. Prog Neuropsychopharmacol Biol Psychiatry. 2008 Feb 15;32(2):451-61.

[30] Bishnoi M, Chopra K, Kulkarni SK. Progesterone attenuates neuroleptic-induced orofacial dyskinesia via the activity of its metabolite, allopregnanolone, a positive GABA(A) modulating neurosteroid. Prog Neuropsychopharmacol Biol Psychiatry. 2008 Feb 15;32(2):451-61.

[31] Giatti S, Caruso D, Boraso M, Abbiati F, Ballarini E, Calabrese D, Pesaresi M, Rigolio R, Santos-Galindo M, Viviani B, Cavaletti G, Garcia-Segura LM, Melcangi RC. Neuroprotective effects of progesterone in chronic experimental autoimmune encephalomyelitis. J Neuroendocrinol. 2012 Jun;24(6):851-61.

[32] Jiang C, Cui K, Wang J, He Y. Microglia and cyclooxygenase-2: possible therapeutic targets of progesterone for stroke. Int Immunopharmacol. 2011 Nov;11(11):1925-31.

[33] Garay L, Tüngler V, Deniselle MC, Lima A, Roig P, De Nicola AF. Progesterone attenuates demyelination and microglial reaction in the lysolecithin-injured spinal cord. Neuroscience. 2011 Sep 29;192:588-97.

[34] Dang J, Mitkari B, Kipp M, Beyer C. Gonadal steroids prevent cell damage and stimulate behavioral recovery after transient middle cerebral artery occlusion in male and female rats. Brain Behav Immun. 2011 May;25(4):715-26.

[35] Wright DW, Kellermann AL, Hertzberg VS, Clark PL, Frankel M, Goldstein FC, Salomone JP, Dent LL, Harris OA, Ander DS, Lowery DW, Patel MM, Denson DD, Gordon AB, Wald MM, Gupta S, Hoffman SW, Stein DG. ProTECT: a randomized clinical trial of progesterone for acute traumatic brain injury. Ann Emerg Med. 2007 Apr;49(4):391-402, 402.e1-2.

[36] Hausmann M, Güntürkün O. Steroid fluctuations modify functional cerebral asymmetries: the hypothesis of progesterone-mediated interhemispheric decoupling. Neuropsychologia. 2000;38(10):1362-74.

[37] Grossman KJ, Goss CW, Stein DG. Effects of progesterone on the inflammatory response to brain injury in the rat. Brain Res. 2004 May 15;1008(1):29-39.

38 Wright DW, Kellermann AL, Hertzberg VS, Clark PL, Frankel M, Goldstein FC, Salomone JP, Dent LL, Harris OA, Ander DS, Lowery DW, Patel MM, Denson DD, Gordon AB, Wald MM, Gupta S, Hoffman SW, Stein DG. ProTECT: a randomized clinical trial of progesterone for acute traumatic brain injury. Ann Emerg Med. 2007 Apr;49(4):391-402, 402.e1-2.

39 Wang Y, Dou X, Li JF, Luo YL. [Brain mechanisms of male sexual function]. Zhonghua Nan Ke Xue. 2011 Aug;17(8):739-43.

40 Schreiber G, Ziemer M. The aging male—diagnosis and therapy of late-onset hypogonadism. J Dtsch Dermatol Ges. 2008 Apr;6(4):273-9. Epub 2008 Jan 21.

41 Holland J, Bandelow S, Hogervorst E. Testosterone levels and cognition in elderly men: a review. Maturitas. 2011 Aug;69(4):322-37.

42 Moffat SD. Effects of testosterone on cognitive and brain aging in elderly men. Ann N Y Acad Sci. 2005 Dec;1055:80-92.

43 Shemisa K, Kunnathur V, Liu B, Salvaterra TJ, Dluzen DE. Testosterone modulation of striatal dopamine output in orchidectomized mice. Synapse. 2006 Oct;60(5):347-53.

44 Gouras GK, Xu H, Gross RS, Greenfield JP, Hai B, Wang R, Greengard P. Testosterone reduces neuronal secretion of Alzheimer's beta-amyloid peptides. Proc Natl Acad Sci U S A. 2000 Feb 1;97(3):1202-5.

45 Carroll JC, Rosario ER. The potential use of hormone-based therapeutics for the treatment of Alzheimer's disease. Curr Alzheimer Res. 2012 Jan;9 (1):18-34.

46 Kujawa KA, Jacob JM, Jones KJ. Testosterone regulation of the regenerative properties of injured rat sciatic motor neurons. J Neurosci Res. 1993 Jun 15;35(3):268-73.

47 Wang X, Stocco DM. The decline in testosterone biosynthesis during male aging: a consequence of multiple alterations. Mol Cell Endocrinol. 2005 Jun 30;238(1-2):1-7.

48 Midzak AS, Chen H, Papadopoulos V, Zirkin BR. Leydig cell aging and the mechanisms of reduced testosterone synthesis. Mol Cell Endocrinol. 2009 Feb 5;299(1):23-31.

CHAPTER EIGHTEEN: ALTERNATIVE THERAPIES, BRAIN STIMULATION, AND BRAIN FUNCTION

1 Field T, Hernandez-Reif M, Diego M, Schanberg S, Kuhn C. Cortisol decreases and serotonin and dopamine increase following massage therapy. Int J Neurosci.2005 Oct;115(10):1397-413.

2 Chu WC, Wu JC, Yew DT, Zhang L, Shi L, Yeung DK, Wang D, Tong RK, Chan Y, Lao L, Leung PC, Berman BM, Sung JJ. Does acupuncture therapy alter activation of neural pathway for pain perception in irritable bowel syndrome?: a comparative study of true and sham acupuncture using functional magnetic resonance imaging. J Neurogastroenterol Motil. 2012 Jul;18(3):305-16.

3   Zhong HZ, Chang JL, Zhu D, Gao Y. [An overview of researches on underlying mechanisms of acupuncture therapy by functional magnetic resonance imaging in recent 5 years]. Zhen Ci Yan Jiu. 2012 Apr; 37(2):161-7.

4   Huang Y, Tang C, Wang S, Lu Y, Shen W, Yang J, Chen J, Lin R, Cui S, Xiao H, Qu S, Lai X, Shan B. Acupuncture regulates the glucose metabolism in cerebral functional regions in chronic stage ischemic stroke patients—a PET-CT cerebral functional imaging study. BMC Neurosci. 2012 Jun 27;13(1):75.

5   An YS, Moon SK, Min IK, Kim DY. Changes in regional cerebral blood flow and glucose metabolism following electroacupuncture at LI 4 and LI 11 in normal volunteers. J Altern Complement Med. 2009 Oct;15(10):1075-81.

6   Sliz D, Smith A, Wiebking C, Northoff G, Hayley S. Neural correlates of a single-session massage treatment. Brain Imaging Behav. 2012 Mar;6(1): 77-87.

7   Lindgren L, Westling G, Brulin C, Lehtipalo S, Andersson M, Nyberg L. Pleasant human touch is represented in pregenual anterior cingulate cortex. Neuroimage. 2012 Feb 15;59(4):3427-32. Villemure C, Laferrière AC, Bushnell MC. The ventral striatum is implicated inthe analgesic effect of mood changes. Pain Res Manag. 2012 Mar-Apr;17(2):69-74.

8   Napadow V, Lee J, Kim J, Cina S, Maeda Y, Barbieri R, Harris RE, Kettner N, Park K. Brain correlates of phasic autonomic response to acupuncture stimulation: An event-related fMRI study. Hum Brain Mapp. 2012 Apr 14.

9   Bolton PS, Budgell B. Visceral responses to spinal manipulation. J Electromyogr Kinesiol. 2012 Mar 20.

10 Ogura T, Tashiro M, Masud M, Watanuki S, Shibuya K, Yamaguchi K, Itoh M, Fukuda H, Yanai K. Cerebral metabolic changes in men after chiropractic spinal manipulation for neck pain. Altern Ther Health Med. 2011 Nov-Dec;17(6):12-7.

11 Taylor HH, Murphy B. Altered central integration of dual somatosensory input after cervical spine manipulation. J Manipulative Physiol Ther. 2010 Mar-Apr;33(3):178-88.

12 Haavik-Taylor H, Murphy B. Cervical spine manipulation alters sensorimotor integration: a somatosensory evoked potential study. Clin Neurophysiol. 2007 Feb;118(2):391-402.

13 Cagnie B, Jacobs F, Barbaix E, Vinck E, Dierckx R, Cambier D. Changes in cerebellar blood flow after manipulation of the cervical spine using Technetium 99m-ethyl cysteinate dimer. J Manipulative Physiol Ther. 2005 Feb;28(2):103-7.

14 Carrick FR. Changes in brain function after manipulation of the cervical spine. J Manipulative Physiol Ther. 1997 Oct;20(8):529-45. Erratum in: J Manipulative Physiol Ther 1998 May;21(4):304.

15 Ouchi Y, Kanno T, Okada H, Yoshikawa E, Shinke T, Nagasawa S, Minoda K, Doi H. Changes in cerebral blood flow under the prone condition with and without massage. Neurosci Lett. 2006 Oct 23;407(2):131-5.

16 Froeliger BE, Garland EL, Modlin LA, McClernon FJ. Neurocognitive correlates of the effects of yoga meditation practice on emotion and cognition: a pilot study. Front Integr Neurosci. 2012;6:48.

17   Kang DH, Jo HJ, Jung WH, Kim SH, Jung YH, Choi CH, Lee US, An SC, Jang JH, Kwon JS. The effect of meditation on brain structure: cortical thickness mapping and diffusion tensor imaging. Soc Cogn Affect Neurosci. 2012 Jun 8.

18   Kozasa EH, Sato JR, Lacerda SS, Barreiros MA, Radvany J, Russell TA, Sanches LG, Mello LE, Amaro E Jr. Meditation training increases brain efficiency in an attention task. Neuroimage. 2012 Jan 2;59(1):745-9.

19   Chiesa A, Brambilla P, Serretti A. Neuro-imaging of mindfulness meditations: implications for clinical practice. Epidemiol Psychiatr Sci. 2011 Jun;20(2):205-10.

20   Zeidan F, Martucci KT, Kraft RA, Gordon NS, McHaffie JG, Coghill RC. Brain mechanisms supporting the modulation of pain by mindfulness meditation. J Neurosci. 2011 Apr 6;31(14):5540-8.

CHAPTER NINETEEN: ESSENTIAL FATTY ACIDS

1   Lands B. Consequences of essential Fatty acids. Nutrients. 2012 Sep;4(9):1338-57. doi: 10.3390/nu4091338.

2   Rao JS, Kellom M, Kim HW, Rapoport SI, Reese EA. Neuroinflammation and synaptic loss. Neurochem Res. 2012 May;37(5):903-10.

3   Haag M. Essential fatty acids and the brain. Can J Psychiatry. 2003 Apr;48(3):195-203.

4   McGahon BM, Martin DS, Horrobin DF, Lynch MA. Age-related changes in synaptic function: analysis of the effect of dietary supplementation with omega-3 fatty acids. Neuroscience. 1999;94(1):305-14.

5   Hamilton JA, Hillard CJ, Spector AA, Watkins PA. Brain uptake and utilization of fatty acids, lipids and lipoproteins: application to neurological disorders. J Mol Neurosci. 2007 Sep;33(1):2-11.

6   Simopoulos AP. The importance of the omega-6/omega-3 fatty acid ratio in cardiovascular disease and other chronic diseases. Exp Biol Med (Maywood). 2008 Jun;233(6):674-88. doi: 10.3181/0711-MR-311. Epub 2008 Apr 11. Review. PubMed PMID: 18408140.

7   Meet Real Free-Range Eggs. Mother Earth News. Oct/Nov 2007.

8   Daley CA, Abbott A, Doyle PS, Nader GA, Larson S. A review of fatty acid profiles and antioxidant content in grass-fed and grain-fed beef. Nutr J. 2010 Mar 10;9:10. doi: 10.1186/1475-2891-9-10. Review. PubMed PMID: 20219103; PubMed Central PMCID: PMC2846864.

9   McAfee AJ, McSorley EM, Cuskelly GJ, Fearon AM, Moss BW, Beattie JA, Wallace JM, Bonham MP, Strain JJ. Red meat from animals offered a grass diet increases plasma and platelet n-3 PUFA in healthy consumers. Br J Nutr. 2011 Jan;105(1):80-9. doi: 10.1017/S0007114510003090. PubMed PMID: 20807460.

10   Grass-fed beef called healthier. By Candy Sagon. The Washington Post. March 15, 2006.

11   Kar S, Webel R. Fish oil supplementation & coronary artery disease: does it help? Mo Med. 2012 Mar-Apr;109(2):142-5.

[12] Hibbeln JR, Nieminen LR, Blasbalg TL, Riggs JA, Lands WE. Healthy intakes of n-3 and n-6 fatty acids: estimations considering worldwide diversity. Am J Clin Nutr. 2006 Jun;83(6 Suppl):1483S-1493S.

[13] McGahon, BM, Martin DS, Horrobin DF, Lunch MA. Age-related changes in synaptic function: analysis of the role of dietary supplementation. Neuroscience. 1999;94(1):305-14.

[14] Fujita S, Ikegaya Y, Nishikawa M, Nishiyama N, Matsuki N. Docosahexaenoic acid improves long-term potentiation attenuated by phospholipase A(2) inhibitor in rat hippocampal slices. Br J Pharmacol. 2001;Apr; 132(7):1417-22.

[15] Kitajka K, Puskas LG, ZVara A, et al. The role of omega-3 polyunsaturated fatty acids in brain: modulation of rat brain gene expression by dietary omega-3 fatty acids. Proc Natl Acad Sci USA. 2002; Mar 5;99(5):2619-24.

[16] Cao D Xue R, Xu J, Liu Z. Effects of docosahexaenoic on the survival and neurite outgrowth of rat cortical neurons in primary cultures. J Nutr Biochem. 2005 Sep 16(9):538-46.

[17] Yehuda S, Rabinovtz S, Carasso RL, Mostofsky DL. Essential fatty acids preparation (SR-3) improves Alzheimer's patient's quality of life. Int J Neurosci. 1996 Nove;87(3-4):141-9.

[18] Morris MC, Evans DA, Bienias JL, et al. Consumption of fish and omega-3 fatty acis and risk of incident Alzheimer's disease. Arch neurol. 2003; 60(7):940-6.

[19] Kalmijn S, Launer LJ, Ott A, Witteman JC, Hofman A, Breteler MM. Dietary fat intake and the risk of incident dementia in the Rotterdam Study. Ann Neurol. 1997;42(5):776-82.

[20] Hashimoto M, Hossain S, Shimada T, et al. Docosahexaenoic acid provides protection from impairment of learning ability in Alzheimer's disease model in rats. J Neurochem. 2002;81(5):1084-91.

[21] Gamoh S, Hashimoto M, Hossain S, Masumura S. Chronic administration of docosahexaenoic acid improves the performance of radial arm maze task in ages rats. Clin Exp Pharmacol Physiol. 2001; 28(4):266-70.

[22] Sugimoto Y, Taga C, Nishiga M, et al. Effect of docosahexaenoic acid-fortified Chlorella vulgaris strain CK22 on the radial maze performance in aged mice. Biol Pharm Bull. 2002;25(8):1090-2.

[23] Gamoh S, Hashimoto M, Sugioka K, et al. Chronic administration of docosahexaenoic acid improves reference memory-related learning ability in young rats. Neuroscience. 1999;93(1):237-41.

CHAPTER TWENTY: TOXINS AND THE BRAIN

[1] Cranor C. The legal failure to prevent subclinical developmental toxicity. Basic Clin Pharmacol Toxicol. 2008 Feb;102(2):267-73.

[2] Houlihan et al. Body burden: the pollution in newborns. July 14, 2005, Environmental Working Group.

[3] Lunder et al. Toxic fire retardants in human breast milk. Sept. 2003. Environmental Working Group.

4   Environmental threats to healthy aging. Stein, J, Schettler, T, Rohrer B, Valenti, M. 2008. Greater Boston Physicians for Social Responsibility and Science and Environmental Health Network.

5   Volk HE, Lurmann F, Penfold B, Hertz-Picciotto I, McConnell R. Traffic-related air pollution, particulate matter, and autism. JAMA Psychiatry. 2013 Jan;70(1):71-7.

6   Calderón-Garcidueñas L, Mora-Tiscareño A, Styner M, Gómez-Garza G, Zhu H, Torres-Jardón R, Carlos E, Solorio-López E, Medina-Cortina H, Kavanaugh M, D'Angiulli A. White matter hyperintensities, systemic inflammation, brain growth, and cognitive functions in children exposed to air pollution. J Alzheimers Dis. 2012;31(1):183-91.

7   Powell JJ, Van de Water J, Gershwin ME. Evidence for the role of environmental agents in the initiation or progression of autoimmune conditions. Environ Health Perspect. 1999 Oct;107 Suppl 5:667-72.

8   Kłys M, Lech T, Zieba-Palus J, Białka J. A chemical and physicochemical study of an Egyptian mummy 'Iset Iri Hetes' from the Ptolemaic period III-I B.C. Forensic Sci Int. 1999 Jan 25;99(3):217-28.

9   Miller CS. The compelling anomaly of chemical intolerance. Ann N Y Acad Sci. 2001 Mar;933:1-23.

10   Miller CS. The compelling anomaly of chemical intolerance. Ann N Y Acad Sci. 2001 Mar;933:1-23.

11   Requejo R, Tena M. Influence of glutathione chemical effectors in the response of maize to arsenic exposure. J Plant Physiol. 2012 May 1;169(7):649-56. doi: 10.1016/j.jplph.2012.01.016.

12   Vojdani A, Lambert J. The onset of enhanced intestinal permeability and food sensitivity triggered by medication used in dental procedures: a case report. Case Rep Gastrointest Med. 2012;2012:265052.

13   Mićović V, Vojniković B, Bulog A, Coklo M, Malatestinić D, Mrakovcić-Sutić I. Regulatory T cells (Tregs) monitoring in environmental diseases. Coll Antropol. 2009 Sep;33(3):743-6.

14   Winder C. Mechanisms of multiple chemical sensitivity. Toxicol Lett. 2002 Mar 10;128(1-3):85-97.

15   Genuis SJ. Sensitivity-related illness: the escalating pandemic of allergy, food intolerance and chemical sensitivity. Sci Total Environ. 2010 Nov 15;408(24):6047-61.

16   Genuis SJ. Sensitivity-related illness: the escalating pandemic of allergy, food intolerance and chemical sensitivity. Sci Total Environ. 2010 Nov 15;408(24):6047-61.

17   Andersen O. Chemical and biological considerations in the treatment of metal intoxications by chelating agents. Mini Rev Med Chem. 2004 Jan;4(1): 11-21.

18   Ewan KB, Pamphlett R. Increased inorganic mercury in spinal motor neurons following chelating agents. Neurotoxicology. 1996 Summer;17(2):343-9.

19   Ibim SE, Trotman J, Musey PI, Semafuko WE. Depletion of essential elements by calcium disodium EDTA treatment in the dog. Toxicology. 1992;73(2):229-37.

20 Flora SJ, Pachauri V. Chelation in metal intoxication. Int J Environ Res Public Health. 2010 Jul;7(7):2745-88.

21 Andersen O. Principles and recent developments in chelation treatment of metal intoxication. Chem Rev. 1999 Sep 8;99(9):2683-710.

22 Andersen O. Chemical and biological considerations in the treatment of metal intoxications by chelating agents. Mini Rev Med Chem. 2004 Jan;4(1): 11-21.

23 Ewan KB, Pamphlett R. Increased inorganic mercury in spinal motor neurons following chelating agents. Neurotoxicology. 1996 Summer;17(2):343-9.

24 Ibim SE, Trotman J, Musey PI, Semafuko WE. Depletion of essential elements by calcium disodium EDTA treatment in the dog. Toxicology. 1992;73(2):229-37.

25 Gardner RM, Nyland JF, Evans SL, Wang SB, Doyle KM, Crainiceanu CM, Silbergeld EK. Mercury induces an unopposed inflammatory response in human peripheral blood mononuclear cells in vitro. Environ Health Perspect. 2009 Dec;117(12):1932-8.

26 Seelbach M, Chen L, Powell A, Choi YJ, Zhang B, Hennig B, Toborek M. Polychlorinated biphenyls disrupt blood-brain barrier integrity and promote brain metastasis formation. Environ Health Perspect. 2010 Apr;118(4): 479-84.

27 Choi YJ, Seelbach MJ, Pu H, Eum SY, Chen L, Zhang B, Hennig B, Toborek M. Polychlorinated biphenyls disrupt intestinal integrity via NADPH oxidase-induced alterations of tight junction protein expression. Environ Health Perspect. 2010 Jul;118(7):976-81.

28 Olsen CE, Liguori AE, Zong Y, Lantz RC, Burgess JL, Boitano S. Arsenic upregulates MMP-9 and inhibits wound repair in human airway epithelial cells. Am J Physiol Lung Cell Mol Physiol. 2008 Aug;295(2):L293-302.

29 Steindel SJ, Howanitz PJ. The uncertainty of hair analysis for trace minerals. JAMA 285:83-85, 1999.

30 Stornello C, Padellaro G. [Observations on the sensibility of many chemical antibodies on the blocks of the Mimeae isolated during the acute respiratory affections (author's transl)]. Ann Sclavo. 1976 Jul-Aug;18(4):541-4.

31 Zhang D, Shen J, Wang C, Zhang X, Chen J. GSH-dependent iNOS and HO-1 mediated apoptosis of human Jurkat cells induced by nickel(II). Environ Toxicol. 2009 Aug;24(4):404-14.

32 Tada-Oikawa S, Kato T, Kuribayashi K, Nishino K, Murata M, Kawanishi S. Critical role of hydrogen peroxide in the differential susceptibility of Th1 and Th2 cells to tributyltin-induced apoptosis. Biochem Pharmacol. 2008 Jan 15;75(2):552-61.

33 Flora SJ, Pachauri V. Chelation in metal intoxication. Int J Environ Res Public Health. 2010 Jul;7(7):2745-88.

34 Chelation in metal intoxication. Int J Environ Res Public Health. 2010 Jul:7(7):2745-2788.

35 Tewthanom K, Janwityanuchit S, Totemchockchyakarn K, Panomvana D. Correlation of lipid peroxidation and glutathione levels with severity of systemic lupus erythematosus: a pilot study from single center. J Pharm Pharm Sci. 2008;11(3):30-4.

36 Won HY, Sohn JH, Min HJ, Lee K, Woo HA, Ho YS, Park JW, Rhee SG, Hwang ES. Glutathione peroxidase 1 deficiency attenuates allergen-induced airway inflammation by suppressing Th2 and Th17 cell development. Antioxid Redox Signal. 2010 Sep 1;13(5):575-87.

37 Yan Z, Banerjee R. Redox remodeling as an immunoregulatory strategy. Biochemistry. 2010 Feb 16;49(6):1059-66.

38 Yan Z, Garg SK, Kipnis J, Banerjee R. Extracellular redox modulation by regulatory T cells. Nat Chem Biol. 2009 Oct;5(10):721-3.

39 Fraternale A, Paoletti MF, Casabianca A, Oiry J, Clayette P, Vogel JU, Cinatl J Jr, Palamara AT, Sgarbanti R, Garaci E, Millo E, Benatti U, Magnani M. Antiviral and immunomodulatory properties of new pro-glutathione (GSH) molecules. Curr Med Chem. 2006;13(15):1749-55.

40 van Ampting MT, Schonewille AJ, Vink C, Brummer RJ, van der Meer R, Bovee-Oudenhoven IM. Intestinal barrier function in response to abundant or depleted mucosal glutathione in Salmonella-infected rats. BMC Physiol. 2009 Apr 17;9:6.

41 Paolicchi A, Dominici S, Pieri L, Maellaro E, Pompella A. Glutathione catabolism as a signaling mechanism. Biochem Pharmacol. 2002 Sep;64(5-6):1027-35.

42 Badaloo A, Reid M, Forrester T, Heird WC, Jahoor F. Cysteine supplementation improves the erythrocyte glutathione synthesis rate in children with severe edematous malnutrition. Am J Clin Nutr. 2002 Sep;76(3):646-52.

43 Odom RY, Dansby MY, Rollins-Hairston AM, Jackson KM, Kirlin WG. Phytochemical induction of cell cycle arrest by glutathione oxidation and reversal by N-acetylcysteine in human colon carcinoma cells. Nutr Cancer. 2009;61(3):332-9.

44 Marsh SA, Laursen PB, Coombes JS. Effects of antioxidant supplementation and exercise training on erythrocyte antioxidant enzymes. Int J Vitam Nutr Res. 2006 Sep;76(5):324-31.

45 Zicker SC, Hagen TM, Joisher N, Golder C, Joshi DK, Miller EP. Safety of long-term feeding of dl-alpha-lipoic acid and its effect on reduced glutathione:oxidized glutathione ratios in beagles. Vet Ther. 2002 Summer;3(2):167-76.

46 Cruzat VF, Tirapegui J. Effects of oral supplementation with glutamine and alanyl-glutamine on glutamine, glutamate, and glutathione status in trained rats and subjected to long-duration exercise. Nutrition. 2009 Apr;25(4):428-35.

47 Mok E, Constantin B, Favreau F, Neveux N, Magaud C, Delwail A, Hankard R. l-Glutamine administration reduces oxidized glutathione and MAP kinase signaling in dystrophic muscle of mdx mice. Pediatr Res. 2008 Mar;63(3):268-73.

48 Johnson AT, Kaufmann YC, Luo S, Todorova V, Klimberg VS. Effect of glutamine on glutathione, IGF-I, and TGF-beta 1. J Surg Res. 2003 May 15;111(2):222-8.

49 Bartfay WJ, Bartfay E. Selenium and glutathione peroxidase with beta-thalassemia major. Nurs Res. 2001 May-Jun;50(3):178-83.

50 Zachara BA, Mikolajczak J, Trafikowska U. Effect of various dietary selenium (Se) intakes on tissue Se levels and glutathione peroxidase activities in lambs. Zentralbl Veterinarmed A. 1993 May;40(4):310-8.

51 Wilke BC, Vidailhet M, Favier A, Guillemin C, Ducros V, Arnaud J, Richard MJ. Selenium, glutathione peroxidase (GSH-Px) and lipid peroxidation products before and after selenium supplementation. Clin Chim Acta. 1992 Apr 30;207(1-2):137-42.

52 Ji DB, Ye J, Li CL, Wang YH, Zhao J, Cai SQ. Antiaging effect of Cordyceps sinensis extract. Phytother Res. 2009 Jan;23(1):116-22.

53 Wang YH, Ye J, Li CL, Cai SQ, Ishizaki M, Katada M. [An experimental study on anti-aging action of Cordyceps extract]. Zhongguo Zhong Yao Za Zhi. 2004 Aug;29(8):773-6.

54 Lee MK, Kim SR, Sung SH, Lim D, Kim H, Choi H, Park HK, Je S, Ki YC. Asiatic acid derivatives protect cultured cortical neurons from glutamate-induced excitotoxicity. Res Commun Mol Pathol Pharmacol. 2000 Jul-Aug;108(1-2):75-86.

55 Pradhan SC, Girish C. Hepatoprotective herbal drug, silymarin from experimental pharmacology to clinical medicine. Indian J Med Res. 2006 Nov;124(5):491-504.

56 Valenzuela A, Aspillaga M, Vial S, Guerra R. Selectivity of silymarin on the increase of the glutathione content in different tissues of the rat. Planta Med. 1989 Oct;55(5):420-2.

57 Maeda T, Miyazono Y, Ito K, Hamada K, Sekine S, Horie T. Oxidative stress and enhanced paracellular permeability in the small intestine of methotrexate-treated rats. Cancer Chemother Pharmacol. 2010 May;65(6):1117-23.

58 Witschi A, Reddy S, Stofer B, Lauterburg BH. The systemic availability of oral glutathione. Eur J Clin Pharmacol. 1992;43(6):667-9.

59 Hagen TM, Wierzbicka GT, Sillau AH, Bowman BB, Jones DP. Bioavailability of dietary glutathione: effect on plasma concentration. Am J Physiol. 1990 Oct;259(4 Pt 1):G524-9.

60 Cacciatore I, Cornacchia C, Mollica A, Pinnen F, Di Stefano A. Prodrug Approach for Increasing Cellular Glutathione Levels. Molecule. 3 March 2010.

61 Vogel JU, Cinatl J, Dauletbaev N, Buxbaum S, Treusch G, Cinatl J Jr, Gerein V, Doerr HW. Effects of S-acetylglutathione in cell and animal model of herpes simplex virus type 1 infection. Med Microbiol Immunol. 2005 Jan;194(1-2):55-9.

62 Ballatori N, Krance SM, Notenboom S, et al. Glutathione dysregulation and the etiology and progression of human diseases. Biol Chem. 2009 Mar;390(3):191-214.

63 Choi YJ, Seelbach MJ, Pu H, Eum SY, Chen L, Zhang B, Hennig B, Toborek M. Polychlorinated biphenyls disrupt intestinal integrity via NADPH oxidase-induced alterations of tight junction protein expression. Environ Health Perspect. 2010 Jul;118(7):976-81.

64 van Ampting MT, Schonewille AJ, Vink C, Brummer RJ, van der Meer R, Bovee-Oudenhoven IM. Intestinal barrier function in response to abundant or depleted mucosal glutathione in Salmonella-infected rats. BMC Physiol. 2009 Apr 17;9:6. doi: 10.1186/1472-6793-9-6.

65 Kelly N, Friend K, Boyle P, Zhang XR, Wong C, Hackam DJ, Zamora R, Ford HR, Upperman JS. The role of the glutathione antioxidant system in gut barrier failure in a rodent model of experimental necrotizing enterocolitis. Surgery. 2004 Sep;136(3):557-66.

66 Bove PF, Wesley UV, Greul AK, Hristova M, Dostmann WR, van der Vliet A. Nitric oxide promotes airway epithelial wound repair through enhanced activation of MMP-9. Am J Respir Cell Mol Biol. 2007 Feb;36(2):138-46.

67 Mendez II, Chung YH, Jun HS, Yoon JW. Immunoregulatory role of nitric oxide in Kilham rat virus-induced autoimmune diabetes in DR-BB rats. J Immunol. 2004 Jul 15;173(2):1327-35.

68 Dijkstra G, van Goor H, Jansen PL, Moshage H. Targeting nitric oxide in the gastrointestinal tract. Curr Opin Investig Drugs. 2004 May;5(5):529-36.

69 Dijkstra G, van Goor H, Jansen PL, Moshage H. Targeting nitric oxide in the gastrointestinal tract. Curr Opin Investig Drugs. 2004 May;5(5):529-36.

70 Keklikoglu N, Koray M, Kocaelli H, Akinci S. iNOS expression in oral and gastrointestinal tract mucosa. Dig Dis Sci. 2008 Jun;53(6):1437-42.

71 Vassallo MF, Camargo CA Jr. Potential mechanisms for the hypothesized link between sunshine, vitamin D, and food allergy in children. J Allergy Clin Immunol. 2010 Aug;126(2):217-22.

72 Kong J, Zhang Z, Musch MW, Ning G, Sun J, Hart J, Bissonnette M, Li YC. Novel role of the vitamin D receptor in maintaining the integrity of the intestinal mucosal barrier. Am J Physiol Gastrointest Liver Physiol. 2008 Jan;294(1):G208-16.

73 Larrey D, Pageaux GP. Genetic predisposition to drug-induced hepatotoxicity. J Hepatol. 1997;26 Suppl 2:12-21.

74 Furness SG, Whelan F. The pleiotropy of dioxin toxicity--xenobiotic misappropriation of the aryl hydrocarbon receptor's alternative physiological roles. Pharmacol Ther. 2009 Dec;124(3):336-53.

75 Griem P, Wulferink M, Sachs B, González JB, Gleichmann E. Allergic and autoimmune reactions to xenobiotics: how do they arise? Immunol Today. 1998 Mar;19(3):133-41.

76 Johnson CH, Patterson AD, Idle JR, Gonzalez FJ. Xenobiotic metabolomics: major impact on the metabolome. Annu Rev Pharmacol Toxicol. 2012;52:37-56.

77 Bethke L, Webb E, Sellick G, Rudd M, Penegar S, Withey L, Qureshi M, Houlston R. Polymorphisms in the cytochrome P450 genes CYP1A2, CYP1B1, CYP3A4, CYP3A5, CYP11A1, CYP17A1, CYP19A1 and colorectal cancer risk. BMC Cancer. 2007 Jul 5;7:123.

78 Cui X, Guo R, Xu Z, Wang B, Li C. Relationship between metabolic phenotype of N-acetylation and bladder cancer. Chin Med J (Engl). 2000 Apr;113(4):303-5.

79 Lee JB, Lee KA, Lee KY. Cytochrome P450 2C19 polymorphism is associated with reduced clopidogrel response in cerebrovascular disease. Yonsei Med J. 2011 Sep;52(5):734-8.

80 Cerne JZ, Pohar-Perme M, Novakovic S, Frkovic-Grazio S, Stegel V, Gersak K. Combined effect of CYP1B1, COMT, GSTP1, and MnSOD genotypes and risk of postmenopausal breast cancer. J Gynecol Oncol. 2011 Jun 30;22(2):110-9.

81 Steventon GB, Heafield MT, Sturman S, Waring RH, Williams AC. Xenobiotic metabolism in Alzheimer's disease. Neurology. 1990 Jul;40(7):1095-8.

82 Steventon GB, Heafield MT, Waring RH, Williams AC. Xenobiotic metabolism in Parkinson's disease. Neurology. 1989 Jul;39(7):883-7.

83 Descotes J, Vial T. Immunotoxic effects of xenobiotics in humans: A review of current evidence. Toxicol In Vitro. 1994 Oct;8(5):963-6.

84 Barbosa ER, Leiros da Costa MD, Bacheschi LA, Scaff M, Leite CC. Parkinsonism after glycine-derivate exposure. Mov Disord. 2001 May;16(3):565-8.

85 Kaye AD, Baluch A, Scott JT. Pain management in the elderly population: a review. Ochsner J. 2010 Fall;10(3):179-87.

86 Faber K. The dandelion Taraxacum officinale. Pharmaize 1958;13:423-436.

87 Susnik F. Present state of knowledge of the medicinal plant Taraxacum officinale. Weber. Med Razgledi 1982;21:323-328.

88 Bohm K. Choleretic action of some medicinal plants. Arzneimittel Forsch 1959;9:376-378.

89 Nassauto G et al. Effects of silbinion on biliary lipid composition. Experimental and clinical study. J Hepatol 1991;12:290-295.

90 Wagnar H. Antihepatotoxic flavonioids. In: CodyV, Middleton E, Harbourne JB, eds. Plant flavonoids in biology and medicine: biochemical, pharmacological, and structure-activity relationships. New York, NY: Alan R Liss. 1986:p545-558

91 Adzet T. Polyphenolic compounds with biological activity and pharmacological activity. Herbs Spices Medicinal Plants 1986;1:167-184

92 Hikino H, Kiso Y, Wagner H. Antihepatotoxic actions of flavanolignans from Silybum marianum fruits. Plant Medica 1984;50:248-250.

93 Fiebrich F, Koch H. Siymarin, an inhibitor of prostaglandin synthetase. Experentia 1979;35:148-152.

94 Palasciano G, Protinacasa P, et al. The effect of silymarin on plasma levels of malonadialdehyde in patients receiving long-term treatment of psychotropic drugs. Curr Ther Res 1994;55:537-545.

95 Sonnenbicher J, Goldberg M, Hane L, et al. Stimulatory effect of silibinin on the DNA synthesis in partially hepatectomized rat livers. Non-responsive in hepatoma and other malignant cell lines. Biochem Pharm 1986;35:538-541.

96 Darnis F, Orcel L, de Saint-Maur PP, Mamaou P. Use of a titrated extract of Centella asiatica in chronic hepatic disorders. Sem Hosp Paris 1979;55:1749-1750.

97   El Zawahry MD, Kahil AM, El Banna MH. Madecassol. A new therapy for hepatic fibrosis. Bull Soc Int Chir (Belgium) 1975;34:296-297.

98   Belcaro GV, Grimaldi R, Guidi G. Improvement of capillary permeability in patients with venous hypertension after treatment with TTFCA. Angiology 1990; 41(7):533-540.

99   Pointel JP, Boccalon H, Cloarec M, et al. Titrated extract of Centella asiatca (TECA) in the treatment of venous insufficiency of the lower limbs. Angiology 1987;38(11):46-50.

100 Hikino H, Kiso Y, Sandah S, Shoji J. Antihepatotoxic actions of ginesenosides form Panax ginseng roots. Planta Medica 1985;52: 62-64.

101 Yammato M, Uemura T, Nakama S, et al. Serum HDL-cholesterol-increasing and fatty liver-improving action of Panax ginseng in high cholesterol diet-feed rats with clinical effects on hyperlipidemia in man. Am J Chin Med 1983;11:96-101.

102 Bombardelli E, Cirstoni A, Lietta A. The effect of acute and chronic (Panax) ginseng saponins treatment on adrenal function; biochemical and pharmacological. Proceedings 3rd International Ginseng Symposium.Seoul: Korean Research Institute. 1980: p 9-16.

103 Oura H, Hiai S, Seno H. Synthesis and characterization of nuclear RNA induced b Radix ginseng extract in rat liver. Chem Pharm Bull 1971;19:1598-1605.

104 Oura H, Hiai S, Nabatini S, Nakagawa H, et al. Effect of ginseng o endoplasmic reticulum and ribosome. Planta Medica 1975;28:76-88.

105 Johnston CJ, Meyer CG, Srilakshmi JC. Vitamin C elevates red blood cell glutathione levels in healthy adults. Am J Clin Nutr 1993; 58: 103-105.

106 Jain A, Buist NR, Keenaaway NG, et al. Effect of ascorbate or N-acetlycysteine treatments in patient with hereditary glutathione synthetase deficiency. J Pediatr 1994; 124: 229-233.

107 Skvortsova RI, Pzniakovski VM, Agarkova IA. Role of vitamin factor in preventing phenol poisoning. Vopr Pitan 1981; 2: 32-35.

108 Brattstoerm L, et al. Plasma homocysteine in women on oral oestrogen-containing contraceptives and in men with oestrogen-treated prostatic carcinoma. Scand J Clin Lab Invest. 52, 1982:283-287.

109 Smithells RW, et al. Possible prevention of neural-tube defects by periconceptional vitamin supplementation. Lancet, Feb 16, 1980:339-342.

110 Butterworth CE, et al. Folate deficiency and cervical dysplasia. JAMA. 1992;267:528-533.

111 Lindenbaum J, et al. Neuropsychiatric disorders caused by cobalamin deficiency in the absence of anemia or macrocytosis. N Eng J Med. 1988;318:1720-1728.

112 Allen RH, et al. Serum beatine, N,N-dimethlyglycine and N-methylglycine levels in patients with cobalamin deficiency and related inborn errors of metabolism. Metab. 1993;42(11):1448-1460.

113 Zingh JM, Jones PA. Genetic and epigenetic aspects of DNA methylation on genome expression, evolution, mutation and carcinogenesis. Carcinogenesis. 1997;18(5):869-882.

114 Smythies JR. The role of the one-carbon cycle in neuropsychatric disease. Biol Psychiatry. 1984;19(5):755-758.

115 Finkelstein JD. Homocysteine: a history in progress. Nutr Rev. 2000;58(7):193-204.

116 Krumdieck CL, Prince CW. Mechanisms of homocysteine toxicity on connective tissues: implications of morbidity of aging. J Nutr. 2000;130:365S-368S.

117 Faber K. The dandelion Taraxacum officinale. Pharmaize 1958;13:423-436.

118 Susnik F. Present state of knowledge of the medicinal plant Taraxacum officinale. Weber. Med Razgledi 1982;21:323-328.

119 Bohm K. Choleretic action of some medicinal plants. Arzneimittel Forsch 1959;9:376-378.

120 Nassauto G et al. Effects of silbinion on biliary lipid composition. Experimental and clinical study. J Hepatol 1991;12:290-295.

121 Wagnar H. Antihepatotoxic flavonoids. In: CodyV, Middleton E, Harbourne JB, eds. Plant flavonoids in biology and medicine: biochemical, pharmacological, and structure-activity relationships. New York, NY: Alan R Liss. 1986:p545-558

122 Adzet T. Polyphenolic compounds with biological activity and pharmacological activity. Herbs Spices Medicinal Plants 1986;1:167-184

123 Hikino H, Kiso Y, Wagner H. Antihepatotoxic actions of flavanolignans from Silybum marianum fruits. Plant Medica 1984;50:248-250.

124 Fiebrich F, Koch H. Siymarin, an inhibitor of prostaglandin synthetase. Experentia 1979;35:150-152.

125 Feibrich F, Koch H. Silymarin an inbitor of lipoxygenase. Experentia 1979;35:148-150.

126 Palasciano G, Protinacasa P, et al. The effect of silymarin on plasma levels of malonadialdehyde in patients receiving long-term treatment of psychotropic drugs. Curr Ther Res 1994;55:537-545.

127 Sonnenbicher J, Goldberg M, Hane L, et al. Stimulatory effect of silibinin on the DNA synthesis in partially hepatectomized rat livers. Non-responsive in hepatoma and other malignant cel lines. Biochem Pharm 1986;35:538-541.

128 Gujral S. Bhumra H. Swaroop M. Effects of ginger (zingebar officinale Roscoe) oleoresin on serum and hepatic cholesterol levels in cholesterol fed rats. Nutr Rep Intl 1978;17:183-189.

129 Giri J, Sakthi Devi TK, Meerarani S. Effect of ginger on serum cholesterol levels. Ind J Nutr Diet 1984;21:433-436.

130 Srinivasan K, Sambaiah K. The effect of spices on cholesterol 7 alpha-hydroxylase activity and the serum and hepatic cholesterol levels in rat. Int J Vitam Nutr Res 1991;61:364-369.

131 Tushilin SA, Drieling DA, Narodetskaja RV, Lukash LK. The treatment of patients with gallstones by lecithin. Am J Gastroenerol 1976:65:231.

132 Hannin I, Ansell GB. Lecithin. Technological, biological, and therapeutic aspects. New York, NY:Plenum Press.1987.

[133] Jenkins SA. Vitamin C and gallstone formation: a preliminary report. Experientia 1977;33:1616-1617.

[134] Wójcikowski J, Daniel WA. The role of the nervous system in the regulation of liver cytochrome p450. Curr Drug Metab. 2011 Feb;12(2):124-38.

[135] Uyama N, Geerts A, Reynaert H. Neural connections between the hypothalamus and the liver. Anat Rec A Discov Mol Cell Evol Biol. 2004 Sep;280(1):808-20.

[136] Wójcikowski J, Daniel WA. The role of the nervous system in the regulation of liver cytochrome p450. Curr Drug Metab. 2011 Feb;12(2):124-38.

[137] Wójcikowski J, Daniel WA. The brain dopaminergic system as an important center regulating liver cytochrome P450 in the rat. Expert Opin Drug Metab Toxicol. 2009 Jun;5(6):631-45.

[138] Wójcikowski J, Daniel WA. Identification of factors mediating the effect of the brain dopaminergic system on the expression of cytochrome P450 in the liver. Pharmacol Rep. 2008 Nov-Dec;60(6):966-71.

[139] Ferguson CS, Tyndale RF. Cytochrome P450 enzymes in the brain: emerging evidence of biological significance. Trends Pharmacol Sci. 2011 Dec;32(12):708-14.

[140] Ravindranath V. Metabolism of xenobiotics in the central nervous system: implications and challenges. Biochem Pharmacol. 1998 Sep 1;56(5):547-51.

[141] Ravindranath V. Metabolism of xenobiotics in the central nervous system: implications and challenges. Biochem Pharmacol. 1998 Sep 1;56(5):547-51.

[142] Dutheil F, Beaune P, Loriot MA. Xenobiotic metabolizing enzymes in the central nervous system: Contribution of cytochrome P450 enzymes in normal and pathological human brain. Biochimie. 2008 Mar;90(3):426-36.

[143] Wahli W. A gut feeling of the PXR, PPAR and NF-kappaB connection. J Intern Med. 2008 Jun;263(6):613-9.

[144] Xie W, Tian Y. Xenobiotic receptor meets NF-kappaB, a collision in the small bowel. Cell Metab. 2006 Sep;4(3):177-8.

[145] Glauert HP, Tharappel JC, Lu Z, Stemm D, Banerjee S, Chan LS, Lee EY, Lehmler HJ, Robertson LW, Spear BT. Role of oxidative stress in the promoting activities of pcbs. Environ Toxicol Pharmacol. 2008 Mar;25(2):247-50.

[146] Pascussi JM, Vilarem MJ. [[Inflammation and drug metabolism: NF-kappB and the CAR and PXR xeno-receptors]. Med Sci (Paris). 2008 Mar;24(3):301-5.

[147] Assenat E, Gerbal-Chaloin S, Larrey D, Saric J, Fabre JM, Maurel P, Vilarem MJ, Pascussi JM. Interleukin 1beta inhibits CAR-induced expression of hepatic genes involved in drug and bilirubin clearance. Hepatology. 2004 Oct;40(4):951-60.

[148] Ke S, Rabson AB, Germino JF, Gallo MA, Tian Y. Mechanism of suppression of cytochrome P-450 1A1 expression by tumor necrosis factor-alpha and lipopolysaccharide. J Biol Chem. 2001 Oct 26;276(43):39638-44.

[149] Al-Sadi RM, Ma TY. IL-1beta causes an increase in intestinal epithelial tight junction permeability. J Immunol. 2007 Apr 1;178(7):4641-9.

[150] Kimura K, Teranishi S, Nishida T. Interleukin-1beta-induced disruption of barrier function in cultured human corneal epithelial cells. Invest Ophthalmol Vis Sci. 2009 Feb;50(2):597-603.

[151] Buhrmann C, Mobasheri A, Busch F, Aldinger C, Stahlmann R, Montaseri A, Shakibaei M. Curcumin modulates nuclear factor kappaB (NF-kappaB)-mediated inflammation in human tenocytes in vitro: role of the phosphatidylinositol 3-kinase/Akt pathway. J Biol Chem. 2011 Aug 12;286(32):28556-66.

[152] Bisht K, Wagner KH, Bulmer AC. Curcumin, resveratrol and flavonoids as anti-inflammatory, cyto- and DNA-protective dietary compounds. Toxicology. 2010 Nov 28;278(1):88-100.

[153] Revel A, Raanani H, Younglai E, Xu J, Han R, Savouret JF, Casper RF. Resveratrol, a natural aryl hydrocarbon receptor antagonist, protects sperm from DNA damage and apoptosis caused by benzo(a)pyrene. Reprod Toxicol. 2001 Sep-Oct;15(5):479-86.

[154] Aktas C, Kanter M, Erboga M, Ozturk S. Anti-apoptotic effects of curcumin on cadmium-induced apoptosis in rat testes. Toxicol Ind Health. 2012 Mar;28(2):122-30.

[155] Roy M, Sinha D, Mukherjee S, Biswas J. Curcumin prevents DNA damage and enhances the repair potential in a chronically arsenic-exposed human population in West Bengal, India. Eur J Cancer Prev. 2011 Mar;20(2): 123-31.

[156] Ahmed T, Pathak R, Mustafa MD, Kar R, Tripathi AK, Ahmed RS, Banerjee BD. Ameliorating effect of N-acetylcysteine and curcumin on pesticide-induced oxidative DNA damage in human peripheral blood mononuclear cells. Environ Monit Assess. 2011 Aug;179(1-4):293-9.

[157] Gradisar H, Keber MM, Pristovsek P, Jerala R. MD-2 as the target of curcumin in the inhibition of response to LPS. J Leukoc Biol. 2007 Oct;82(4):968-74.

INDEX

CPSIA information can be obtained at www.ICGtesting.com
Printed in the USA
BVOW05s1231171215

430087BV00006B/40/P